# ATLAS of MICROSCOPIC ANATOMY

## a companion to Histology and Neuroanatomy

Ronald A. Bergman, Ph.D.

Associate Professor,
Department of Anatomy
The Johns Hopkins University
School of Medicine
Baltimore, Maryland

Adel K. Afifi, M.D., M.Sc.

Associate Professor and Chairman,
Department of Human Morphology;
Consultant in Neurology
American University of Beirut
School of Medicine
Beirut, Lebanon

1974   W. B. SAUNDERS COMPANY   PHILADELPHIA   LONDON   TORONTO

W. B. Saunders Company:  West Washington Square
Philadelphia, Pa.  19105

12 Dyott Street
London, WC1A  1DB

833 Oxford Street
Toronto 18, Ontario

Atlas of Microscopic Anatomy: A Companion to Histology and Neuroanatomy        ISBN 0-7216-1687-9

Print No.:    9    8    7    6    5    4    3    2    1

# Preface

This atlas of microscopic anatomy was prepared with the student as the foremost consideration. It is hoped that this collection of photomicrographs will materially aid the student in his initial and continuing efforts to recognize and, most importantly, to understand the structure and function of cells, tissues and organs as revealed by light microscopy.

The student of microscopic anatomy usually begins his study by examining tissue slices which are stained with dyes of various colors or impregnated with soluble metallic salts. These methods have been developed during the past 200 years to reveal structural details of cells, tissues and organs which cannot be recognized or investigated by any other means. New techniques are being developed continually to further our understanding. Routine and special methods employed by the light microscopist have defined biological structures and are the foundation from which biochemical and physiological studies arise and are correlated.

Staining is an essential part of the methods used by the light microscopist, and the student must recognize and understand the use of the more important techniques, if he is to gain more than a superficial understanding of biological tissues. It is for this reason that the illustrations in this atlas are in color; insofar as these staining techniques are understood, they reveal very precise and specific information about structure.

No single staining method available to the microscopist can adequately reveal each and every detail of biological structure. It is important, therefore, that the student understand that if a complete picture is to be obtained several staining methods must be employed. Because it is recognized that students will experience some difficulty in remembering the various methods available, the photographs in this atlas have been selected to demonstrate some of the most important and useful techniques. It is hoped that this atlas will be a continuing source of reference during and beyond the elementary courses of study.

Loan collections to which most students have access are varied in their completeness and in the staining methods which have been employed. The authors have included photomicrographs of cells, tissues and organs which may not be included in basic student loan collections in order to provide additional reference material.

This book is not intended to replace comprehensive textbooks of histology or neuroanatomy or other original sources of information but rather to complement them and to be the basis for additional in-depth inquiry into details of structure and function.

Although the light microscopic structures of both man and animal have been thoroughly investigated, detailed structural-functional correlations remain as an important field for continuing research. The light microscope and the varied methods available to the student of cell anatomy and physiology will yield much new information. In conjunction with the electron microscope, the light microscope will continue as a primary tool in unifying and clarifying our understanding of anatomy, biochemistry, physiology and pathology.

We are indebted to many, most of whom are unknown to us personally, whose extraordinary talent has resulted in this atlas. Many of the slides which were photographed have been handed down through several generations of microscopic anatomists. The oldest slide in our possession was prepared 80 years ago. Other slides were prepared specifically for this book. It is to these master craftsmen and to those researchers whose genius has given us the methods we use in the study of microscopic anatomy that this atlas is dedicated. Some of the names of these individuals appear in the text and appendices.

More directly involved in the preparation of this atlas were M. Z. M. Ibrahim, Tamir Nassar, Nuha Nuwayri-Salti, Farid Khuri, Raif Nassif, Nadia Bahuth, Vazken der Kaloustian, Elbert Ruth, Eduard Gfeller, Jerry Sutton, Nancy Tountas, Linda Ziemer and Phyllis S. Bergman, whose special contributions were generously given and gratefully received. To our wives and children, who relieved us from innumerable daily responsibilities so that we might complete this work, we owe a particular debt of gratitude. The encouragement, cooperation and interest shown by John Hanley and Raymond Kersey of the W. B. Saunders Company in the production of this book are sincerely appreciated. The advice and counsel of George Smar, Phototype Engraving Company, are acknowledged.

We earnestly solicit constructive criticism from students and teachers alike so that the usefulness of this atlas can be extended and improved to its maximum potential.

RONALD A. BERGMAN
ADEL K. AFIFI

# Contents

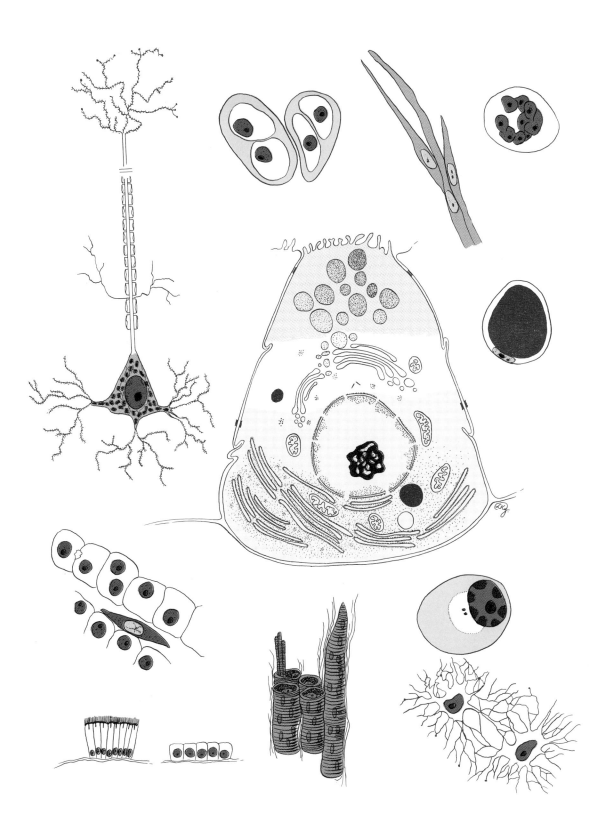

# Cells

From a single cell (the fertilized ovum), through cell division and differentiation or specialization, four basic tissues arise which carry out the diverse functions essential for life: the epithelial, connective, muscular and nervous tissues. The cells which comprise these basic tissues have certain characteristics in common, but they also differ strikingly in their size, shape, organelle content and function. General and special techniques have been developed by the biologist to visualize cellular structure and function. The photomicrographs in this section were selected to demonstrate various methods which reveal specific organelles and inclusions common to most cell types. Cytological considerations will continue into subsequent sections, which deal with specialized cells and organs. The understanding of cellular function depends upon the recognition of the role played by each component part of the cell.

In general, all cells possess: (1) an outer limiting membrane (the cell membrane, or plasmalemma); (2) one or more nuclei with nucleoli containing deoxyribonucleic acid (DNA) and ribonucleic acid (RNA), respectively; (3) cytoplasmic RNA; (4) a Golgi apparatus; (5) membranes in the form of vacuoles or sacs; (6) mitochondria; and (7) energy stored in the form of glycogen and lipid.

The outer limiting membrane can only be seen with the light microscope under special circumstances, since it has been demonstrated by electron microscopy to be about 100 Ångstroms (Å) in thickness. Because the light microscope can only resolve structures larger than 2750 Å, or 0.275 $\mu$, the cell membrane will not be seen unless it is intimately associated with connective tissue elements or if it is artificially thickened to become stainable. The outer limiting membrane can be seen in Plates 14, 17 and 62.

The nucleus is of special importance for an understanding of cell function. Because it is large enough for a detailed examination by the light microscope when stained even by routine methods, such as hematoxylin and eosin (H. & E.), its varying functional states can be assessed. It has been demonstrated that active deoxyribonucleic acid (DNA) does not stain with the nuclear stain hematoxylin. Inactive DNA is readily stained with hematoxylin, toluidine blue and other similar basic dyes. Most nuclei contain varying amounts of functional and inactive DNA. The stainable DNA may appear in clumps or in a reticulated pattern. The functional DNA is termed euchromatin, whereas the non-functional, or inactive, DNA is called heterochromatin. The nerve cell nucleus seen in Plate 1 contains no stainable DNA, which indicates its active involvement in the metabolism of the cell. The densely stained heterochromatin seen in the nucleus of the maturing red blood cell (Plate 1) signals the termination of nuclear function in the synthesis of hemoglobin which takes place in the cytoplasm. In the case of the red blood cell, the useless nucleus is eventually ejected from the cell. During cell division, the stainable, inactive DNA appears in the form of threads or rods called chromosomes (Plates 3 and 4).

The nucleus also contains one or more nucleoli which stain routinely with the nuclear stains cited above. The nucleolus is composed, most importantly, of RNA and it is the source of cytoplasmic RNA (Plates 1 and 25).

The cytoplasm of most cells contains some RNA which may not be detectable by routine methods. In these instances, it is likely that the protein synthesis related to this RNA is associated mainly with the maintenance and repair of cellular structures or organelles. In certain instances, however, the cytoplasm contains a significant amount of RNA which is readily stained and can be directly related to some specific function, such as the elaboration of digestive enzymes (Plate 5).

In certain nerve cells cytoplasmic RNA appears as specific blue-staining (basophilic) patches called Nissl bodies (Plate 1). In these two examples, the staining pattern is a permanent and recognizable feature of the normal cell. The electron microscope has revealed that in these cases the RNA is bound to cytoplasmic membranes. In the developing red blood cell and muscle fiber, however, the RNA is not membrane-bound and gradually disappears when these cells become structurally and functionally mature (Plate 1).

The Golgi apparatus seen in Plate 7 is well developed in cells actively engaged in protein synthesis, and its role is best understood in the case of the enzyme-producing pancreatic acinar cell. Proteins synthesized through the interaction of nuclear, nucleolar and cytoplasmic nucleic acids are first concentrated in the sacs of the Golgi apparatus in the form of granules or droplets. Except for glycoprotein and protein polysaccharide synthesis, it is unlikely that the Golgi apparatus is directly involved enzymatically in synthetic activity, but its relative size changes directly in relation to the synthetic activity of the cell. Although this organelle was first convincingly demonstrated by Golgi in nerve cells, its precise role in these cells is not completely understood.

The cytoplasm of many mature cells contains little RNA, and when these cells are stained with hematoxylin and eosin the cytoplasm binds the eosin and appears red. In these cells functions other than protein synthesis predominate. The parietal cell of the stomach which elaborates hydrochloric acid is an example of such an eosinophilic (acidophilic) cell (Plate 5). The cytoplasm of this cell contains numerous mitochondria and cytoplasmic membranes.

Mitochondria are found in all cells except the mature red blood cell. They vary in number, size, shape and distribution, depending upon the cell type and its specific energy requirements. Mitochondria are membranous sacs to which enzymes are both permanently and loosely bound. This organelle produces the energy-rich adenosine triphosphate necessary for synthetic and other cellular functions. Additional details can be found in the legends to Plate 6.

The substrates utilized by the mitochondrial enzymes in the elaboration of energy-yielding compounds include stored glycogen and lipid droplets. These cellular inclusions are seen in Plates 8, 9 and 12. Other inclusions found in certain cells are pigment granules (Plates 11 and 12), protein granules (Plates 50 and 122) and phagocytized dust (Plate 29).

Other specialized organelles are associated with specific cell types, and these will be discussed in subsequent sections of this atlas.

## NUCLEUS
### A. Motor neuron
### B1. Basophilic & B2. Orthochromatic erythroblasts

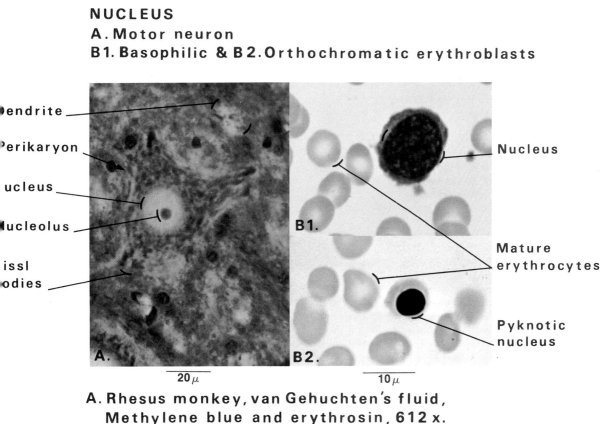

Dendrite

Perikaryon

Nucleus

Nucleolus

Nissl bodies

B1.

Nucleus

Mature erythrocytes

Pyknotic nucleus

A.

B2.

20 μ

10 μ

### A. Rhesus monkey, van Gehuchten's fluid, Methylene blue and erythrosin, 612 x.
### B. Human, Air dried smear, Wright's stain, 1416 x.

The fact that nuclei of certain cells differ in appearance and staining properties can be directly related to nuclear function. Compare the appearance of the functionally active nucleus of the motor neuron with that of the functionally inactive nucleus of the maturing red blood cell.

**A:** This plate shows a motor neuron characterized by a multipolar perikaryon, cytoplasm rich in Nissl bodies (ribonucleoproteins) and a stout dendrite which can be identified because it is structurally similar to the cell body from which it arises. The nucleus, centrally placed within the cell body, is spherical and unstained (contains euchromatin) and has a prominent densely staining basophilic nucleolus rich in ribonucleic acid. This cell body is located within the spinal cord but its elongated axon leaves the cord to terminate on striated skeletal muscle fibers.

**B1:** This figure shows a basophilic erythroblast (also known as a prorubricyte), one of the early cells in the development of the red blood corpuscle. Note that the nucleus occupies a significant portion of the cell and that its stainable inactive chromatin is coarse. A nucleolus is present but obscured by stainable heterochromatin. The cytoplasm of this cell contains ribonucleic acid, giving it a lavender hue. Compare the cytoplasm of this cell with a mature non-nucleated red blood cell.

**B2:** This figure shows the small pyknotic nucleus of an orthochromatic erythroblast. This cell is also known as a metarubricyte or a normoblast. The chromatin (heterochromatin) is very compact and densely stained. Such a nucleus is functionless and is ultimately discarded, resulting in a mature non-nucleated erythrocyte.

# NUCLEUS
## Female sex chromatin
### peripheral blood smear, buccal epithelium, and corpus luteum

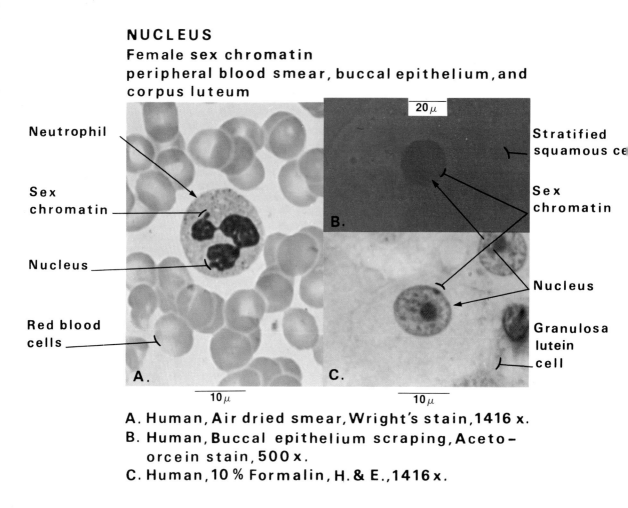

A. Human, Air dried smear, Wright's stain, 1416 x.

B. Human, Buccal epithelium scraping, Aceto-orcein stain, 500 x.

C. Human, 10 % Formalin, H. & E., 1416 x.

This figure shows the appearance of female sex chromatin in a neutrophil (A), a buccal smear (B) and corpus luteum cells (C). Sex chromatin (Barr body), composed of one of the X chromosomes that remains condensed in interphase, is usually seen as a discrete structure in the nucleus. Sex chromatin is presumably present in all cells in the female, but in the majority of cells it is obscured within the nucleus.

**A:** Portion of a peripheral blood smear showing abundant red blood cells and a single polymorphonuclear neutrophilic granulocyte. The deeply stained chromatin of the mature neutrophil nucleus is characteristically segmented or multilobed. The lobes are attached by thin chromatin threads. Attached to one of the lobes is a small "drumstick" appendage, the sex chromatin. This appendage is found in about 3 per cent of the neutrophils in females.

**B:** A buccal smear was prepared by scraping the stratified squamous epithelium of the oral cavity. The stratified squamous cell is poorly delineated but the nucleus of the cell is stained and shows a sex chromatin body (reddish-brown coloration) on the nuclear membrane. The sex chromatin body may appear convex or triangular in shape. It may also lie near the center of the nucleus.

**C:** A section of the corpus luteum, showing a nucleus of the granulosa lutein cell with a sex chromatin body adhering to the nuclear membrane.

## CHROMOSOMES
### A. Metaphase chromosomes
### B. Karyotype

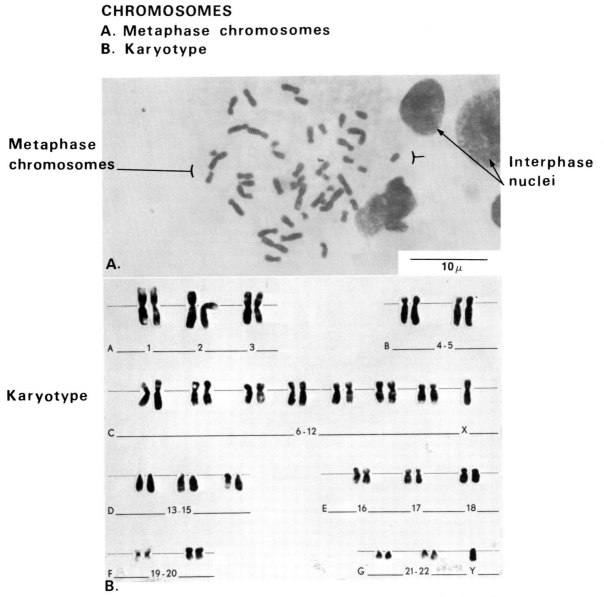

**Metaphase chromosomes**

**Interphase nuclei**

A.

10 μ

**Karyotype**

A ___ 1 ___ 2 ___ 3 ___    B ___ 4-5 ___

C ___ 6-12 ___ X ___

D ___ 13-15 ___    E ___ 16 ___ 17 ___ 18 ___

F ___ 19-20 ___    G ___ 21-22 ___ Y ___

B.

**Human, Peripheral lymphocyte culture, Air dried trypsin-banded, Giemsa stain, 2142 x.**

68-hour peripheral lymphocyte culture, phytohemagglutinin-stimulated to induce lymphocyte transformation and mitosis.

In *A*, the mitosis has been arrested in metaphase with colchicine, and the chromosomes dispersed with hypotonic potassium chloride. Interphase nuclei are seen adjacent to the dispersed chromosomes.

*B* is an analysis of male chromosomes seen in *A*. This arrangement of the chromosomes is known as a karyotype. Note the dark and light areas (bands) that characterize each chromosome. Note the 22 pairs of autosomes (Nos. 1 to 22) and the pair of sex chromosomes (XY in this case). The 22 pairs of chromosomes have been classified on morphological grounds into seven groups (A to G).

The chromosomes seen here are judged to be normal. Abnormal, duplicated or missing chromosomes can be related to defective somatic and mental development in man.

# CELL DIVISION
## Lymph node

Early
prophase (B)

Interphase (A)

Late
prophase (C)

Metaphase (

Telophase (F

Anaphase (E)

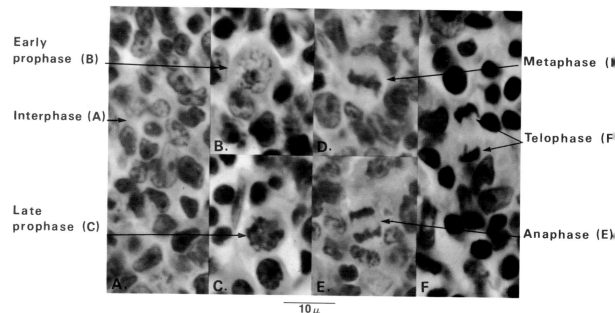

10μ

## Rat, Helly's fluid, Mallory's stain, 1416 x.

This Plate illustrates the nuclear events in mitosis. They will be described in the sequence in which they occur.

**Interphase (A):** Non-dividing or resting stage. The chromatin appears as an irregular reticular meshwork. The nuclear membrane, or envelope, and the nucleolus are distinctly seen. Chromosomes are not visible.

**Early prophase (B):** Nuclear membrane and nucleolus disappear. Granularity of the nucleus is markedly increased, and filamentous structures are seen. These granules and filaments represent the chromosomes, which become shorter and thicker in this stage.

**Late prophase (C):** The thread- or rod-like character of the chromosomes is more apparent. Each chromosome consists of two coiled chromatids which are not visible in this preparation. The disappearance of the nuclear membrane allows mixing of nuclear and cytoplasmic material.

**Metaphase (D):** Chromosomes appear condensed and line up in the equatorial plane of the cell. Each chromosome is still composed of two chromatids.

**Anaphase (E):** The daughter chromosomes (chromatids) separate and are drawn to opposite poles of the cell. They remain separate and tightly coiled, and appear at this magnification to be fused. Cytoplasmic division begins.

**Telophase (F):** The two distinct groups of daughter chromosomes (chromatids) appear fused and tightly packed. Cytoplasmic division is completed. Nuclear membranes re-form and nucleoli reappear.

## CHIEF and PARIETAL CELLS
### Stomach
### fundus

Chief
cells

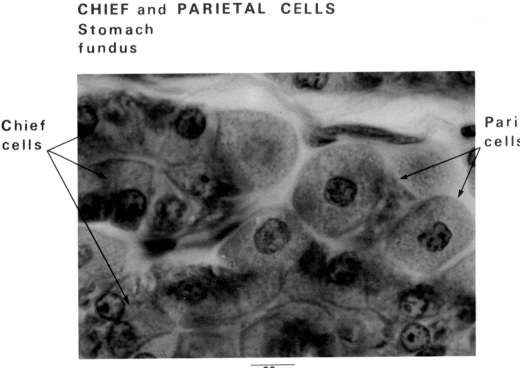

Parietal
cells

$\overline{20\,\mu}$

## Dog, Helly's fluid, H. & E., 612 x.

**Chief cell:** Pyramidal shape. Basal nucleus. Granular apex contains zymogen granules. Basophilia of base is due to cytoplasmic ribonucleic acid (RNA). Secretes pepsinogen and rennin, and may be the source of the anti-pernicious anemia factor.

**Parietal cells:** Wedged between and larger than chief cells. Centrally placed nuclei surrounded by a finely granular acidophilic cytoplasm. Cytoplasm granularity is due to abundant but unstained mitochondria. Secrete hydrochloric acid, which converts pepsinogen to pepsin, a proteolytic digestive enzyme active at very low pH. See Plate 166.

Cells whose cytoplasm stains intensely blue with hematoxylin are primarily involved in protein synthesis (*e.g.,* chief cells). Cytoplasm that is eosinophilic (stained with eosin) contains little RNA and is engaged in other kinds of cellular activity (e.g., muscular contraction, active transport or the elaboration of hydrochloric acid, as in this preparation). See Appendix IV for a brief discussion of the staining mechanism and the hematoxylin and eosin dyes.

# MITOCHONDRIA
## Liver cells

Nucleus

Nucleolus

Mito-
chondria

Sinusoid

Red blood
cell

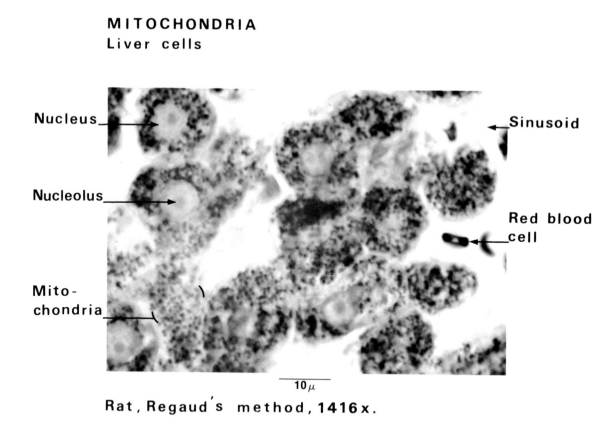

10 μ

Rat, Regaud's method, 1416x.

**Nucleus:** Spherical, centrally located. Contains deoxyribonucleic acid (DNA) and nucleolar ribonucleic acid (RNA).

**Nucleolus:** Prominent. Contains ribonucleic acid (RNA) and is the source of cytoplasmic RNA.

**Mitochondria:** Spheroid, rod-shaped or filamentous. The mitochondria are rich in oxidative enzymes and provide the energy for numerous chemical reactions (*e.g.,* muscular contraction, active transport). Utilizing absorbed nutrients from the diet, energy-rich adenosine triphosphate is produced and made available to the cell for its energy needs. Mitochondria also contain enzymes concerned with protein synthesis and lipid metabolism.

**Sinusoids:** Vascular channels larger in diameter than capillaries but, like capillaries, the walls are one cell thick. These specialized capillaries, or sinusoids, are found in the liver, spleen, bone marrow, adrenal and pituitary glands.

**Red blood cell:** The red blood cell delivers oxygen to the cells and tissues at the capillary or sinusoid level. As the red cell passes through these smallest of vascular channels carbon dioxide is absorbed and transported to the lungs, where it is eliminated.

Mitochondria were described probably for the first time by Kölliker in 1857 in striated muscle. The fixation and staining method used in this preparation can be routinely employed for demonstrating mitochondria.

PLATE 7

## GOLGI APPARATUS
### Dorsal root ganglion cells

Nucleus 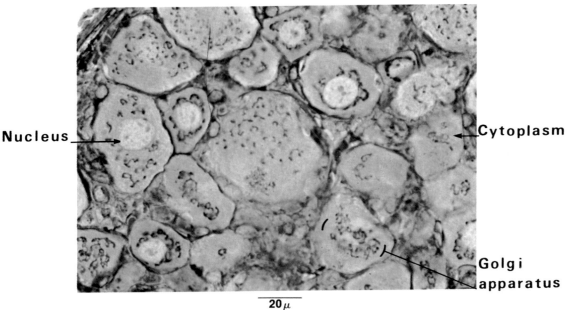 Cytoplasm

Golgi apparatus

20 μ

### Guinea pig, Kopsch's method, 612 x.

**Nucleus:** Vesicular. Prominent nucleolus.

**Cytoplasm:** The Golgi apparatus is the only cytoplasmic organelle seen in this preparation.

**Golgi apparatus:** Reticulated appearance and highly developed in a perinuclear network. The Golgi apparatus is known to play an important role in packaging and concentrating protein-rich secretory products elaborated by glandular cells; in general, it does not appear to play a role in the synthetic mechanism. The Golgi apparatus is also found in cells which are not secretory, and its function in these cells is uncertain.

This organelle was discovered by Camillo Golgi in 1896. The method used here and modifications of it are the best available for revealing this important cell organelle.

## GLYCOGEN
### Liver

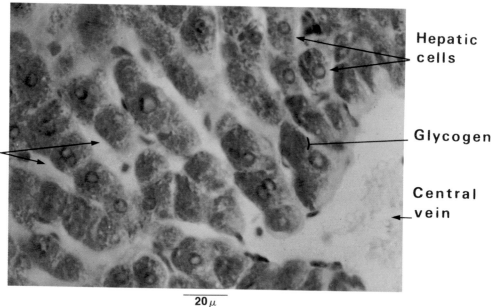

**Hepatic cells**

**Sinusoids**

**Glycogen**

**Central vein**

20 μ

### Rabbit, Absolute alcohol, Best's carmine & hematoxylin stains, 612 x.

**Sinusoids:** Vascular channels larger in diameter than ordinary capillaries but composed of a single layer of fenestrated endothelial cells separating sheets of hepatic cells.

**Hepatic cells:** Arranged in cords. Each cell has a distinct central nucleus. These cells may contain more than one nucleus.

**Glycogen:** Stored throughout the cytoplasm. Glycogen is normally stored in hepatic cells whose content varies with the functional state of the liver and the dietary intake. Glycogen is a polysaccharide, a polymer composed of many molecules of glucose.

**Central vein:** Center of the hepatic lobule. Smallest radicle of the hepatic vein which receives the contents of all the sinusoids comprising the hepatic lobule.

The stain used here is specific for glycogen, although the rationale for its selectivity is uncertain. For another glycogen stain see Plate 75.

## LIPID
### Striated muscle of diaphragm
### longitudinal and cross section

Lipid
droplets

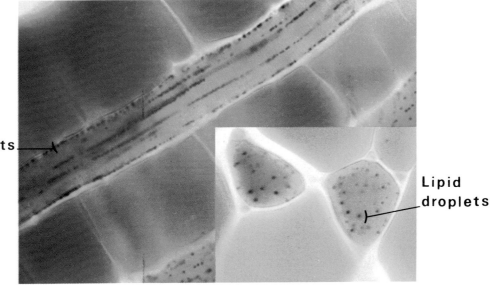

Lipid
droplets

20 μ

### Rat, Frozen section, Osmium tetroxide fixation
### and stain, 612 x.

Cells contain lipid droplets, neutral fats which are liquid at body temperature. Lipids are metabolized for energy or incorporated in cell membranes and other structures. In routine preparations lipid is extracted and is not seen. In well-fixed tissues clear round holes may sometimes be seen which mark the site of lipid droplets within the cytoplasm of cells. The lipid in this preparation was fixed with osmium tetroxide, which renders it insoluble and appears black.

**Lipid droplets:** Irregularly distributed within smaller muscle fibers. In contrast, larger fibers are devoid of lipid droplets.

# CYTOPLASMIC FIBRILS
## Multipolar nerve cells
## spinal cord

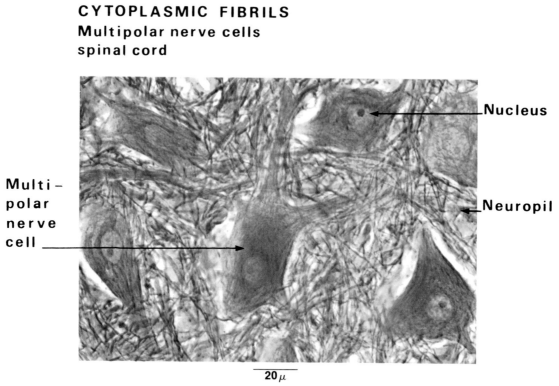

Nucleus

Multi-
polar
nerve
cell

Neuropil

20 μ

## Guinea pig, Alcohol, Bielschowsky's method, 612 x.

**Multipolar nerve cell:** Cell body and multiple processes (axon and dendrites) which contain neurofibrils in the cytoplasm and a prominent nucleus. Muscle fibers also contain fibrillar structures within their cytoplasm. See Plate 68.

**Nucleus:** Centrally located within the cell body with a large deeply stained nucleolus.

**Neuropil:** Region between neurons filled with processes of nerve cells and neuroglia.

## MELANOCYTES
### Skin
### scalp

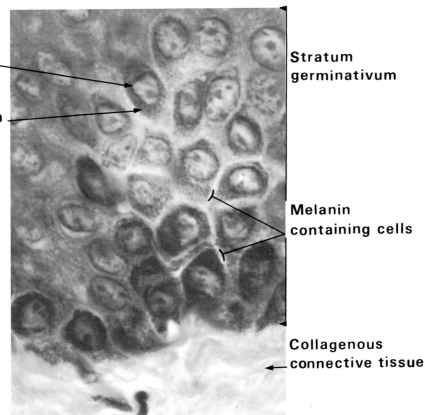

Nucleus

Cytoplasm

Stratum
germinativum

Melanin
containing cells

Collagenous
connective tissue

$10\,\mu$

**Human , 10% Formalin, H. & E., 1416 x.**

Melanocytes (melanin-containing cells) are found in the basal layer of the epidermis (stratum germinativum) in some sites of the body. The pigment is practically absent from the palms and soles, while the areola of the mammary gland, the circumanal region, the labia majora and the scrotum are more richly pigmented. The melanin pigment is found as granules primarily within the cells of the basal layer. Some granules appear to be scattered among the cells but are actually located in melanocyte processes. Note the reduction in melanin pigment in more superficial layers. The collagenous connective tissue shown is in the dermis of the skin.

## LIPOCHROME PIGMENT
## Spinal cord
## lower motor neuron

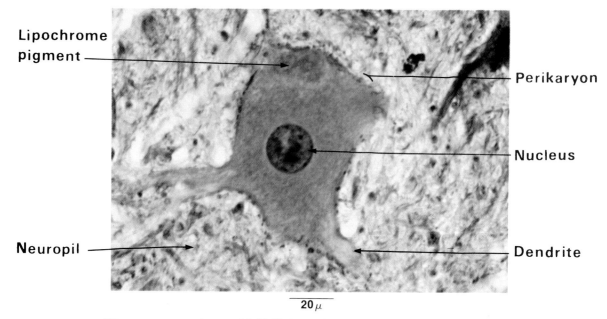

Lipochrome
pigment

Perikaryon

Nucleus

Neuropil

Dendrite

20 μ

**Rhesus monkey, 10% Formalin, Glees' method, 612 x.**

This plate shows a large multipolar motor neuron in the anterior horn of the spinal cord. Note the characteristic large, rounded central nucleus, the prominent nucleolus and processes which extend from the cell body (perikaryon). Note also the stout dendrite. A collection of lipochrome pigment (lipofuscin) is seen in one corner of the cytoplasm. Lipochrome pigment is believed to be a product of normal metabolic activity.

## FOUR BASIC TISSUES
Epithelium, Connective, Muscular and Nervous tissues.

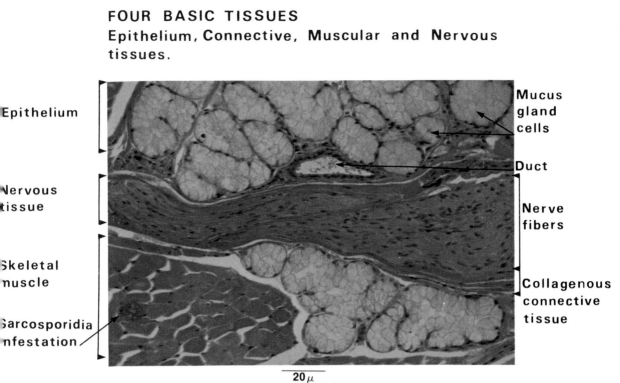

Epithelium

Nervous tissue

Skeletal muscle

Sarcosporidia infestation

Mucus gland cells

Duct

Nerve fibers

Collagenous connective tissue

20μ

**Rhesus monkey, Helly's fluid, H. & E., 612 x.**

This figure shows the four basic tissues in one section.

Epithelial tissue is seen as secretory mucous gland cells. Note the formation of acini, a circular cluster of cells with a central lumen which is in continuity with the external free surface. The nuclei are flattened against the cell membrane at the base of the cell by the mucous droplets, which are tightly packed within the cytoplasm. The cytoplasm appears clear, or unstained, because the mucus is lost during tissue processing. A portion of the duct which links the gland cells with surface epithelium is seen in cross section.

Nervous tissue is represented by bundles of nerve fibers. Elongated nuclei associated with the nerve fibers are those of Schwann cells, which elaborate the myelin sheath around axons.

A dense collagenous connective tissue sheath encloses the nerve fiber bundle and mucous glands.

A bundle of skeletal muscle fibers is seen in cross section. The muscle is infested with sarcosporidia. This parasite is commonly found in the muscle of monkeys, and more rarely in man. Note the polygonal shape of individual muscle fibers and the peripherally located nuclei.

In subsequent sections, the structure of the four basic tissues will be considered in detail.

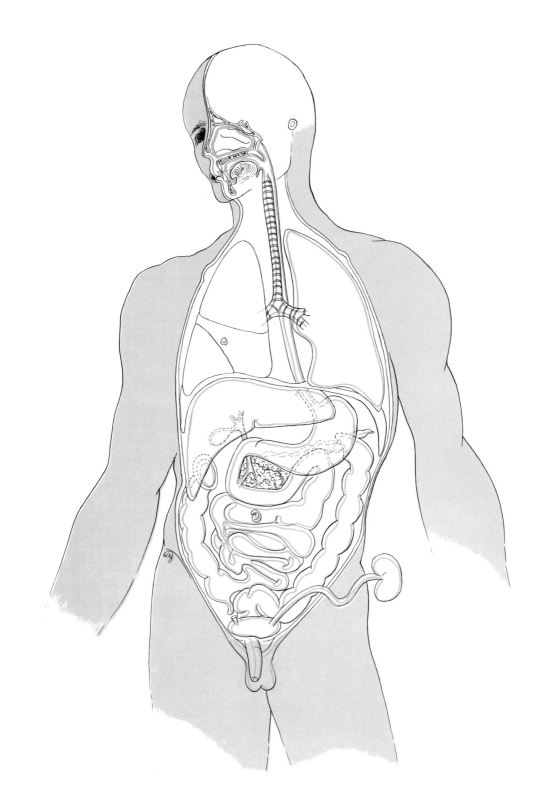

# Epithelial Tissue

The layer of cells which covers the outer and lines the inner body surfaces is designated as epithelium. In general, many of these cells have a free surface which is exposed to the external environment (skin, and the respiratory, digestive, genital and urinary tracts). Other epithelial cells, the glands, found in underlying connective tissue, are in continuity with the surface epithelium by epithelial duct cells. The glandular epithelium secretes diverse products which are carried to the external surface. The products of these glands include sweat, mucus, milk, digestive enzymes, hydrochloric acid, bile, urine, reproductive cells and others. Some epithelial cells have become separated from the free or exposed surface and form distinctive cell masses, the endocrine glands. The secretory products of these glands are delivered to the vascular system to be carried to their specific site or sites of activity. The endocrine glands will be considered in another section of this atlas.

It is important to remember that everything that enters or leaves the body is either modified or synthesized by epithelial cells or has passed through epithelial cells. The various functions of epithelium include: protection, secretion, excretion, digestion, absorption, lubrication, sensory reception and reproduction. These diversified functions depend upon structurally diverse cell types and cell groupings.

The epithelia are classified by histologists according to cell layering and cell shape. Three distinct types of epithelium are recognized: (1) simple, which is a single cell layer; (2) pseudostratified, which is a single cell layer but which appears to be two or more layers; and (3) stratified, which is composed of several to many cell layers. Only the simple and stratified epithelia have important subgroupings which are classified according to the shape of the surface cells. The simple epithelia are described as *squamous* (sheets of flattened cells), *cuboidal* (in which the cells are roughly equal in height and width) and *columnar* (in which the cells are greater in height than in width). The stratified epithelia include *stratified squamous* (in which the superficial cells are flattened), *stratified cuboidal* (in which the superficial cells are cuboidal) and *stratified columnar* (in which the superficial cells are columnar).

From a functional point of view, the simple epithelia carry out the most diverse activities including absorption, excretion, synthesis, secretion and sensory reception, whereas the stratified epithelia serve protective, transport and reproductive roles. In order to serve their distinctive functional roles, epithelial cells often display distinctive cell membrane or surface modifications and appendages.

The epithelial types demonstrated in this section are meant to represent the morphological varieties of simple and stratified epithelia. The structural features of many other epithelial cell types and groupings are found in other sections of this atlas, where their functional role will be considered.

A classification of epithelial cell types and some of their locations in the body are tabulated for convenience as follows.

A. Simple epithelium
   1. Squamous
      Innermost lining of blood and lymph vessels and the heart (the endothelium).

Lining the pleural, cardiac and abdominal cavities.
Initial segments of the ducts of glands.
Air sacs or alveoli of the respiratory system.
Kidney glomeruli.
Kidney tubules (thin segment of the loop of Henle of the nephron).
2. Cuboidal
"Germinal" epithelium covering the ovary.
Ducts of many glands.
Ciliary body of the eye.
3. Columnar
Stomach, intestines and gallbladder of the digestive system.
Small bronchi of the respiratory system.
Uterine tubes.
The secretory cells of many glands (endocrine and exocrine) vary from
cuboidal or pyramidal to columnar. Size and shape may vary with the
functional state.
4. Pseudostratified
Pharynx, trachea and large bronchi.
Male sexual duct (vas deferens).
Parts of the male and female urethra.
5. Specialized
Glands of the intestinal tract, nasal cavity, bronchi and uterine tubes.
6. Pigmented
Epithelium of the retina.
7. Neuroepithelium
Receptor cells of taste, hearing and vestibular system.
B. Stratified epithelium
1. Stratified squamous
Keratinized and non-keratinized epithelium of the skin, conjunctiva (eye-
lid), oral cavity, esophagus and anus.
Urethra near external orifice.
Vagina.
2. Stratified cuboidal
Ducts of sweat and sebaceous glands of the skin.
Graafian follicle of the ovary.
3. Stratified columnar
Pharynx, larynx, urethra and portions of the excretory ducts of salivary
and mammary glands.
4. Transitional
Renal calyx, ureter and bladder of the urinary system.

Several specializations of epithelial cells which occur at their free or exposed surface include: the brush or striated border of absorbing cells of the
intestine and kidney; motile cilia of the pseudostratified epithelium of the respiratory system; and non-motile stereocilia of the pseudostratified epithelium
lining the epididymis of the male reproductive tract. Specializations which
structurally and functionally link adjacent cells together include the terminal
bars illustrated in Plate 22 and the "intercellular bridges" or desmosomes
associated with the prickle cells found in stratified squamous epithelium (Plate
123). Marked infoldings of the basal cell membrane, termed basal striations,
are seen in certain actively transporting cells such as those of the proximal
convoluted tubule cells of the kidney and ducts of certain glands (see Plates
15 and 182). Between the basal surface of epithelial cells and the underlying
connective tissue is the so-called basement membrane. This extracellular
structure has been shown by electron microscopy to have several components
which are produced both by epithelial cells and underlying connective tissue
fibroblasts (see Plates 19 and 20).

# SQUAMOUS & CUBOIDAL EPITHELIAL CELLS
## Kidney tubules
### medulla

Henle's loop;
thin segment

Squamous
epithelium

Collecting
tubule

Cuboidal
epithelium

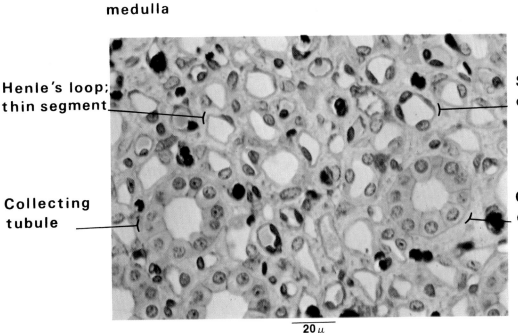

20 μ

## Rabbit, Helly's fluid, Iron hematoxylin – orange G, 612 x.

**Squamous epithelium:** Single layer of flattened or squamous cells with ovoid nuclei bulging into the lumen of the thin loop of Henle. The thin loop of Henle serves an essential role in concentrating urine, rendering it hypertonic with respect to blood plasma.

**Cuboidal epithelium:** Single layer of cuboidal cells (height and width of cells about equal) lining the collecting tubule. Spherical, darkly staining nuclei; clear cytoplasm.

A diagnostic feature of the collecting tubules of the kidney is the appearance of distinct cell boundaries. The collecting tubules, under the influence of the antidiuretic hormone which is secreted into the vascular system in the posterior lobe of the pituitary gland (hypophysis), become permeable to water, which is reabsorbed into the vascular system, thereby concentrating the urine. In the absence of the antidiuretic hormone, the urine is dilute or hypotonic with respect to the blood.

## CUBOIDAL EPITHELIUM
### Brush border, basal striations
### proximal tubules
### kidney

Nucleus

Nucleolus

Brush border

Brush border

Basal striations

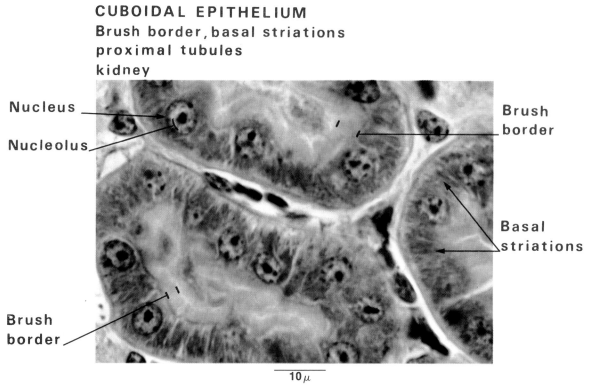

10 μ

### Rhesus monkey, Helly's fluid, Iron hematoxylin & Orange G stains, 1416 x.

**Nucleus:**   Round and large with prominent nucleolus.

**Brush border:**   On the luminal surface of the tubule cells. Consists of microvilli which vastly increase its absorptive surface.

**Basal striations:**   Consist of rod-shaped mitochondria contained within compartments formed by specialized infoldings of the basal cell membrane.

The cells of the proximal tubule with their apical and basal specializations have the capacity to reabsorb selectively and transport metabolically valuable substances from the glomerular filtrate (*e.g.*, glucose and amino acids), returning them to the vascular system. They also transport and secrete other substances into the lumen of the proximal tubule to be eliminated in the urine.

# COLUMNAR EPITHELIUM
# UNICELLULAR GLAND

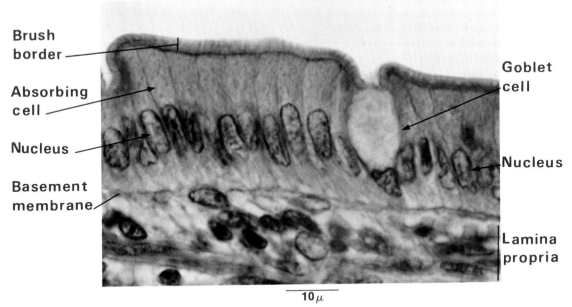

Brush border

Absorbing cell

Nucleus

Basement membrane

Goblet cell

Nucleus

Lamina propria

10 μ

## Cat, Helly's fluid, Mallory's stain, 1416 x.

**Absorbing cell:** Single cell layer of tall columnar cells. Basal ovoid nucleus. Although the cells appear rectangular in this section, they are actually five- or six-sided when they are cross sectioned (see Plate 17). When the underlying tissue folds or bends, these cells may have a pyramidal appearance.

**Nucleus:** Ovoid. Situated in lower half of the columnar cell. The nuclei in tightly packed cells may appear elongated and staggered at different levels within the cell. This is readily seen in pseudostratified ciliated columnar epithelium (see Plate 18).

**Brush border:** Also known as the striated border. Made up of fine, closely packed microvilli which vastly increase the surface area of the cell. Characteristic of absorptive surfaces. Adequate absorption of digestive products is dependent upon this cell surface specialization of absorbing columnar epithelial cells.

**Goblet cell:** Unicellular mucous glands scattered among the tall columnar cells appear empty because mucin is extracted during tissue processing. See Plate 19 for goblet cell mucus. These unicellular gland cells are a specialization of simple epithelium and serve a protective function for the principal epithelial cell type.

**Basement membrane:** Delicate in appearance but a firm support for the columnar cells. See also Plate 19.

**Lamina propria:** Connective tissue stroma. Reticular framework containing a variety of wandering cells as well as vascular and lymphatic channels. Cells commonly found in the lamina propria include lymphocytes, plasma cells, eosinophils and mast cells. See also Plate 173.

## COLUMNAR EPITHELIAL CELLS
## GOBLET CELLS
### Cross section

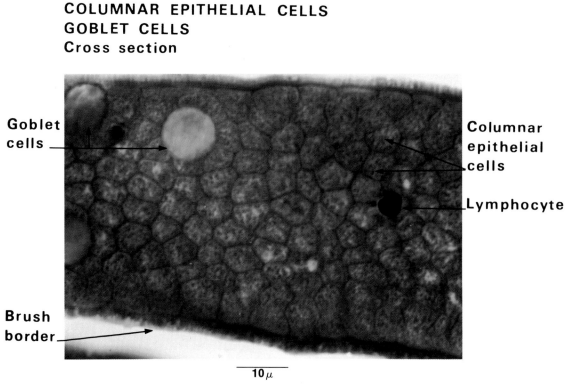

Goblet cells

Columnar epithelial cells

Lymphocyte

Brush border

10μ

**Cat, Helly's fluid, Mallory's stain, 1416 x.**

This is a cross section of unicellular secretory cells and absorbing intestinal epithelial cells. The secretory goblet cells are interspersed between the more numerous columnar absorptive cells. Mucus in the goblet cells stains light blue. Cell boundaries or limiting membranes are distinctly seen. The goblet cells are round while the columnar absorptive cells are multifaceted (five or six sides) in cross section. The presence of a brush border (striated border) on epithelial cells characterizes absorptive surfaces. A lymphocyte nucleus is seen among the columnar cells.

Goblet and columnar epithelial cells can be seen in Plate 16 in longitudinal section.

## PSEUDOSTRATIFIED COLUMNAR EPITHELIUM WITH STEREOCILIA
### Ductus epididymis

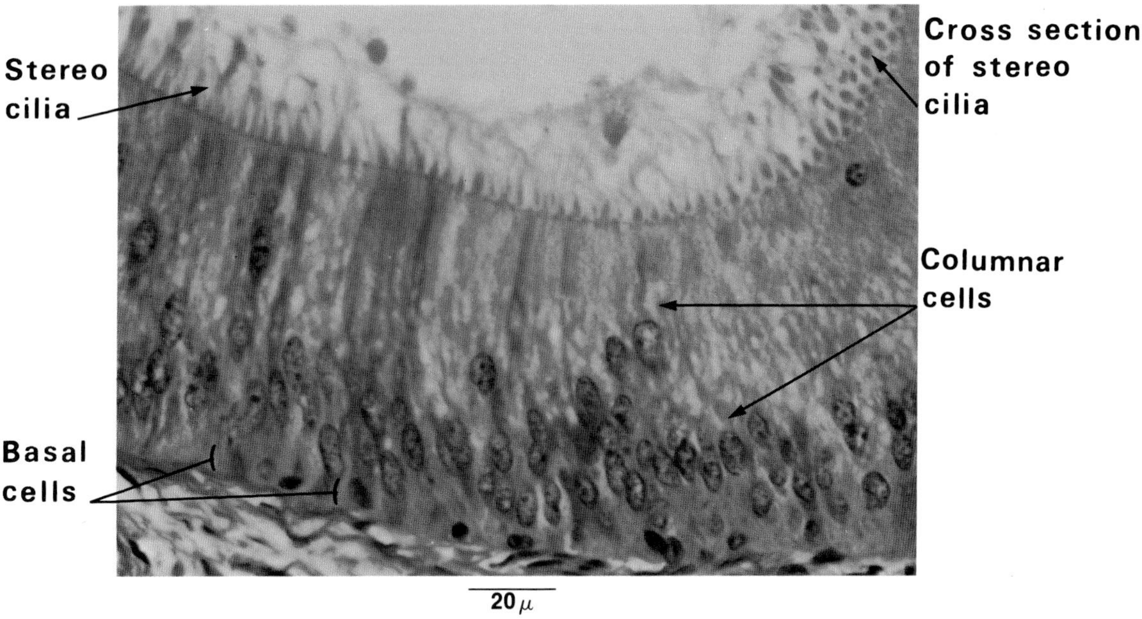

Stereo cilia

Cross section of stereo cilia

Columnar cells

Basal cells

20 μ

**Rhesus monkey, Helly's fluid, H. & E., 612 x.**

The ductus epididymis is lined by a pseudostratified columnar epithelium containing two types of cells: tall columnar cells bearing so-called stereocilia and rounded basal cells. The cells forming a pseudostratified epithelium deceptively appear to be stratified in two or more layers. The cells actually vary in height, but all are in contact with the basement membrane.

**Columnar cells:** Tall cells bearing stereocilia. These are non-motile processes of the columnar cells projecting into the lumen. Although they are called cilia, electron micrographs show that they lack the structural characteristics of cilia, and they resemble greatly elongated microvilli. In this figure they are seen in the cross section and longitudinal section. Nuclei of columnar cells are elongated and lie at different levels.

**Basal cells:** Rounded or triangular cells, lying against the basement membrane, form a discontinuous layer around the duct.

## BASEMENT MEMBRANE
### Pseudostratified columnar ciliated epithelium & Goblet cells
### trachea

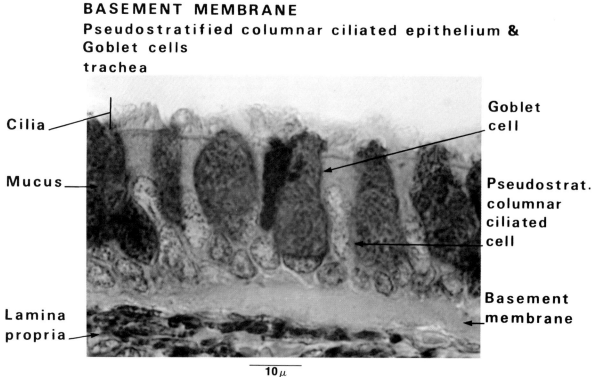

Cilia

Mucus

Lamina propria

Goblet cell

Pseudostrat. columnar ciliated cell

Basement membrane

10 μ

### Rhesus monkey, Helly's fluid, Modified aldehyde fuchsin stain, 1416 x.

**Pseudostratified columnar ciliated cell:**   Epithelial lining of the trachea contains tall, ciliated columnar cells, non-ciliated goblet cells and short basal cells.

**Goblet cells:**   Non-ciliated, flask-shaped mucus-secreting cells.

**Mucus:**   Mucopolysaccharide droplets seen here filling goblet cells. When the mucus is discharged the cell collapses only to become distended once again as mucus is synthesized.

**Cilia:**   Arising from basal bodies which appear here as a thin dark line just below the surface of the tall columnar cells. Basal bodies  are modified centrioles which are synthesized in great numbers during development and from which the cilia arise. These motile structures carry cells, debris and inhaled foreign material away from the respiratory surfaces.

**Basement membrane:**   This structure is unusually thick and prominent, underlying the epithelium in the trachea. The basement membrane is an extracellular "homogeneous" structure composed of mucopolysaccharides in which reticular fibers are embedded. Electron microscopists include the basal lamina (500 to 800 Å thick) as a part of this complex structure. The basement membrane is elaborated by both epithelial and connective tissue cells.

**Lamina propria:**   Thin but rich in elastic fibers.

# STRATIFIED GERMINAL EPITHELIUM
## Seminiferous tubules

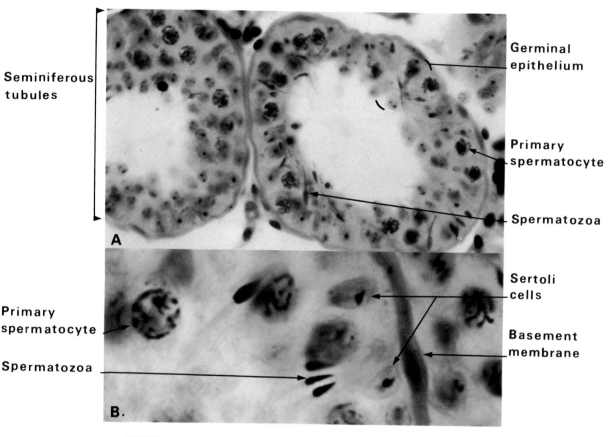

Seminiferous tubules

Germinal epithelium

Primary spermatocyte

Spermatozoa

A

Primary spermatocyte

Spermatozoa

Sertoli cells

Basement membrane

B.

A. $\overline{20\,\mu}$  B. $\overline{10\,\mu}$

**Rhesus monkey, Helly's fluid, Iron hematoxylin and orange G stains, A. 162 x., B. 1416 x.**

The germinal epithelium of the seminiferous tubules is composed of several layers of spermatogenic cells disposed between the basement membrane of the tubule and the lumen. (See Plate 225.)

**Primary spermatocyte:** Largest germ cell. Nuclei are large, vesicular and have condensed chromatin. Chromatin may appear as elongated threads.

**Spermatozoa:** Mature germinal cell consisting of a head and a tail. The heads are in close association with Sertoli cells, and the tails project into the lumen of the seminiferous tubule. Condensed nuclei forming the heads of spermatozoa contain a single set of chromosomes. Spermatozoa are the source of testicular hyaluronidase, an enzyme which may play a role in fertilization.

**Sertoli cell:** These are supporting cells of the testicular epithelium. Tall columnar cells extend from the basement membrane to the lumen. These cells possess an ovoid nucleus with a prominent nucleolus. Cell borders not well outlined in this preparation. Proximity to heads of spermatozoa is characteristic.

**Basement membrane:** Connective tissue sheath of the seminiferous tubules. The basement membrane is reinforced by outer layers of connective tissue.

# STRATIFIED SQUAMOUS EPITHELIUM
## A. Nonkeratinized
## B. Keratinized

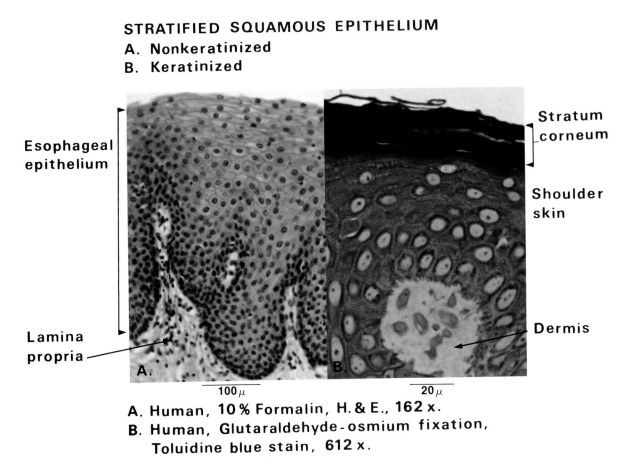

Esophageal epithelium

Lamina propria

Stratum corneum

Shoulder skin

Dermis

A. 100 μ      B. 20 μ

A. Human, 10% Formalin, H. & E., 162 x.
B. Human, Glutaraldehyde-osmium fixation, Toluidine blue stain, 612 x.

Stratified squamous epithelium is made up of several layers of cells. The deepest layer is composed of cuboidal or low columnar cells, the middle layer of polygonal cells and the superficial layers of flattened cells. The epithelium caps connective tissue papillae (lamina propria or dermis). The stratified squamous epithelium located internally (esophagus) is non-keratinized, while that located externally (skin) is keratinized (*i.e.*, possesses a stratum corneum). The stratum corneum is made up of flattened non-viable, non-nucleated epithelial cells containing keratin. (See also Plate 121.)

## STRATIFIED COLUMNAR EPITHELIUM
### Mucous gland duct
### tongue

Duct
lumen

Terminal
bars

Columnar
cell

Basal
cell

Plasma
cell

Collagen

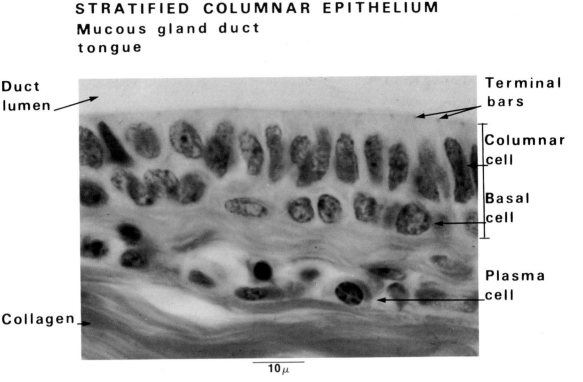

10 μ

### Human, Zenker's fluid, Iron hematoxylin & carmine stain, 1416 x.

**Columnar cells:**  Columnar cells form the superficial layer of the stratified columnar epithelium.

**Basal cell:**  These cells are irregularly polyhedral and form the deep layers of this stratified epithelium.

**Terminal bars:**  Darkly stained, thickened zone is the specific attachment site of the lateral surface of adjacent superficial columnar cells (so-called junctional complex from electron microscopic studies).

**Collagen:**  A component of the connective tissue stroma.

**Plasma cell:**  Eccentrically placed, prominent and structurally characteristic nucleus in an abundant basophilic cytoplasm. Plasma cells produce antibodies. (See also Plates 28 and 173).

## TRANSITIONAL EPITHELIUM
### Ureter

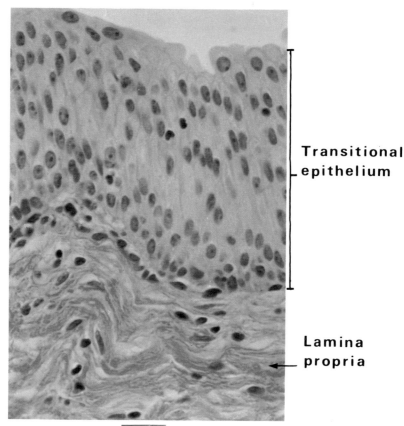

Transitional
epithelium

Lamina
propria

20 μ

## Human, Helly's fluid, H. & E., 612 x.

**Transitional epithelium:** This stratified epithelium is found lining the urinary tract from the renal calyces to the urethra. It is in direct continuity with the simple epithelium of the ducts and collecting tubules of the kidney and the stratified squamous epithelium of the urethra. Superficial cells are cuboidal and large, and the basal cells are cuboidal to columnar. The surface cells of this epithelium vary in shape from squamous when stretched to columnar when contracted. Note the convex luminal border of the surface cells. These cells may be multinucleated and polyploid.

**Lamina propria:** Predominantly reticular and collagenous connective tissue fibers with some elastic fibers. The lamina propria contains many cells, including lymphocytes, plasma cells, eosinophils and mast cells, in addition to blood capillaries and lymphatic vessels.

The term transitional epithelium does not imply that this epithelium is in actual transition from one type to another, but rather refers to the appearance of the cells, which changes as the organs with which they are associated are stretched or relaxed.

## PIGMENT EPITHELIUM
### Eye
### choroid layer

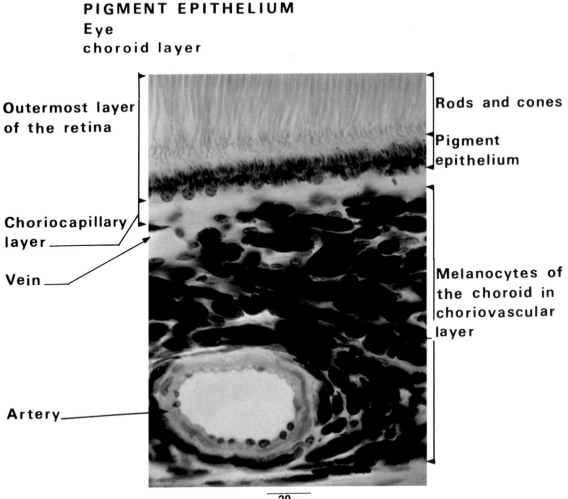

Outermost layer of the retina

Rods and cones

Pigment epithelium

Choriocapillary layer

Vein

Melanocytes of the choroid in choriovascular layer

Artery

20 μ

### Rhesus monkey, Helly's fluid, H. & E., 612 x.

The choroid layer of the eye is a highly vascular and pigmented coat surrounding the retina. Shown in this figure is a part of the retina adjoining the choroid layer, as well as the major choroid layers. In the outermost layer of the retina, the following structures are seen:

**Rods and cones:** Neuroepithelial cells sensitive to light, arranged vertically and parallel. (See also Plates 254, 255 and 256.)

**Pigment epithelium:** Single layer of pigmented cuboidal epithelial cells firmly bound to the choroid layer. Contains melanin pigment. In retinal detachments, the pigment epithelium remains attached to the choroid.

The two major layers of the choroid seen in this plate are the following:

**Choriocapillary layer:** Composed of a network of wide lumen capillaries disposed in one plane and separated by delicate connective tissue fibers. Note that pigmented cells are essentially lacking in this layer. This layer supplies nutrition to the cells of the outermost layers of the retina.

**Choriovascular layer:** Filled with pigmented cells (melanin) and large size vessels.

## GLANDULAR EPITHELIUM
### Zymogen
### pancreatic acinar cells

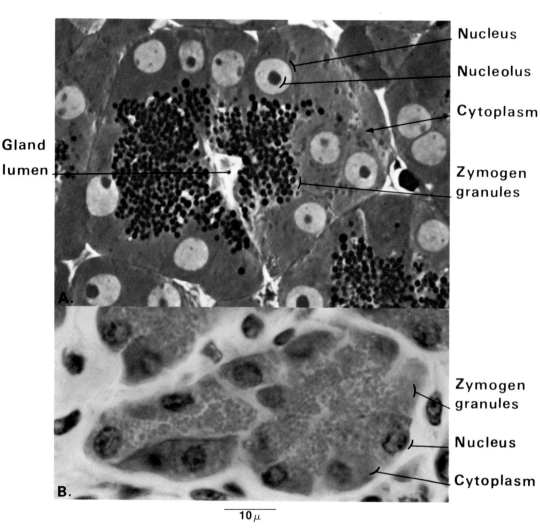

Nucleus

Nucleolus

Cytoplasm

Zymogen granules

Gland lumen

Zymogen granules

Nucleus

Cytoplasm

10 μ

Rhesus monkey; **A.** Glutaraldehyde-osmium fixation; Toluidine blue and Periodic acid-Schiff stains; **B.** Helly's fluid, Gomori's chrom alum hematoxylin; **1416 x.**

The configuration of pancreatic acinar cells is seen in these two preparations.

Note the pyramidal shape of the acinar cell, the basally located round nuclei with distinct nucleoli and two discrete zones of the cytoplasm. The apical zone near the lumen contains zymogen granules; the basal zone is intensely basophilic and free of granules. Electron microscopy has shown that the intense basophilia of the basal zone is due to its rich content of ribonucleoprotein bound to membrane (endoplasmic reticulum). It is known that the zymogen granules are synthesized in the basal cytoplasm and transported to the apical zone, to be discharged into the pancreatic duct.

# Connective Tissue

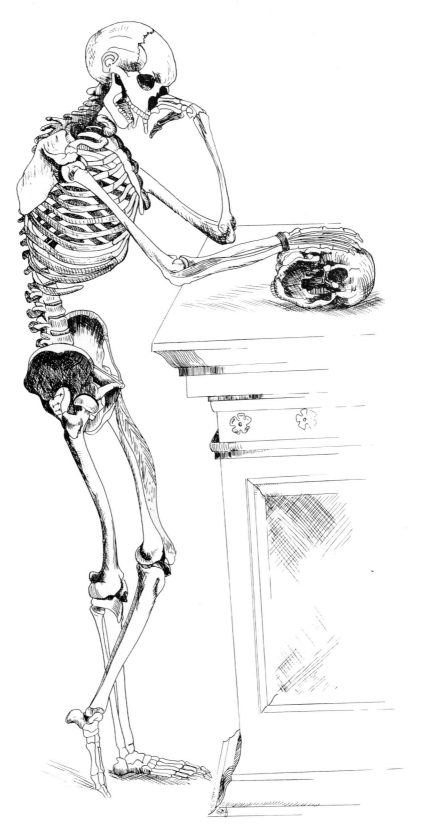

# Connective Tissue

The connective tissues include a variety of cells, non-living cell products and blood. One classification for the various connective tissues is as follows.

1. Adult Connective Tissue
    I. Connective tissue proper
        A. General
            1. Loose (areolar)
            2. Dense
        B. Special
            1. Elastic
            2. Reticular
            3. Adipose
            4. Pigmented
    II. Cartilage
        A. Hyaline
        B. Fibrous
        C. Elastic
    III. Bone
    IV. Blood and lymph
2. Embryonic Connective Tissue
    I. Mesenchyma
    II. Mucous tissue

## 1. Adult Connective Tissue

### I. Connective tissue proper

The *loose or areolar connective tissue* is made up of many of the cell types and intercellular materials (matrix) which compose the other connective tissues. It is widely distributed in the body and is found most readily beneath the skin, where it is termed the superficial fascia. This connective tissue binds cells and organs together but permits these cells and organs to move as necessary in relationship to each other. Because of the large amount of ground substance, it allows cells to move freely, and other structures, such as blood vessels and nerve fibers, to pass. This connective tissue is important because of its cellular content, for defense against infections and repair of damaged tissues.

Students of gross anatomy have a vivid memory of the *loose connective tissue* because they usually dissect it when removing the skin from the underlying muscle and the muscles from each other.

The most important cells of the *loose connective tissue* include the following. *Fibroblasts* synthesize connective tissue fibers. *Macrophages,* or *histiocytes,* and *monocytes* ingest, digest or store certain microscopic particles, such as debris of dead cells, bacteria and other materials. Capable of ameboid movement, these cells wander throughout the connective tissue and concentrate in regions requiring their necessary functional role. *Mast cells* synthesize and release substances of physiological importance, heparin and histamine. Heparin is a potent anticoagulant of blood, while histamine increases the permeability of blood capillaries. *Eosinophils,* also present in this connective tissue, produce and release histamine in small quantities. Their numbers increase in parasitic infections and in allergic hypersensitivity, *e.g.,* hayfever and asthma. *Lymphocytes* and *plasma cells* are also inhabitants of loose connective tissue and play an important role in the defense mechanism by producing antibodies, the immunoglobulins of the blood. In addition, *fat cells* may occur singly and in small or large groups. When fat cells predominate, the tissue is called *adipose tissue.* One of the special connective tissues (I,B,3 of our classification), *adipose tissue* serves as a reservoir of energy and as a soft packing in potential spaces (*e.g.,* axilla). It also invests glands (*e.g.,* mammary glands) which undergo cyclic or functional variation in size and activity, and surrounds highly mobile organs (*e.g.,* eye), blood vessels and nerve fiber bundles.

The more important intercellular components of the *loose connective tissue* include *collagenous, elastic* and *reticular* fibers and *amorphous ground substance.* Of these, *collagen* is usually found in greatest abundance and is strong and inelastic. It joins muscles to bone and skin and its distribution determines the limits of movement or expansion of tissues and organs. Within the limits set by collagenous connective tissue, *elastic fibers* permit extension, retraction and dynamic support of tissues and organs. They are highly refractile, and special histological methods reveal their presence. *Reticular fibers* are very fine and highly branched collagenous fibers. They form supporting networks around blood vessels and cells in some organs. They are in continuity with collagenous fibers and are inelastic. These fibers are only revealed by special histological methods. *Amorphous ground substance,* in which the connective tissue fibers are embedded, has a viscosity which varies from fluid to gel. The ground substance is only seen under very special circumstances of tissue preparation. The ground substance stains metachromatically with toluidine blue, and this suggests that it belongs to a class of chemical compounds called protein polysaccharides (mucopolysaccharides).

*Dense connective tissue* contains fewer cells but they are similar in type to those found in loose connective tissue. Collagenous fibers predominate in this type of connective tissue. *Dense connective tissue* appears in two forms, *dense irregular* and *dense regular* connective tissue. The irregular type is found in the dermis of the skin, deep fascia, the capsules or coverings of organs and nerve sheaths. *Dense regular* connective tissue is found in many tendons which provide a flexible but inelastic union between bone and skeletal muscle. Other examples of dense regular connective tissue include most ligaments, aponeuroses and the cornea of the eye.

Connective tissues with special characteristics of structure and function include *elastic, reticular* and *pigmented* types. *Adipose tissue,* which belongs with this group, has already been mentioned. *Elastic fibers* in dense parallel bands (elastic tissue) can be found associated with the vertebral column (ligamentum flava), in the suspensory ligament of the penis and in the vocal cords. A connective tissue sheet or fascia of the abdominal wall (Scarpa's fascia) is predominantly elastic tissue. Elastic fibers are functionally important components of skin and the hollow organs which include the large elastic arteries of the vascular system, trachea and bronchi of the respiratory system and elsewhere. *Reticular connective tissue fibers* are found in abundance in lymph nodes, blood-forming organs, spleen, liver and elsewhere, but, as mentioned before, cannot be seen unless special techniques are employed to reveal their presence. This type of connective tissue fiber is associated with phagocytic reticular cells. *Pigment tissue* is a cellular connective tissue rather than a fibrous non-living connective tissue and has many melanin-containing connective tissue cells. It is found predominantly in the choroid of the eye.

## II. Cartilage

*Cartilage* is a non-vascular tissue containing fibrous connective tissue embedded in an abundant and firm matrix. The cells which produce cartilage are called chondroblasts, and in mature cartilage they are termed chondrocytes. In the early fetus, the greater part of the skeleton is cartilaginous and, during later stages of development, the cartilage model is transformed into bone (endochondral ossification). Three types of cartilage are most frequently encountered. *Hyaline cartilage* is found at the ventral ends of the ribs, in the nose, larynx, trachea and the articular surfaces of adjacent bones of movable joints. The matrix or ground substance is strongly basophilic and stains metachromatically with toluidine blue and other similar basic dyes. It is the acidic sulfate groups of the protein polysaccharides comprising the ground substance of the matrix that are responsible for the staining reactions noted.

*Fibrocartilage* has a limited distribution. It is found in the intervertebral discs, the symphysis pubis, the menisci and ligaments of the knee and other joints and in the tendons of some muscles where they glide over bones (*e.g.,* the tendons of the peroneus longus and tibialis posterior). Fibrocartilage is composed predominantly of collagenous fibers arranged in bundles, with cartilage cells surrounded by a sparse cartilage matrix between the bundles. The collagenous fibers provide flexibility and strength and the cartilage gives it firmness.

*Elastic cartilage* is found in the external ear (pinna), the auditory tube, the epiglottis and in the corniculate and cuneiform cartilages of the larynx. It is yellow in color and is more flexible and elastic than the other cartilage types due to abundant branching elastic fibers in the matrix. Elastic fibers often concentrate in the walls of the lacunae which surround the cartilage cells.

## III. Bone

*Bone* is a tissue which forms the greatest part of the skeleton and is one of the hardest structures of the body; only the dentin and enamel of teeth are harder. It is tough and slightly elastic, withstanding tension and compression. Bone differs from cartilage in having its collagenous connective tissue matrix impregnated with inorganic salts, primarily calcium phosphate and lesser amounts of calcium carbonate, calcium fluoride, magnesium phosphate and sodium chloride. The osteoblasts which form the osseous tissue become encapsulated in lacunae but maintain contact with the vascular system via microscopic processes located in canaliculi. They are then referred to as osteocytes. A characteristic feature of the shaft (diaphysis) of a long bone is its organization in concentric circles or lamellae around a central canal containing a blood vessel. This is called the Haversian system. Between neighboring Haversian systems are non-concentric lamellae, devoid of Haversian canals, termed interstitial lamellae. Vascular canals, called Volkmann's canals, traverse the long axis of the bone, linking adjacent Haversian systems with each other and with the exterior of the bone.

The outer perimeter of a long bone, beneath the osteogenic connective tissue layer (called the periosteum), is composed of circumferential lamellae which also lack Haversian canals. This thick-walled hollow shaft of compact bone (the diaphysis) contains bone marrow. The distal ends of long bones, where Haversian systems are not found, appear spongy and are called cancellous or spongy bone. The epiphyses at the ends of the diaphysis or shaft contain the spongy bone covered by a thin layer of compact bone. The cavities of the epiphyseal spongy bone are in continuity with the bone marrow core of the diaphysis except during the period of growth of long bones in young animals. Interposed between the epiphysis and the diaphysis is the cartilaginous epiphyseal plate. The epiphyseal plate is joined to the diaphysis by columns of cancellous bone.

When bone is formed in and replaces a cartilaginous model the process is called endochondral ossification. Some parts of the skull develop from osteogenic mesenchymal connective tissue without a cartilage model having been formed first. This is termed intramembranous ossification, and these bones are called membrane bones. In both instances, three types of cells are associated with bone formation and growth: osteoblasts, osteocytes and osteoclasts. The osteoblasts produce osseous tissue, become embedded in the matrix formed, and are then renamed osteocytes. The osteoclasts actively resorb and remodel bone as required for growth. The osteoclasts are giant multinucleated phagocytic cells.

### IV. Blood and lymph

This type of connective tissue is peculiar because its matrix is liquid. The blood is carried in blood vessels and is moved throughout the body by the contractile activity of the heart. Lymph is found in lymphatic vessels but originates in the extracellular spaces. Distinctive cell types are found in blood and lymph vessels and will be considered in detail in subsequent sections of this atlas.

## 2. Embryonic Connective Tissue

### I. Mesenchyma

Derived from embryonic mesoderm, mesenchyma is the first connective tissue formed. The cells are widely spaced, with an abundance of intercellular matrix. The primitive mesenchymal cells differentiate into all the supporting tissues of the body. The cells derived from the mesenchyma include blood cells, megakaryocytes, endothelium, mesothelium, reticular cells, fibroblasts, mast cells, plasma cells, reticuloendothelial cells, cartilage cells, bone cells and smooth muscle.

### II. Mucous tissue

Widely distributed in the embryo as a loose connective tissue, mucous tissue is composed of large stellate fibroblasts in an abundant intercellular substance which is homogeneous and soft. In the umbilical cord it is known as Wharton's jelly.

# AREOLAR CONNECTIVE TISSUE
## Subcutaneous

Elastic
fibers

Fibroblasts

Collagenous
fibers

Lymphocyte

Mast cell

$20\mu$

## Rat, 10 % Formalin, H. & E., 612 x.

Areolar connective tissue is so named because of the many small areas or potential spaces that are seen within this tissue. It is the most widely encountered type of connective tissue and contains most of the connective tissue components.

**Collagenous fibers:**  Coarse interlacing bundles of fibers that run in all directions in the connective tissue.

**Elastic fibers:**  Slender network of branching fibers irregularly dispersed in the connective tissue. Smaller than the collagen fiber bundles.

**Mast cell:**  A large cell with a small spherical nucleus and abundant cytoplasm containing coarse granules. Produces heparin and histamine. In some animals 5-hydroxytryptamine (serotonin) is also produced by this cell.

**Fibroblasts:**  Only nuclei are seen in this preparation. Nuclei are ovoid and larger than other connective tissue nuclei. Fibroblasts are the most common cell type found in areolar connective tissue. They synthesize and deposit collagen.

**Lymphocytes:**  Only nuclei are seen in this preparation. Smaller than fibroblast nuclei, rounder and more deeply stained. They are not as abundant as fibroblasts.

## MAST CELLS

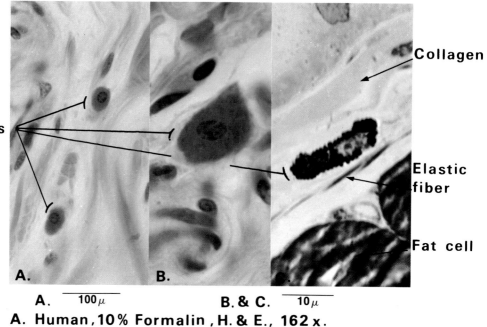

**Mast cells**

**Collagen**

**Elastic fiber**

**Fat cell**

A.

B.

**A.** ‾‾100 μ‾‾    **B. & C.** ‾‾10 μ‾‾
**A. Human, 10% Formalin, H. & E., 162 x.**
**B. Rat, Helly's fluid, Toluidine blue and erythrocin stains, 1416 x.**
**C. Rat, Glutaraldehyde - osmium fixation, Toluidine blue stain, 1416 x.**

Mast cells are found in areolar connective tissue and along the course of small blood vessels. They have a spheroid nucleus and abundant cytoplasm. The cytoplasm is filled with coarse granules that stain red in H. & E. preparations (A), but stain metachromatically with toluidine blue and other basic aniline dyes (B and C). Granules may be so abundant as to obscure the nucleus.

In man, mast cells produce heparin, a substance used as an anticoagulant to prevent blood clots. They also produce histamine, which increases the permeability of capillaries and influences the blood pressure.

In rats, mast cells also contain serotonin (5-hydroxytryptamine), which causes vasoconstriction and elevation of blood pressure.

Collagen and elastic fibers are scattered in the interstices between mast cells. Two fat cells stained black by osmium tetroxide fixation are seen in C.

## PLASMA CELLS
Lamina propria
jejunum

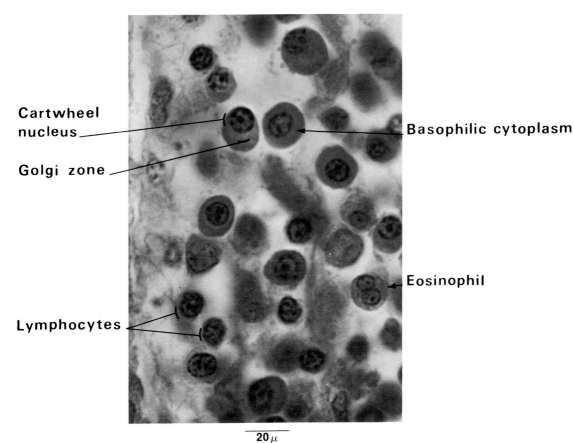

Cartwheel nucleus

Golgi zone

Basophilic cytoplasm

Eosinophil

Lymphocytes

$20\,\mu$

**Human, 10% Formalin, H. & E., 612 x.**

Plasma cells, although uncommon in loose connective tissue, are plentiful in the lamina propria of the digestive tract. Note the ovoid shape of the cell, the eccentric round or oval nucleus and the intensely basophilic cytoplasm. The less densely stained area of the cytoplasm in juxtaposition to the nucleus contains the Golgi complex and centrioles. Nuclear chromatin is characteristically clumped around the periphery of the nucleus and produces, in negative image, a radial pattern resembling the spokes of a wheel. The basophilia of the cytoplasm is shown by electron microscopy to be due to an extensive system of membrane-bound ribonucleoprotein. These cells produce antibodies.

Note the bilobed nucleus characteristic of human eosinophils in loose connective tissue. Eosinophils reach the lamina propria from the blood capillaries. The coarse, intensely eosinophilic granules of this cell are shown in Plate 57.

Compare the size of lymphocytes and plasma cells. Note that the nucleus of the lymphocyte fills most of the cell, with only a thin rim of basophilic cytoplasm around it. Some of the lymphocytes in the lamina propria migrate through the epithelium to the lumen, where they are eliminated.

## MACROPHAGES
## Lung
## terminal bronchiole

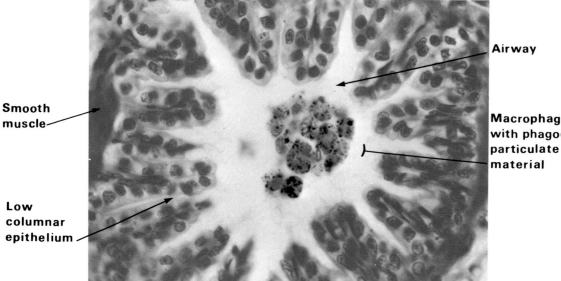

Airway

Smooth
muscle

Macrophages
with phagocytized
particulate
material

Low
columnar
epithelium

100 μ

## Cat, 10% Formalin, H. & E., 162 x.

This illustration shows a cross section of a terminal bronchiole with phagocytized material (black) in macrophages within the lumen of the bronchiole (airway). The pleating of the epithelial lining denotes a constricted bronchiole. Note the low columnar epithelial lining of the wall of the bronchiole and the smooth muscle bundle adjacent to the lining epithelium. (See also Plate 195.)

## TENDON
Embryonic triceps muscle tendon

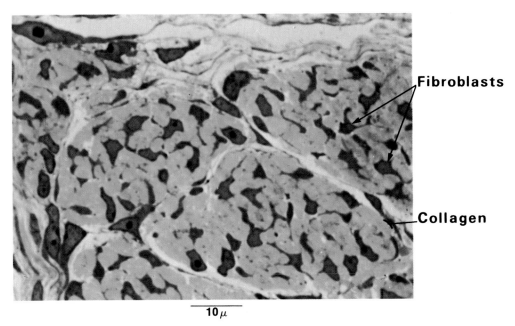

Human, Glutaraldehyde - osmium fixation,
Toluidine blue stain, 1416 x.

**Fibroblasts:**   Also known in mature tendons as tendon cells, they are the only cell type present. They are stellate in shape with cytoplasmic processes extending between and around the collagen bundles.

**Collagen:**   In thick bundles or fascicles, separated by tendon cells and loose connective tissue.

# COLLAGENOUS CONNECTIVE TISSUE
## Tendo calcaneus (Tendon of Achilles)
### longitudinal section

Fibrocyte nuclei

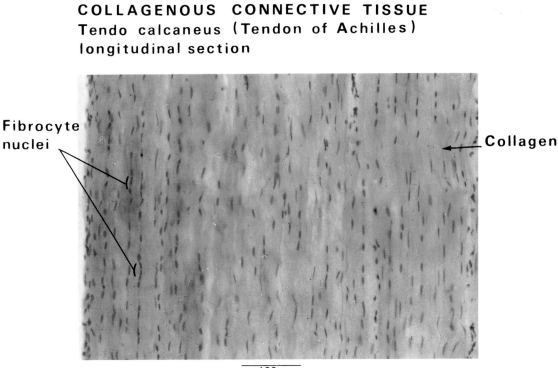

Collagen

100 μ

## Human,10% Formalin,H.&E.,162x.

**Collagen:** Fibers oriented in one direction and in dense aggregates and bundles separated by a small amount of areolar connective tissue containing vessels and nerves. Collagen fibrils are flexible, have high tensile strength and are inelastic. This large tendon links the gastrocnemius and soleus muscles with the calcaneus bone at the rear of the foot.

**Fibrocyte nuclei:** The predominant cell in this type of connective tissue (dense collagenous type) is oriented primarily in the longitudinal axis, in rows between the bundles of collagenous fibers.

## LIGAMENT
### Temporal bone and stapes

Anterior
crus of
stapes

Haversian
canal

Tympanic
cavity

Temporal
bone

Annular
ligament

Base of
stapes

Vestibule

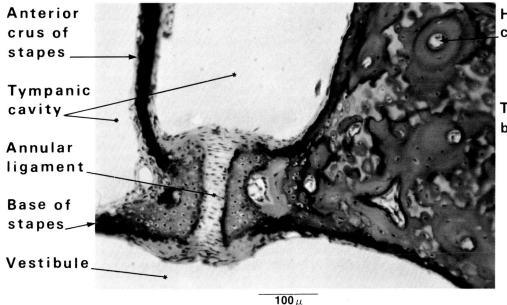

$$\overline{100\,\mu}$$

### Cat, Müller's fluid, Iron hematoxylin, 162x.

**Tympanic cavity:**  Air-containing space in the middle ear. Limited laterally by the tympanic membrane and medially by the osseous labyrinth. Although not illustrated here, the cavity contains the chorda tympani nerve, the auditory ossicles and the small tendons of the stapedius and tensor tympani muscles, which are connected to the bony ossicles.

**Stapes:**  One of the three auditory ossicles in the tympanic cavity. It was so named by Ingrassias, who described it in 1546. The name is derived from Latin (*stare,* to stand; *pes,* foot; the thing in which the foot stands) because of its resemblance to a stirrup. The ossicle consists of a head, neck, two limbs, or crura, and a base. The two crura are connected to the base. This figure shows only the anterior crus of the stapes and part of the base.

**Anterior crus of the stapes:**  Shorter and less curved than the posterior crus with which it is connected by the base.

**Base of the stapes:**  Also called foot plate of the stapes. Fixed to the margin of the fenestra vestibuli (ovalis) by the annular ligament. Also connects the two crura of the stapes.

**Annular ligament:**  A ring of fibroelastic tissue which fixes the base of the stapes to the fenestra vestibuli but permits the stapes to rock or move in response to vibrations of the eardrum. The sound waves are transmitted to the stapes by the incus and malleus (the other two auditory ossicles).

**Vestibule:**  Large bony cavity medial to the tympanic cavity. In its lateral wall is the fenestra vestibuli, to which the foot of the stapes is fixed.

**Temporal bone:**  Surrounding the ear cavities and containing the vestibular and sound receptor organs (semicircular canals and the cochlea). See Plates 260, 262 and 263.

# ELASTIC MEMBRANES
# COLLAGENOUS FIBERS
### Aorta

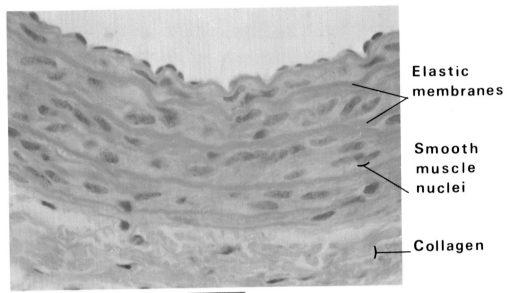

Elastic membranes

Smooth muscle nuclei

Collagen

100 μ

### Rat, Helly's fluid, H. & E., 162 x.

**Elastic membranes:** Abundant in the media of elastic arteries. The elastic fibers anastomose to form a fenestrated "membrane" which is circularly arranged in layers.

**Smooth muscle nuclei:** Smooth muscle fibers are located between the elastic fiber networks. Circularly disposed.

**Collagen:** In the adventitia, collagen forms a loose irregular connective tissue layer surrounding the blood vessel. Elastic fibers, not distinguishable by this method, are also found in this connective tissue coat.

Compare this general staining method with that used in Plate 34. The general method used in this preparation allows differentiation of the various vessel wall components only by the variations in the intensity of staining. The pronounced eosinophilia of the elastic fibers reflects their high content of basic amino acids. See also Plates 135 and 139.

## ELASTIC MEMBRANES
## COLLAGENOUS FIBERS
### Aorta

Elastic
membranes

Elastic
membranes

Collagen

Collagen

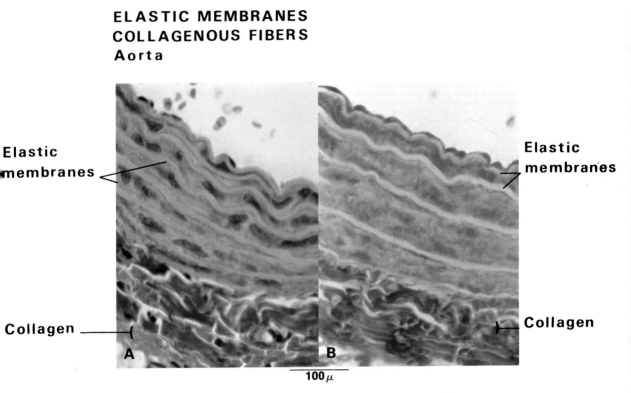

A   B

100 μ

## Rat, Helly's fluid, Mallory's stain (A), Mallory-
## azan stain (B), 162 x.

**Elastic membranes:**  Elastic membranes are a striking feature of the aorta. Located within the tunica media of the vessel wall, they serve as "shock absorbers." Elastic arteries are subject to the greatest and most rapid changes in blood pressure. The elastic membranes or laminae are separated from each other by smooth muscle fibers, fibroblasts and collagenous and reticular connective tissue fibers. Note that the elastic laminae are unstained by the methods employed here. Elastic tissue stains can be seen in Plates 119, 135, 137 and 139.

**Collagen:**  Primarily located external to the outermost elastic lamina, it stains a bright blue with Mallory and Mallory-azan stains. Note the collagenous connective tissue immediately adjacent to the elastic laminae. The methods employed here selectively stain collagenous fibers. Compare with Plate 33.

See Plates 135 and 136 to compare the structure of this rat aorta with those of rabbit and man.

## RETICULAR CELLS
### Lymph node
### subcapsular sinus

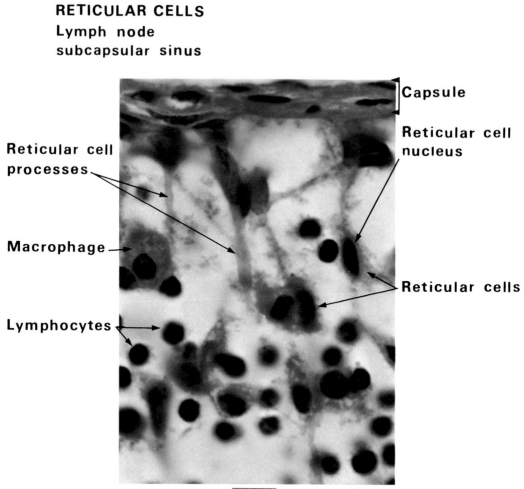

Capsule

Reticular cell nucleus

Reticular cell processes

Macrophage

Reticular cells

Lymphocytes

20 μ

**Rhesus monkey, Helly's fluid, H. & E., 612 x.**

The subcapsular sinus of a lymph node is a lymph channel beneath the capsule of the node (see Plate 146). The component elements of the sinus are seen in this figure: reticular cells and their processes which form a meshwork. Reticular cells are star-shaped, with lightly staining cytoplasm and processes that are in contact but not continuous with processes of adjacent cells. These cells and their processes form the reticular tissue mesh-work of the node in which lymphocytes and free macrophages are found.

# RETICULAR FIBERS
## Liver

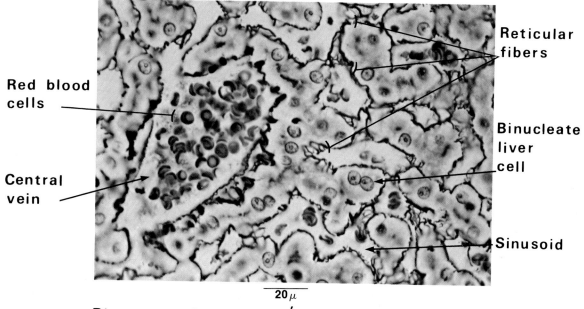

Red blood cells

Central vein

Reticular fibers

Binucleate liver cell

Sinusoid

20 μ

Rhesus monkey, Wilder's method, 612 x.

**Reticular fibers:** Branch and anastomose in a delicate fibrous network delineating the sinusoids. Small diameter and resistance to dyes make them difficult to demonstrate except by special techniques such as the method employed in this preparation.

**Binucleate liver cells:** Polyhedral cells with centrally placed nuclei and prominent nucleoli. Occasionally multinucleate.

**Sinusoids:** Constitute the intralobular system of specialized vascular channels. Carry blood from interlobular branches of the portal vein centripetally to the central vein. They anastomose and separate adjacent hepatic cellular plates.

**Central vein:** In the center of the hepatic lobule. Smallest radicle of hepatic veins. Receives the contents of all the sinusoids of the hepatic lobule.

**Red blood cells:** Filling the central vein, they carry oxygen to the hepatic cells and remove carbon dioxide. The red blood cell is approximately 7.5 μ in diameter and can be used as a rough internal micron marker.

## RETICULAR FIBERS
### Duodenum smooth muscle

**Inner layer of muscularis**

**Outer layer of muscularis**

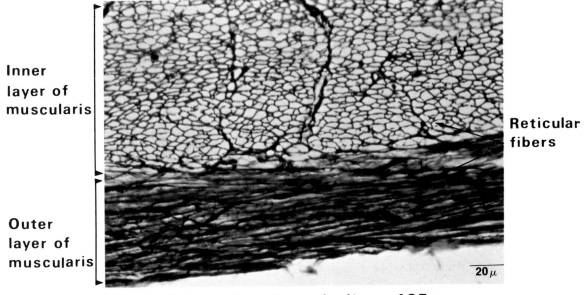

**Reticular fibers**

20 μ

### Rat, 10% Formalin, Gomori silver, 435x.

This is part of the muscular coat of the duodenum, stained with a special silver technique to demonstrate reticular fibers. Note the abundance of reticular fibers between muscle fibers. The latter are not stained by this method. The negative outlines of the transversely sectioned muscle fibers of the inner circular coat are well delineated by the stained reticular fibers.

## FAT CELLS
### Panniculus adiposus

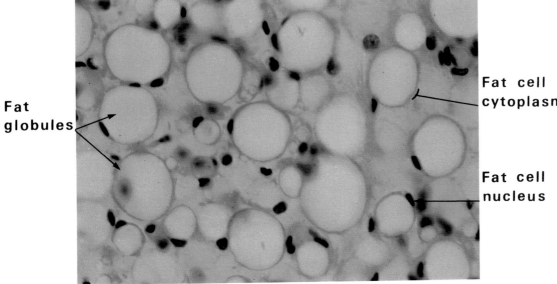

Fat globules

Fat cell cytoplasm

Fat cell nucleus

**Human, 10% Formalin, H. & E., 612 x.**

20 μ

**Fat cell cytoplasm:** Appears as a thin rim at the periphery of the cell. Stored fat is the predominant component of cytoplasm.

**Fat cell nucleus:** The nucleus is flattened in the cytoplasm, permitting maximum storage of fat globules.

**Fat globules:** Appear as empty spaces because the fat has been dissolved out by solvents used in the preparation of tissues. Special fixatives and stains are needed to demonstrate lipid droplets (see Plate 9). At body temperature the fat is liquid.

The fat cell lipid is in the form of a single droplet and these cells are described as unilocular. In brown fat (Plate 39) the lipid appears as small multiple droplets, and these cells are described as multilocular.

## BROWN FAT
### Mediastinum

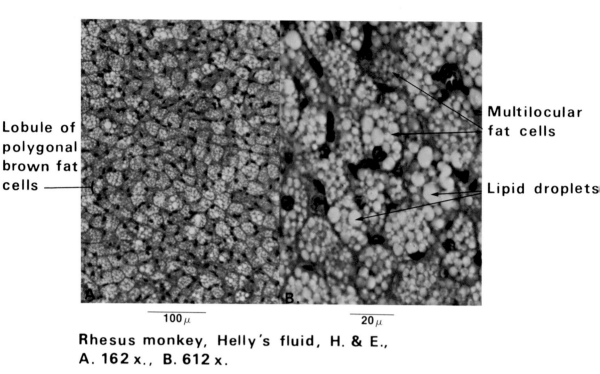

Lobule of polygonal brown fat cells

Multilocular fat cells

Lipid droplets

100 μ          20 μ

**Rhesus monkey, Helly's fluid, H. & E.,**
**A. 162 x., B. 612 x.**

Brown fat is an uncommon variety of fat found in specific locations in the body. Unlike the more common white fat, brown fat cells contain a number of small lipid droplets, hence the name multilocular fat. White fat cells, in contrast, contain a single lipid droplet (Plate 38).

# HYALINE CARTILAGE
## Trachea

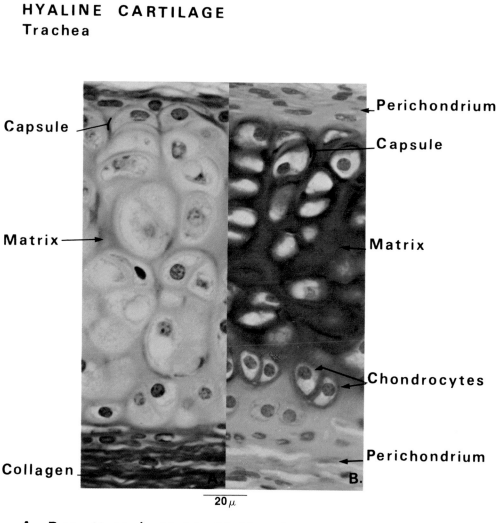

Capsule

Matrix

Collagen

Perichondrium

Capsule

Matrix

Chondrocytes

Perichondrium

A.

B.

$20\,\mu$

A. Rat, Helly's fluid, Mallory's stain, 612 x.
B. Rat, Helly's fluid, Toluidine blue and erythrosin, 612 x.

**Perichondrium:** A dense layer of irregular fibrous connective tissue which always invests hyaline cartilage except at the free surfaces of articular cartilage. Note how the perichondrium in *A* is better shown by a connective tissue stain (Mallory) specific for collagen.

**Chondrocytes:** Two or more cartilage cells enclosed within smooth-walled spaces or lacunae. Note the centrally placed, large spherical nuclei (isogenous grouping). The vacuolation noted in the cytoplasm of chondrocytes is an artifact of processing resulting from poor preservation of fat droplets and glycogen. Note the rounded appearance of chondrocytes centrally located and the flattened appearance of cells near the perichondrium.

**Matrix:** Derived from a Latin word meaning womb, a place where something is formed and a medium enclosing other bodies. The matrix is composed of ground substance (protein polysaccharide) and connective tissue fibers. It fills the space between chondrocytes. In *B*, note the metachromasia of the matrix stained with toluidine blue. The metachromasia is due to the high content of chondroitin sulfate.

**Capsule:** The wall of the lacunae is referred to as a capsule. The capsule is a condensation of the matrix surrounding the lacunae.

PLATE 41

## ELASTIC CARTILAGE
### Epiglottis

Dog, Zenker's fluid, H. & E., 162 x.

**Cartilage cells:** Large, pleomorphic and housed in lacunae of the matrix. One or more cells may be found in one lacuna.

**Capsules:** Condensed matrix surrounding cartilage cells. Stains intensely and represents the most recent deposition of matrix.

**Matrix:** Contains collagenous and elastic fibers embedded in a highly acidic ground substance consisting of chondroitin sulfate and protein.

**Elastic fibers:** Oriented in all directions within the matrix, elastic fibers give flexibility to the cartilage.

## ENDOCHONDRAL OSSIFICATION
Finger
phalanx

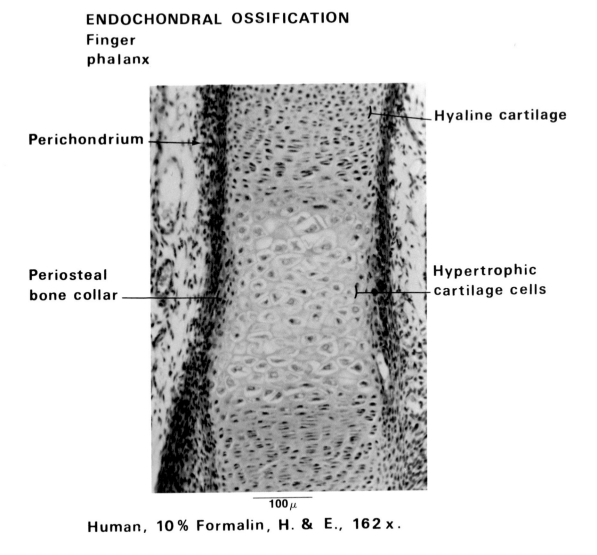

Perichondrium

Hyaline cartilage

Periosteal
bone collar

Hypertrophic
cartilage cells

100 μ

Human, 10% Formalin, H. & E., 162 x.

Endochondral bone is a form of ossification in which an embryonal type of hyaline cartilage precedes the formation of bone. In this figure, note the change from the zone of reserve cartilage cells to the zone of hypertrophic cartilage cells. Lacunae are increased in size and the interlacunar space is reduced in the region of the hypertrophic cells. Note the concomitant change in the perichondrium in which the inner cells change into osteogenic cells (osteoblasts) leading to the formation of the periosteal (perichondral) bone collar.

## ENDOCHONDRIAL BONE FORMATION
Middle phalanx

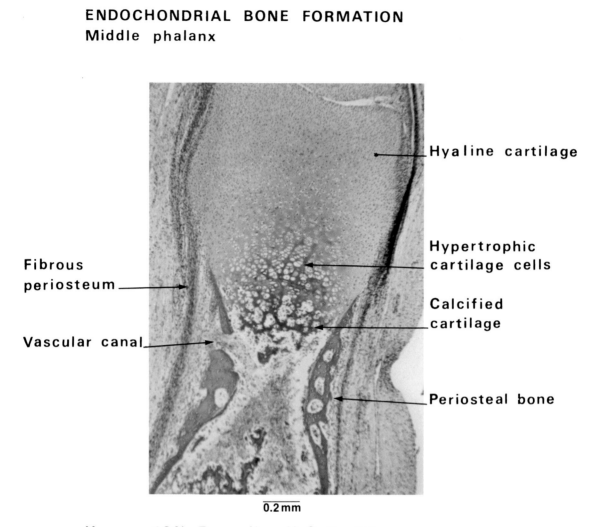

Hyaline cartilage

Hypertrophic cartilage cells

Fibrous periosteum

Calcified cartilage

Vascular canal

Periosteal bone

0.2mm

**Human, 10% Formalin, H. & E., 50 x.**

Stages of intracartilaginous bone formation are shown in this figure. Note the transition from the intact large area of hyaline cartilage to the region of hypertrophic cartilage cells. In the latter zone, there is an obvious increase in the number and size of lacunae. The interlacunar matrix is reduced in size. This zone is continuous with the zone of calcified cartilage, in which calcium salts are added to the matrix. Note that the calcified matrix in this zone stains more intensely. Also note the concomitant changes taking place in the periosteum. Two layers of periosteum are seen: fibrous, forming an outer collar, and osteogenic (periosteal bone), forming an inner collar around the ossification center. Periosteal ossification begins in the inner layer of the periosteum, where cells become osteogenic and form osteoblasts. Note that the bony collar is fenestrated to allow passage of vascular connective tissue (vascular canal) carrying blood vessels and osteogenic cells from the periosteum.

## MEMBRANE BONE
### Mandible

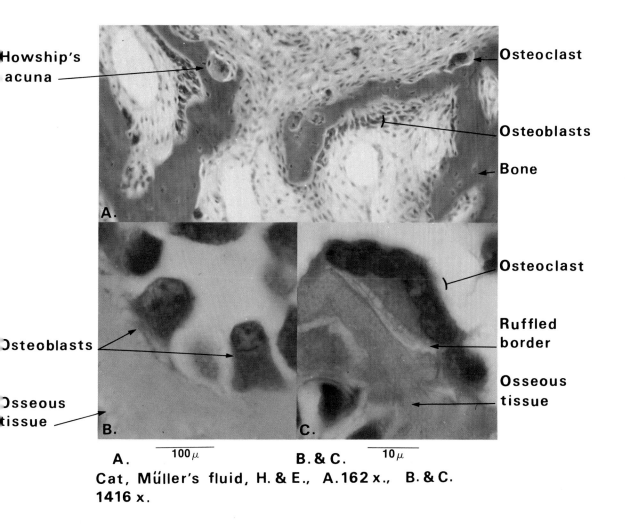

Howship's acuna

Osteoclast

Osteoblasts

Bone

Osteoblasts

Osteoclast

Ruffled border

Osseous tissue

Osseous tissue

A. 100 μ    B. & C. 10 μ

**Cat, Müller's fluid, H. & E., A.162 x., B. & C. 1416 x.**

**Howship's lacuna:** Resorption depressions in the bone surface in which osteoclasts are lodged.

**Osteoclast:** A multinucleated giant cell associated with areas of bone resorption. The surface adjacent to bone being resorbed has numerous cytoplasmic processes, giving the ruffled border appearance.

**Osteoblasts:** Responsible for bone matrix formation and present wherever osseous tissue is elaborated. In membranous bone, osteoblasts arise as differentiated mesenchymal cells.

# ENDOCHONDRAL BONE AND FIBROCARTILAGE
Tibia
knee joint

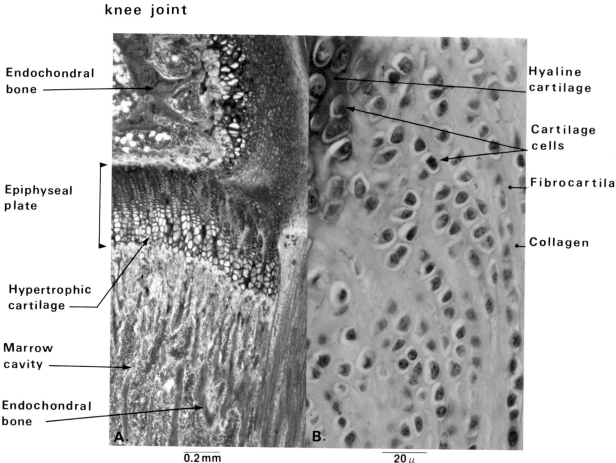

Endochondral bone

Epiphyseal plate

Hypertrophic cartilage

Marrow cavity

Endochondral bone

Hyaline cartilage

Cartilage cells

Fibrocartila

Collagen

A.

B.

0.2 mm

20 μ

Rat, 10% Formalin, A. H. & E., 50x., B. Gomori's aldehyde fuchsin, 612x.

Endochondral bone formation is a process in which an embryonal type of hyaline cartilage precedes bone formation. In *A*, a stage in the endochondral ossification in a long bone (tibia) is shown. Note the cartilaginous epiphyseal plate which separates the epiphysis (above) from the diaphysis (below). The epiphyseal plate is the source of new cartilage, which is replaced by bone during growth in length. Note the zone of hypertrophic cartilage within the epiphyseal plate. This is a stage in endochondral bone formation preceding calcification. Islands of formed endochondral bone are seen above and below the epiphyseal plate in the epiphysis and diaphysis. Note the marrow cavity between plates of endochrondral bone in the diaphysis. This cavity is formed by resorption of endochondral bone.

In *B*, note the characteristic grouping of fibrocartilage cells and their arrangement in rows separated by dense collagenous connective tissue. Adjacent to fibrocartilage, note the hyaline cartilage cells.

## BONE
### Fibula

Haversian
canal

Blood
pigment

Lacunae
and
canaliculi

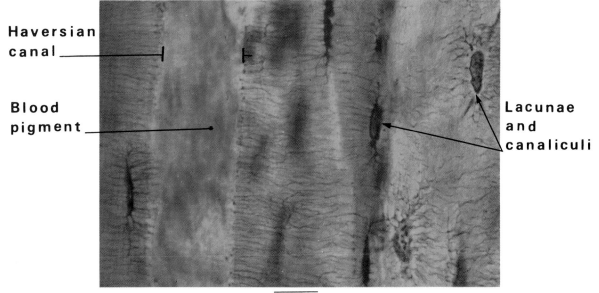

20 μ

**Human, Ground bone, Unstained, 612 x.**

**Haversian canal:** Conduct blood vessels, lymphatics and nerves through bone. Haversian canals surrounded by concentric lamellae of compact bone form the Haversian system. These canals are named after Clopton Havers, an English physician, who described them in his *Osteologia Novia,* published in London in 1691.

**Blood pigment:** From disintegrated blood elements in the vessels within the Haversian canals.

**Lacunae and canaliculi:** The former are cell spaces that housed osteocytes, and the latter are channels extending out of the lacunae that accommodated cell processes of osteocytes.

# BONE
## Compact
## cross section

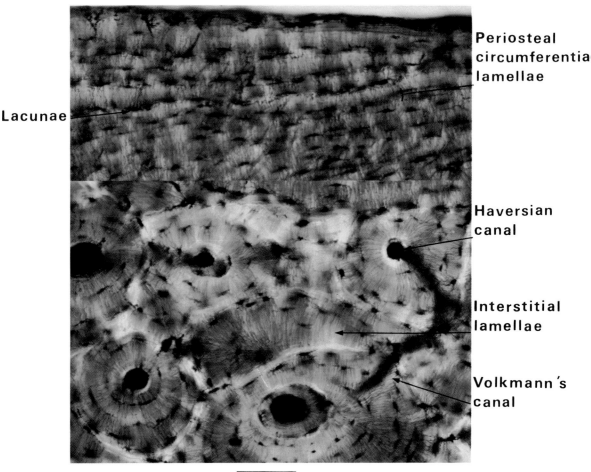

Lacunae

Periosteal
circumferentia
lamellae

Haversian
canal

Interstitial
lamellae

Volkmann's
canal

100 μ

## Human, Ground bone, 162 x.

**Lacunae:**  Cavities housing the osteocytes.

**Periosteal circumferential lamellae:**  Series of parallel lamellae lying next to the periosteum.

**Haversian canals:**  Abundant, and chacteristic of compact bone. Their course follows the main axis of long bone. Conduct blood vessels, lymphatics and nerves throughout the bone. They branch and anastomose and become continuous with Volkmann's canals. Haversian canals surrounded by concentric lamellae of compact bone form the Haversian system.

**Volkmann's canals:**  Cross connections between Haversian canals. They pierce the lamellae of two Haversian systems. Contain blood vessels, lymphatics and nerves. Supply the interstitial lamellae.

**Interstitial lamellae:**  A set of bone lamellae that fill the spaces between Haversian systems. Vary in shape and orientation.

## MESENCHYMAL CONNECTIVE TISSUE

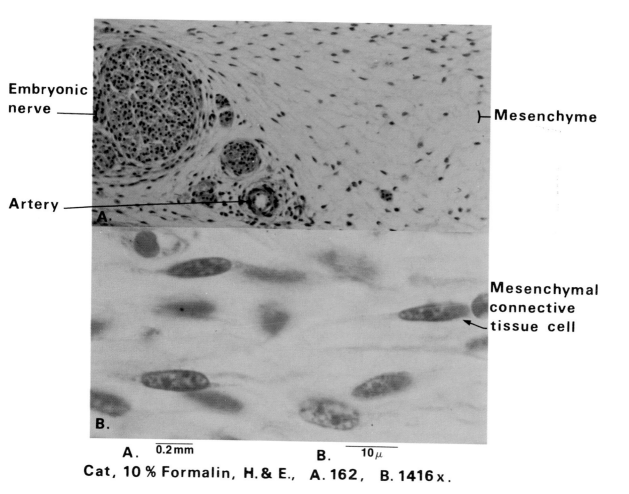

Embryonic nerve

Mesenchyme

Artery

A.

B.

Mesenchymal connective tissue cell

A. 0.2 mm    B. 10 μ

Cat, 10 % Formalin, H. & E.,   A. 162,   B. 1416 x .

**Mesenchyme:**   Unspecialized connective tissue having a delicate spongy structure that characterizes embryonic life. Consists of cells and matrix. The matrix contains ground substance and scanty fine fibrils. Mesenchymal cells differentiate into the supporting tissues, vascular tissues, blood and smooth muscle.

**Mesenchymal connective tissue cell:**   Spindle-shaped, tapering processes, large nucleus and scanty cytoplasm. Processes appear continuous with those of adjacent cells (syncytium). In reality, these processes are in contact but are not continuous.

An embryonic nonmyelinated nerve and artery are also seen in the mesenchyme.

# MUCOUS CONNECTIVE TISSUE
## Umbilical cord

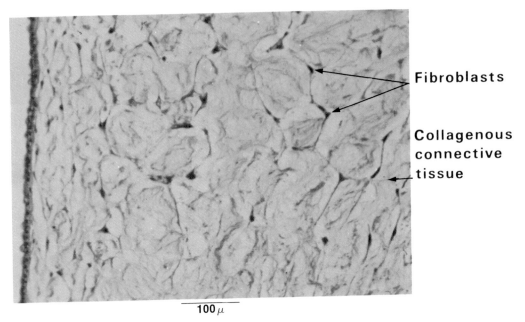

Fibroblasts

Collagenous
connective
tissue

100 μ

Rhesus monkey, Helly's fluid, H. & E., 162 x.

Mucous connective tissue is characteristically found in the umbilical cord. It also is transiently encountered as a stage in the differentiation of mesenchyme into connective tissue.

The distinctive cell of mucous connective tissue is a primitive fibroblast, which may be spindle or stellate in shape. In H. & E. preparations, only nuclei of fibroblasts are evident. Fine collagenous fibrils aggregate in the ground substance, which is characteristically abundant and gelatinous.

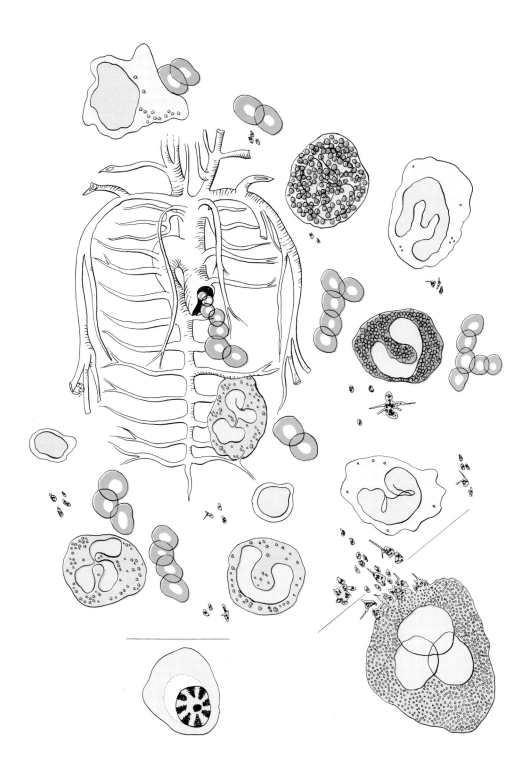

# Blood

Blood is a connective tissue in which the matrix is fluid. It is composed of red blood corpuscles, white cells and a fluid, the blood plasma, and is transported throughout the body within blood vessels.

A. Red blood corpuscles are also known as erythrocytes or red blood cells. In man, the mature red blood corpuscle does not contain a nucleus and is therefore an incomplete cell incapable of cell division or reproduction. The red blood corpuscle is a biconcave disc. This shape favors the rapid absorption and release of oxygen and carbon dioxide. The absence of a nucleus also facilitates respiratory function. Circulating red blood corpuscles average about 8.5 $\mu$, while in dried blood smears they are approximately 7.5 $\mu$, and in fixed and sectioned tissues they may shrink still further. In tissue sections they can be used as a "rough" internal measure for size estimation.

In human males, there are approximately 5.5 million red corpuscles per cubic mm of blood. In females, the normal number is about 5.0 million per cubic mm of blood. It is estimated that a 150 pound man has about 5 liters of blood. Massed red blood corpuscles are red in color due to the presence of the respiratory pigment hemoglobin. The mature red blood corpuscle is membrane-bound and contains a homogeneous cytoplasm normally devoid of a nucleus and cell organelles. A small number (about 0.5 to 1.5 per cent) of immature red blood corpuscles (reticulocytes) contain some ribonucleoprotein (ribosomes), which is stainable with nuclear dyes such as brilliant cresyl blue and appears as a reticulum.

It is estimated that the life span of the red blood corpuscle is around 120 days. This means that about $25 \times 10^{10}$ corpuscles are replaced daily; a turnover rate of 2.5 million corpuscles a second. Both damaged and normal erythrocytes are removed from the vascular system by macrophages, which are found primarily in the liver, spleen and bone marrow. The breakdown products of hemoglobin are excreted in the bile (bilirubin), but the iron is conserved and used in new red corpuscles.

A red blood corpuscle is filled with the respiratory pigment hemoglobin, which combines with oxygen in the lungs and carries it to the tissues, where it is exchanged for carbon dioxide. The carbon dioxide is carried to the lungs, where it is replaced by oxygen. The cycle is repeated continuously throughout the life of the corpuscle.

Red corpuscles, normally devoid of nucleic acids, stain with acid dyes because of their strongly basic hemoglobin. They stain red with the hematoxylin and eosin (H. & E.) stains (eosinophilic). Red blood cells are uniform in diameter and, in tissue sections, they are normally found within blood vessels. Extravascular red blood corpuscles may arise from tissue preparation (artifact) or from the rupture of blood vessels resulting from disease or accident.

B. White blood cells or leucocytes are complete cells containing nuclei and the usual cell organelles. Two distinct groups are recognized. The so-called agranular leucocytes include the lymphocytes and the monocytes. The granular leucocytes include the neutrophilic, eosinophilic and basophilic granulocytes.

The agranular leucocytes normally contain some nonspecific granules (Plates 51 and 52), whereas the granular leucocytes always contain specific granules in their cytoplasm. See Plate 50. The relative proportion of leucocytes in normal adult human blood is as follows: neutrophil, 40 to 75 per cent; eosinophil, 1 to 3 per cent; basophil, 0.5 to 1 per cent; lymphocyte, 20 to 45 per cent; and monocyte, 2 to 10 per cent.

The normal average number of leucocytes varies between 5000 and 9000 per cubic mm in adults. If the number of white blood cells is increased (above 12,000) or decreased (below 5000), disease is indicated. An increase from normal values is termed leucocytosis and a decrease is termed leucopenia. For example, neutrophils are known to increase in number in pus-forming infections, and eosinophils increase in allergies and parasitic infestations. Other diseases may result in changes in the number of one or more of the other leucocytes.

The life span of white blood cells is considered to be shorter than that of red blood cells but exact timing is difficult because they normally leave the vascular system to enter the tissue spaces to perform their special functions. Aging leucocytes are removed from the circulation by the macrophages of the liver and spleen, or they may die and disintegrate in the connective tissue or migrate through the epithelia of the gastrointestinal and respiratory tracts and be eliminated.

Some leucocytes can be identified in tissue sections (*e.g.,* lymphocytes and eosinophils are most readily seen in routine sections), but others are not seen to advantage by this method. The peripheral blood smear is the preferred method of identification of cell types. Leucocytes tend to be relatively inactive while in the blood stream but are capable of ameboid movement and concentrate in sites of infection in the tissues and organs. Neutrophils and monocytes are the most phagocytic of the white blood cells, and ingest foreign particles, bacteria and degenerating cells and cell fragments. The monocyte is considered to be the most active phagocyte. Neutrophils provide the first line of defense against invading foreign bodies and organisms, and lymphocytes are believed to form antibodies, a function shared with the plasma cells.

C. The lymphocyte varies widely in size. Small lymphocytes are 7 to 10 $\mu$ in diameter, and large lymphocytes are approximately 14 to 20 $\mu$ in diameter. Intermediate sizes are frequently encountered. The nuclei of lymphocytes are usually round but may also be slightly indented. The nuclear chromatin is clumped, and stains intensely with Wright's stain. The cytoplasm immediately adjacent to the nucleus is agranular, is poorly stained and appears as a perinuclear halo. The remainder of the cytoplasm is basophilic and stains variable shades of blue. Some lymphocytes possess azurophilic granules which stain a reddish or purple hue and are not evenly distributed. See Plates 51 and 147. Lymphocytes are produced in lymphoid tissues.

D. Monocytes are approximately 15 to 25 $\mu$ in diameter. The nuclei of monocytes are usually kidney-shaped, indented or lobed. The cytoplasm of the monocyte is gray-blue and contains azurophilic granules which are evenly distributed. Vacuoles are often demonstrable in the cytoplasm. Monocytes often show evidence of ameboid movement and are voracious phagocytes. Monocytes are produced by the lymphoid organs. See Plate 52.

E. Blood platelets are fragments of the cytoplasm derived from the megakaryocyte. Platelets are small discs about 2 to 4 $\mu$ in diameter and number between 200,000 to 350,000 per cubic mm of blood. In general, two to six blood platelets or thrombocytes are seen in an oil immersion field but their distribution is variable and they may appear in large clumps. Their specific function is related to the clotting of blood both inside and outside blood vessels.

F. Blood plasma is the fluid in which the blood cells reside within the blood vessels. Plasma constitutes 55 per cent of whole blood, while cellular components total 45 per cent. Blood plasma contains gases, proteins, carbohydrates, amino acids, lipids, inorganic salts, enzymes, hormones and antibodies. It is slightly alkaline. Blood plasma serves an important role in coagulation, temperature regulation, respiration, regulation of blood pH (buffer) and fluid balance. Hormones, absorbed nutrients and metabolic wastes are carried in the plasma to sites of action, utilization or elimination.

## Origin of Blood Cells

Inasmuch as blood cells have a short life span, they must be constantly replaced in vast numbers. The term applied to this process is hemopoiesis and takes place in the bone marrow and lymphoid tissues of adults. In the embryo and fetus various organs are involved in blood cell formation. These organs include the yolk sac, liver, spleen, thymus and lymph nodes, as well as the bone marrow.

## Erythropoiesis

Red blood corpuscles undergo their maturation within the bone marrow, and several stages can be recognized. The earliest cells of this series have a large round nucleus. The chromatin is reticulated, and one or more small nucleoli can be recognized. The cytoplasm is seen as a thin rim which stains a royal blue color with Wright's stain. These cells unfortunately are called by several names: rubriblast, proerythroblast, pronormoblast or megaloblast. As the rubriblast matures, the nucleus become smaller, the chromatin coarsens and nucleoli become ill-defined or disappear. The cytoplasm is still basophilic (blue). These cells are termed prorubricytes, basophilic erythroblasts, basophilic normoblasts or early erythroblasts. The next recognizable stage involves further coarsening and reduction in nuclear size. Nucleoli are absent. Relatively, the cytoplasm appears to occupy more of the cell and is seen to contain a mixture of eosinophilic (red) and basophilic (blue) cytoplasm. These cells are named rubricytes, polychromatophilic erythroblasts, normoblasts, intermediate erythroblasts or intermediate normoblasts. The nucleus of the next stage is still smaller than the preceding stage and is a solid blue-black color. The nucleus is now non-functional. The cytoplasm is predominantly acidophilic with some residual basophilia. The hemoglobin, which is eosinophilic, dominates with only minimal amounts of residual ribonucleoprotein staining the cytoplasm a bluish tint. The nucleus is ejected from the cell in the next stage, and the cytoplasm still retains a slight bluish tint, but the predominant color is reddish, signifying the increased synthesis of hemoglobin. These cells are termed diffusely basophilic erythrocytes or polychromatophilic erythrocytes. In the final stage, the cytoplasmic ribonucleoprotein disappears and the corpuscles appear as biconcave discs, 6 to 8 $\mu$ in diameter and reddish in color when stained with Wright's stain. These structures are termed red blood corpuscles, erythrocytes or red blood cells. Erythropoiesis can be seen in Plate 55.

## Granulocytic System

Granular leucocytes develop in the bone marrow from undifferentiated cells called myeloblasts. Myeloblasts are approximately 20 $\mu$ in diameter. The nucleus is round, stains a purple color and contains two or more nucleoli. The cytoplasm is basophilic and when stained with Wright's stain appears agranular and pale blue. In the next recognizable stage, the nucleus is reduced in size and the chromatin becomes more coarse and unevenly stained. This cell contains granules which stain variably from red to purple-blue and is designated a progranulocyte or a promyelocyte. A progranulocyte becomes a myelocyte when the granules become sufficiently differentiated in size, color and shape to be recognizable as the specific granules of neutrophils, eosinophils or basophils. The subsequent developmental changes are similar for the three types of granulocytes.

The primary changes are a reduction in cell size and alterations in nuclear shape. The nucleus of the myelocyte tends to be slightly flattened. The chromatin becomes increasingly coarse, and nucleoli are usually indistinct or absent. The next stage, the metamyelocyte, contains an indented kidney-shaped nucleus. Additional folding results in a horseshoe-shaped nucleus, which stains deeply with basic dyes. The overall cell size continues to decrease. These cells are called bands. The final developmental stage results in a cell with a segmented or lobed nucleus. The lobes are united by narrow filaments or chromatin strands. The cytoplasm contains the specific granules characteristic of the three types. These cells are called segmented granulocytes or polymorphonuclear granulocytes. The mature polymorphonuclear granulocyte is approximately 15 $\mu$ in diameter.

The developmental stages of the neutrophil, eosinophil and basophil are seen in Plates 56, 57, and 58. Mature granulocytes are seen in Plate 50.

## WHITE BLOOD CELLS
### Granulocytes

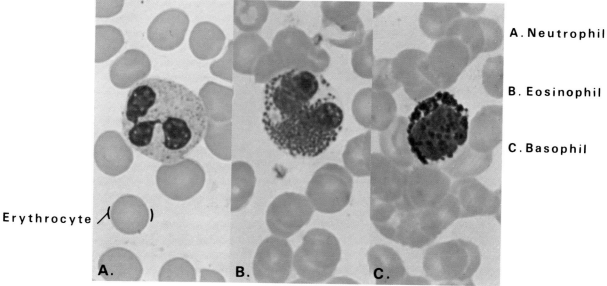

A. Neutrophil

B. Eosinophil

C. Basophil

Erythrocyte

A.   B.   C.

10 μ

### Human, Air dried blood smear, Wright's stain, 1416 x.

**Erythrocyte:** Biconcave and circular outline, devoid of a nucleus. Number in man varies between 5 and 5.5 million per cubic mm of blood. Erythrocytes carry oxygen from the lungs to the tissues and carbon dioxide from the tissues to the lungs.

**Neutrophil:** Compare sizes of the neutrophil and the erythrocyte. Lobulated nucleus, individual lobes connected by thin bridges. Cytoplasmic granules are small. Constitute 40 to 75 per cent of the total white blood cell count. Number of neutrophils increases in inflammation and they act as the first line of defense against invading pyogenic organisms.

**Eosinophil:** Nucleus bilobed. Cytoplasmic granules are large, uniform in size and stain intensely with acid dyes. Constitute 1 to 3 per cent of total white count. Increase in number in allergic states and in parasitic infections.

**Basophil:** Nucleus is large but less lobated than other white blood cells. Cytoplasmic granules are large, variable in size and have a strong affinity for basic dyes. Constitute 0.5 to 1 per cent of white count. They are believed to synthesize the heparin and histamine found in circulating blood.

## LYMPHOCYTES
### Small and large lymphocytes

Small
lymphocytes

Large
lymphocytes

Nucleus

Nucleus

Cytoplasm

Cytoplasm with
azurophilic
granules

Erythrocyte

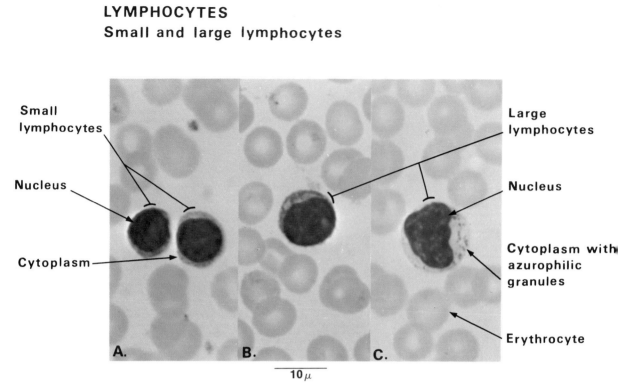

A.          B.          C.

10 μ

### Human, Air dried blood smear, Wright's stain, 1416 x.

**Small lymphocytes:** The most common type in normal blood. Has a large, dense, round nucleus and thin basophilic cytoplasm. Capable of ameboid movement and the production of antibodies.

**Large lymphocytes:** Not very common in normal blood. Nucleus indented. Cytoplasm more abundant than in small lymphocytes. Azurophilic granules are frequently found in large lymphocytes, less commonly in small lymphocytes.

## MONOCYTES

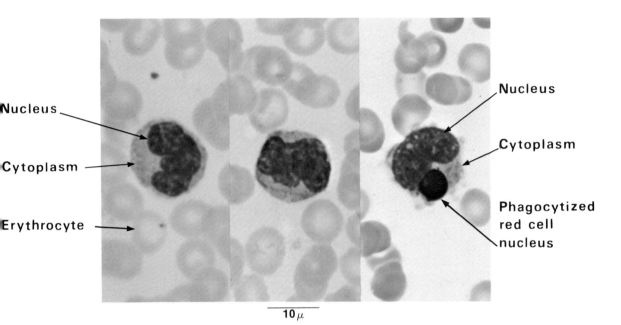

Human, Air dried blood smear, Wright's stain, 1416 x.

Monocytes are the largest cells found in normal blood. The nucleus is centrally or peripherally located, indented and ovoid or horseshoe-shaped; the nuclear chromatin is not as dense as that of lymphocytes. Cytoplasm is abundant and contains azurophilic granules which are usually smaller than those seen in lymphocytes. Monocytes are voracious phagocytes. The monocyte seen on the extreme right shows pseudopodia extending from the cell body and contains a phagocytized red cell nucleus.

Note the comparative size of erythrocytes and monocytes.

# BONE MARROW
# PERIPHERAL BLOOD

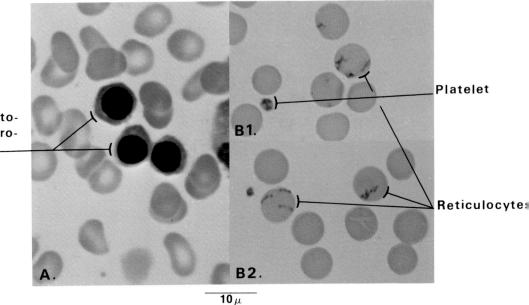

Polychromato-
philic erythro-
blasts

Platelet

B1.

Reticulocytes

A.

B2.

10μ

A. Human, Air dried marrow smear, Wright's
stain, 1416 x.
B. Human, Air dried blood smear, Brilliant cresyl
blue, 1416 x.

**Polychromatophilic erythroblasts (rubricytes):** Derivatives of basophilic erythroblasts (prorubricytes). Dense nuclear chromatin with polychromatophilic cytoplasm due to a declining RNA content and an increase in newly synthesized hemoglobin.

**Reticulocytes:** Immature red blood cells seen in the circulating blood. Clumping of ribosomes gives them a reticulated appearance.

**Platelets:** Also called thrombocytes, minute round or ovoid structures. Important in blood coagulation. Derived from bone marrow megakaryocytes.

## RED BONE MARROW
### In situ

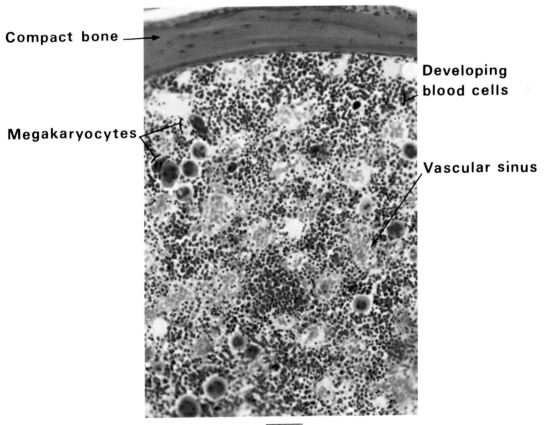

Compact bone

Developing blood cells

Megakaryocytes

Vascular sinus

0.2 mm

**Human, Müller's fluid, H. & E., 50 x.**

In this plate, a layer of compact bone surrounds the red bone marrow cavity.

Red or hemopoietic marrow is the characteristic variety of marrow until middle childhood. By late adolescence most red marrow is replaced by fatty or yellow bone marrow. In adults, red marrow occurs in the sternum, ribs, vertebrae, heads of long bones and cranium.

Red marrow is characterized by high cellularity and sinuses filling spaces between a delicate reticular supporting tissue. The cells seen are giant megakaryocytes and developing red and white blood cells.

## BONE MARROW
### Developing red blood cells

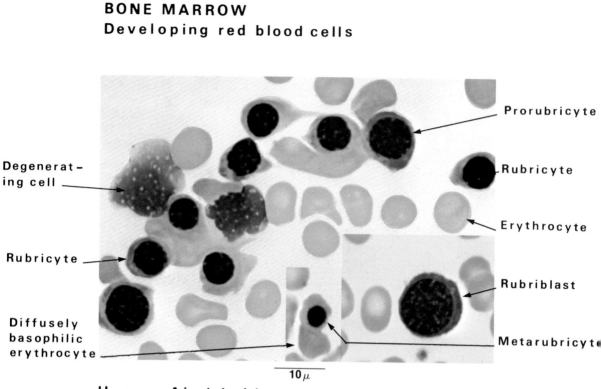

Human, Air dried bone marrow smear, Wright's stain, 1416 x.

**Rubriblast (proerythroblast, hemocytoblast, myeloblast):**  Stem cell of the erythroid series. Large rounded nucleus, basophilic cytoplasm.

**Prorubricyte (basophilic erythroblast):**  Develops from the rubriblast. Smaller than the stem cell, nucleus has coarser chromatin. RNA-rich cytoplasm is densely basophilic. Basophilia obscures hemoglobin content. Undergoes mitotic division, giving rise to rubricytes.

**Rubricyte (polychromatophilic erythroblast):**  Product of mitotic division of prorubricytes. Smaller than mother cell. Nuclear chromatin more compact. Cytoplasmic basophilia less marked and hemoglobin content greater than in mother cell. Mixed affinity for both acid and basic dyes (due to their content of hemoglobin and RNA, respectively) determines their polychromatophilic staining characteristics.

**Metarubricyte (normoblast):**  Arises by mitotic division of rubricyte. Nucleus small and pyknotic. Cytoplasm distinctly acidophilic due to increased hemoglobin content.

**Erythrocyte:**  Non-nucleated (nuclei of metarubricytes have been extruded) circular outline. In side view, they appear dumbbell-shaped because of the biconcave nature of their surfaces. Number varies in man from 5 to 5.5 million per cubic mm. Carry oxygen from lungs to tissue, and carbon dioxide from tissue to lungs. Filled with hemoglobin. Immature stages in development (reticulocytes) have a diffusely basophilic cytoplasm because of the residual content of RNA.

**Degenerating cell:**  Often found in bone marrow. Remnants of damaged corpuscles, megakaryocytes or myeloblasts. These are primarily artifacts of a marrow smear preparation.

## BONE MARROW
### Developing neutrophils

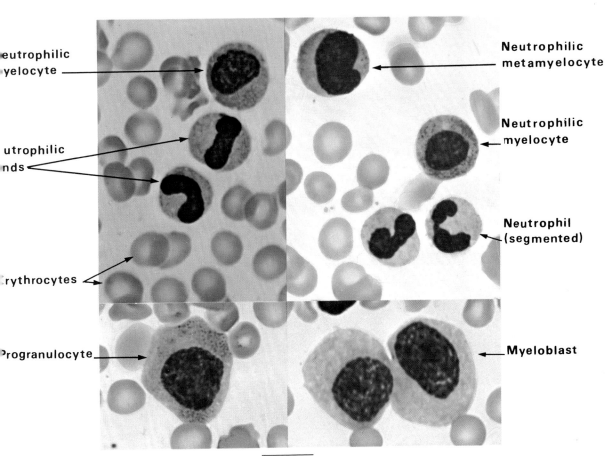

eutrophilic
yelocyte

Neutrophilic
metamyelocyte

utrophilic
nds

Neutrophilic
myelocyte

Neutrophil
(segmented)

rythrocytes

Progranulocyte

Myeloblast

10 μ

## Human, Air dried marrow smear, Wright's stain, 1416 x.

**Myeloblast:**   The stem cell of the leucocytic series. Lightly basophilic cytoplasm. Nuclei large and rounded. The chromatin is in the form of moderately coarse interconnected strands. Constitutes 0.3 to 0.5 per cent of marrow cells. Myeloblasts increase in leukemia.

**Progranulocyte:**   Also called promyelocyte. Arises and differentiates from myeloblasts. Large cells, nuclei rounded with coarse chromatin. Cytoplasm basophilic with some azurophilic granules. This cell type constitutes about 4 per cent of marrow cells.

**Neutrophilic myelocyte:**   Arises from progranulocytes. Smaller, less basophilic cytoplasm containing differentiated granules and a more compact nuclear chromatin.

**Neutrophilic metamyelocyte:**   Kidney-shaped nucleus. Not capable of division. Differentiates into mature neutrophilic myelocytes.

**Neutrophilic bands:**   Immature neutrophils. Nuclei are horseshoe- or drumstick-shaped.

**Neutrophil (segmented):**   Mature cell. Nucleus markedly lobated. The lobes may be connected with a thin chromatin thread. Chromatin is compact. Abundant cytoplasm. Granules in the cytoplasm are small and may be inconspicuous.

## BONE MARROW
### Developing eosinophils

Myeloblasts

Eosinophilic metamyelocyt

Eosinophilic myelocyte

Myeloblast

Eosinophil segmented

Eosinophilic band

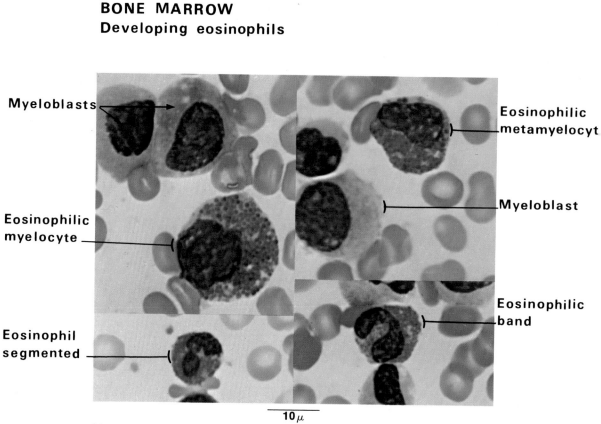

10 μ

Human, Air dried marrow smear, Wright's stain, 1416 x.

**Myeloblast:** Stem cell of the leucocytic series. Rounded large nucleus. Lightly basophilic agranular cytoplasm. See also Plate 56.

**Eosinophilic myelocyte:** Develop from myeloblasts. Specific acidophilic granules appear in cytoplasm. Nucleus is rounded or oval. Chromatin of nucleus is coarser than in the myeloblast. This cell is capable of division.

**Eosinophilic metamyelocyte:** This cell is no longer capable of cell division. Nucleus is kidney-shaped or indented. Cytoplasm contains acidophilic granules.

**Eosinophilic band:** Immature or juvenile eosinophil. Nucleus horseshoe- or drumstick-shaped. Eosinophilic granules in cytoplasm.

**Eosinophilic segmented:** Mature eosinophil. Nucleus is loblated. Lobes are connected with thin chromatin threads. Abundant granular cytoplasm.

# BONE MARROW
## Developing basophils

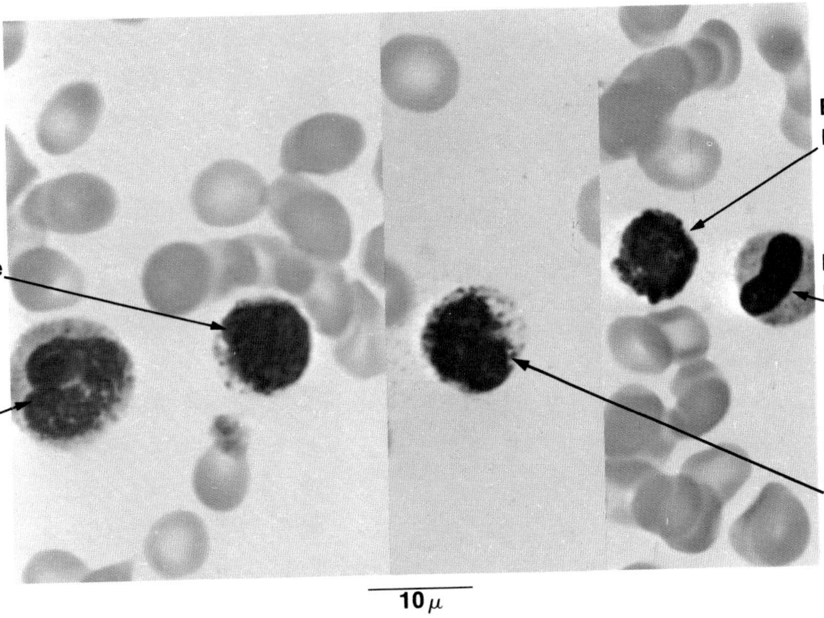

Basophilic
band

Basophilic
metamyelocyte

Neutrophilic
band

Segmented
neutrophil

Basophilic
metamyelocyte

10 μ

**Human, Air dried marrow smear, Wright's stain, 1416 x.**

**Basophilic metamyelocyte:** Derived from basophilic myelocyte, which is not represented in this figure. Basophilic myelocytes are scarce and may not be seen in a single marrow smear preparation. It is believed that their granules are water-soluble. This cell is no longer capable of cell division. Nucleus oval to kidney-shaped. Cytoplasm has basophilic granules.

**Basophilic band:** Immature basophil. Nucleus horseshoe-shaped. Basophilic granules in cytoplasm.

**Neutrophilic band:** See Plate 56. Note the difference in cytoplasmic granularity between the neutrophilic band and the basophilic band.

**Segmented neutrophil:** See Plate 56.

## BONE MARROW
### Wandering cells

Phagocytized nucleus

Nucleus

Erythrocytes

Nucleus

Nucleus

Phagocytic histiocyte

Pseudopods

Monocyte

Lymphocyte

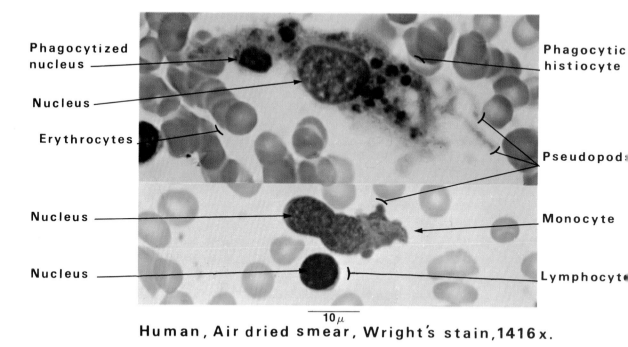

10 μ

**Human, Air dried smear, Wright's stain, 1416 x.**

**Phagocytic histiocyte:**   Large cell. Irregular cell outline with many short cell processes (pseudopods). Abundant cytoplasm containing phagocytized material. Nucleus oval-shaped.

**Monocyte:**   Large cell with a prominent eccentric nucleus. Highly ameboid cytoplasm containing various inclusions.

**Lymphocyte:**   Spherical, dense nucleus with a thin, inconspicuous rim of basophilic cytoplasm.

**Erythrocytes:**   See Plate 55.

# BONE MARROW

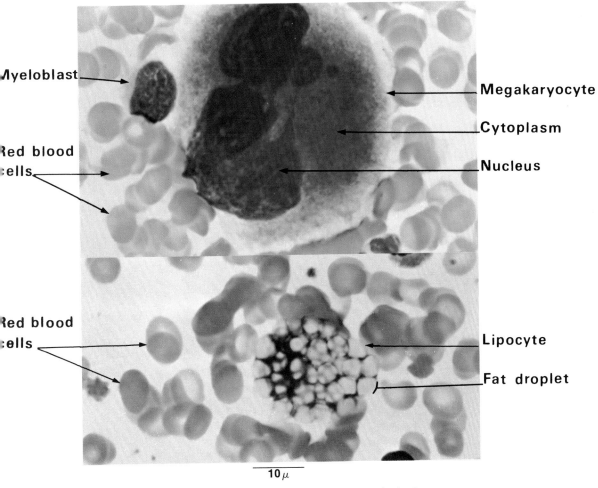

Myeloblast

Megakaryocyte

Cytoplasm

Red blood cells

Nucleus

Red blood cells

Lipocyte

Fat droplet

10 μ

Human, Air dried marrow smear, Wright's stain, 1416 x.

**Megakaryocyte:** Giant cell characteristic of bone marrow. Conspicuous multilobed nucleus. Cytoplasm contains fine granules. Pseudopodia extend from the cell surface and later detach to form the blood platelets. Blood platelets participate in the blood clotting mechanism by contributing to the formation of thromboplastin, by "plugging" abnormal breaks in the endothelium of blood vessels, and by inducing the constriction of damaged blood vessels.

**Red blood cells:** Non-nucleated corpuscles having a circular or dumbbell-shaped appearance. Contain hemoglobin.

**Lipocyte:** Fat cells are constantly present in bone marrow. They have irregular outlines and are filled with lipid droplets.

# Muscular Tissue

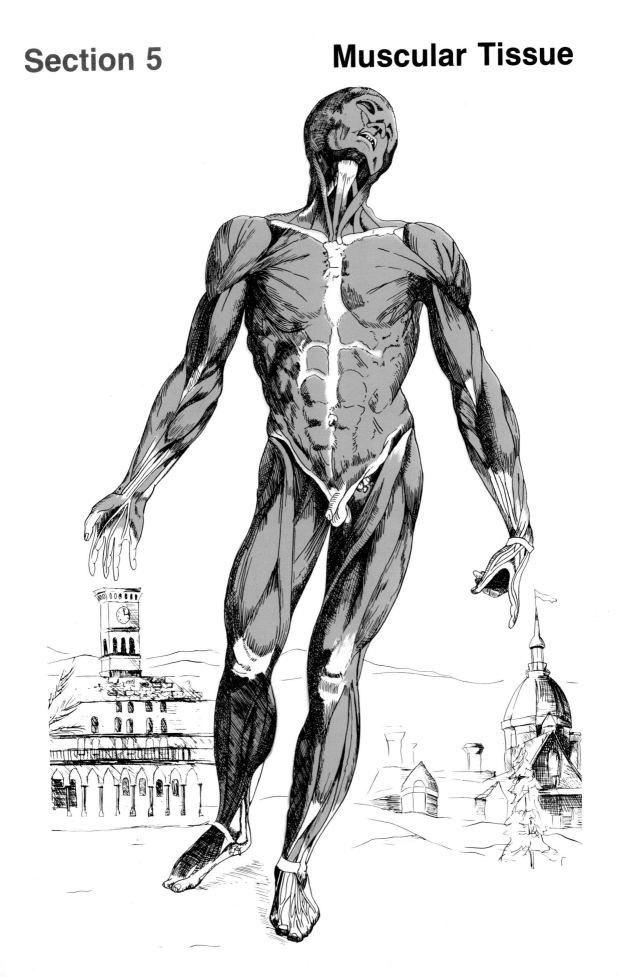

# Muscular Tissue

Muscle fibers are elongated cells with distinctive shapes specialized for shortening or contraction. These contractile fibers provide the means of movement for minute body hairs, air in respiration, ingested food and liquid, reproductive cells, blood and lymph, and small and large parts of the body. Muscular contractions which may be coarse or extremely refined and graded between fast and slow are controlled by the nervous system, which is devoted in large measure to these essential activities. Muscle fibers in vertebrates may be classified structurally as nonstriated, plain, or smooth; striated cardiac; and striated skeletal. A broadened classification which considers function is: smooth, involuntary; striated cardiac, involuntary; and striated skeletal, voluntary. The structural-functional classification indicates whether the contractile activity is under intentional or reflex control. Another facet of functional consideration is concerned with the ability of smooth and cardiac muscle to contract spontaneously in the absence of a nerve supply (myogenic contraction). The contractile activity of involuntary muscle is normally regulated by the autonomic (sympathetic and parasympathetic) nervous system. Striated skeletal muscle fibers are totally dependent upon the nervous system for their structural integrity and function. Each striated skeletal muscle fiber is supplied by a nerve fiber ending on a specialized region of the sarcolemma (the motor end plate). If the nerve supply to a muscle is interrupted, the muscle atrophies rapidly (denervation atrophy).

Smooth muscle fibers are in general small, fusiform fibers which vary from about 15 to 200 $\mu$ in length and from 3 to 10 $\mu$ in diameter. Each muscle fiber possesses a single, elongated nucleus, which characteristically becomes shorter and broader and tends to coil when the muscle fiber contracts. Smooth muscle fibers may occur singly, as in the scrotum (tunica dartos); in small bundles or fascicles associated with hair follicles (arrector pili muscle); in well defined, layered sheets which are coiled, as in muscular arteries, or arranged at right angles to each other, as in the intestines; or in an irregular pattern, as in the stomach, bladder and uterus. Branched fibers can be found in the nipple of the mammary glands and in the endocardium of the atrium of the heart.

Smooth muscle fibers usually contract slowly but are capable of sustained contractile activity. Most of the smooth muscle fibers of the gastrointestinal and genitourinary tracts are linked to each other by specialized contacts (tight junction or nexus) which transmit electrical excitatory stimuli from cell to cell. This structural-functional arrangement permits large numbers of smooth muscle fibers to be activated by a minimal nerve supply. The excitatory nerve impulse is transmitted to a smooth muscle fiber and is conducted from fiber to fiber, resulting in a sustained and coordinated contraction (peristalsis).

Cardiac muscle fibers are generally larger than smooth muscle fibers and appear cross striated when stained or examined with polarized light. Cardiac muscle fibers are joined serially end to end, and characteristically branch to unite with adjacent fibers. Cardiac muscle fibers form a functional but not a protoplasmic syncytium. The junctional site between fibers is called the intercalated disc. The intercalated disc is composed of two important components; the adhesion plate (desmosome) between adjacent cells and the tight junction, or nexus, which allows the electrical excitatory impulse to be transmitted from cell to cell, resulting in a coordinated contraction essential to normal heart function. The branched cardiac fibers possess one or two nuclei which are centrally located. The contractile substance of the cardiac fiber is organized into subunits called myofibrils, which are cross striated. The cross striations will be discussed below in relation to striated skeletal muscle. The myofibril characteristic of cardiac and skeletal muscle is not seen in smooth muscle although the myofilaments of which the myofibril is composed are found in all three muscle fiber types. Myofilaments cannot be resolved by the light microscope.

Striated skeletal muscle fibers vary in length between 2 and 25 cm, depending on the muscle. The diameter of a single muscle fiber is also variable but is usually between 10 and 100 $\mu$. These multinucleated giant cells, unlike smooth and cardiac muscle fibers, are not structurally or functionally uniform. Two or more distinct muscle fiber types have been identified in man and other species by light and electron microscopy and histochemistry. Characteristically, the nuclei of skeletal muscle fibers are located peripherally, adjacent to the outer limiting membrane or sarcolemma. In certain skeletal muscle fibers, namely the red or slow contracting muscle fibers, the nuclei may be found scattered throughout the sarcoplasm. Based upon structural-functional studies, living muscle fibers which appear red are designated, in man, as Type I muscle fibers. These muscle fibers contain many mitochondria, store lipid, are rich in myoglobin and contract slowly. Muscle fibers which appear white contain few mitochondria, store glycogen, are relatively devoid of myoglobin and contract rapidly but fatigue quickly. In man, these are designated as Type II muscle fibers.

In cross section, skeletal muscle fibers are seen to be composed of numerous small aggregates (1 to 2 $\mu$) of contractile substance, the myofibrils. Myofibrils are composed of myofilaments, but these cannot be resolved by the light microscope. In longitudinal section, the muscle fiber and the myofibril appear cross striated. The darkly staining segment, 1.6 $\mu$ in length, is designated the A band (anisotropic band) which is a region of high refractive index and is birefringent when examined with a polarizing microscope. Alternating with the A bands is a lightly staining region of variable length, the I band (isotropic band), which is a region of low refractive index. The I band is bisected by a thin dark-staining Z line. When a muscle fiber contracts the A bands move toward each other, meeting at the Z line, and the I bands disappear. Additional details of the contractile process will be considered in the legend of Plate 66.

## STRIATED MUSCLE
### Embryonic tissue
### cross section

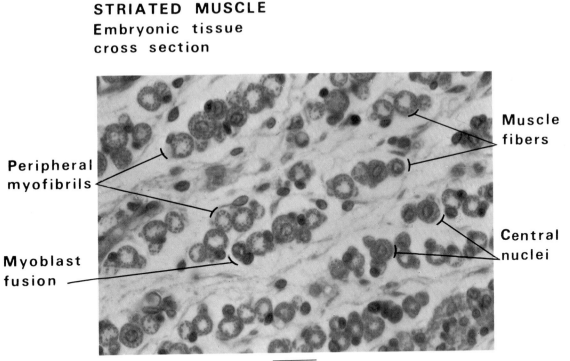

Peripheral
myofibrils

Muscle
fibers

Central
nuclei

Myoblast
fusion

20 μ

## Human, Helly's fluid, H. & E., 612 x.

Developing muscle fibers are seen in different stages of development. Embryonic muscle fibers are characterized by centrally placed nuclei and peripherally disposed myofibrils. These fibers grow in length and diameter by myoblast fusion. No nuclear divisional figures are ordinarily seen at this stage. As the muscle fiber matures, the nuclei become located primarily beneath the sarcolemma at the periphery of the fiber.

A congenital disorder of skeletal muscle seen in children (centrovacuolar myopathy) is characterized by a histologic picture identical with that seen in embryonic skeletal muscle.

## STRIATED MUSCLE
### Sarcolemma

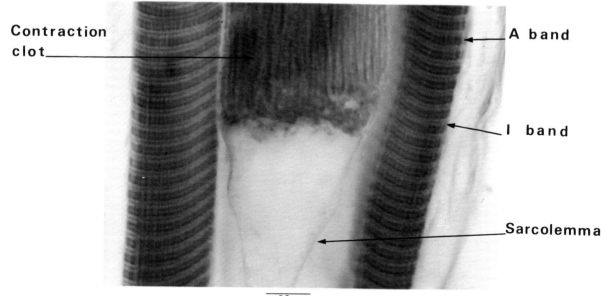

Contraction clot

A band

I band

Sarcolemma

20 μ

Human, Zenker's fluid, Verhoeff & Van Gieson's stain, 612 x.

**Sarcolemma:** External limiting membrane of muscle fibers. Not ordinarily seen in light microscopic preparations. Seen here because of artifactual retraction of contractile elements. This artifact permitted Bowman, in 1840, to demonstrate the membrane and to name it the sarcolemma. The true sarcolemma, very much thinner than seen here, is responsible for the conduction and spread of electrical impulses from the motor end plate over the entire muscle surface, resulting in contractile activity. Electron microscopy has shown the sarcolemma to be 100 Å in thickness. The apparent increase in thickness rendering it visible in this preparation is due to adherent stainable sarcoplasm and, externally, to a thin basement membrane and associated reticular connective tissue fibers.

# STRIATED MUSCLE
## Polarization microscopy

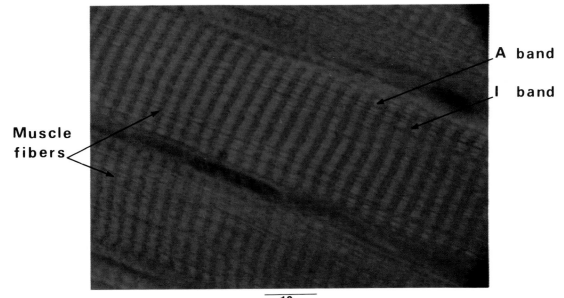

A band

I band

Muscle
fibers

10 μ

### Human, Helly's fluid, H. & E., 1416 x.

The names given to the two major transverse striations of skeletal and cardiac muscle are derived from the studies of Brücke (1858). With routine light microscopic techniques, alternating dark and light bands are seen within striated muscle fibers (Plates 64, 65 and 66). Polarization microscopy reverses the appearance of the dark band, which becomes bright, and the light band, which appears dark. The dark band of routine light microscopy, exhibiting birefringence with polarized light, is anisotropic and is called the A band. The light band of routine light microscopy is poorly refractile and relatively isotropic and is called the I band.

**Muscle fibers:** Showing cross striations formed by alternating segments of high and low refractive index resulting from their submicroscopic structure, which is revealed by electron microscopy.

**A band:** Anisotropic band.

**I Band:** Isotropic band. Note the birefringence or anisotropy of the Z line in the center of the I band.

## STRIATED MUSCLE
### Transverse striations
### longitudinal section

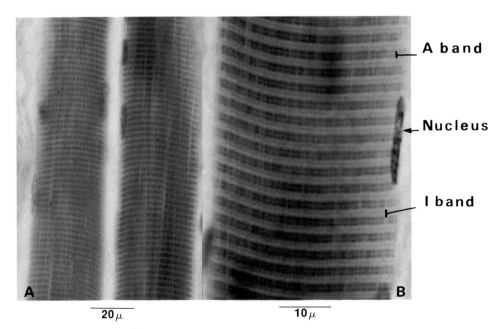

**Human , Helly 's fluid , Phosphotungstic acid hematoxylin stain , A 612 x., B 1416 x.**

Phosphotungstic acid hematoxylin is a stain particularly suited for the demonstration of striations in skeletal muscle. Iron hematoxylin and Mallory-azan are also effectively used for this purpose. Note that at low magnification only the two major cross striations can be seen. The dark band is the A band, and the light band is the I band. Higher magnifications are usually required to see the light-staining area in the center of the A band, which is known as the H zone, and the thin, dark line bisecting the I band, which is named the Z line. The repeating structural unit between two Z lines is called a sarcomere.

# STRIATED MUSCLE
## Tongue

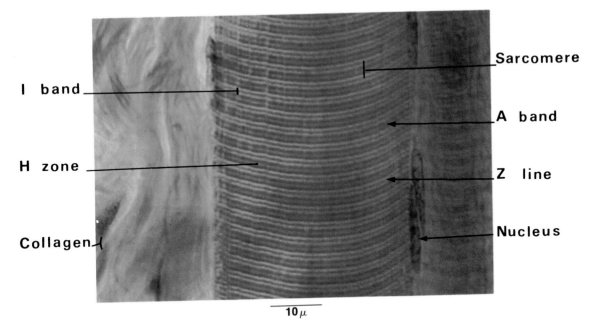

Sarcomere

I band

A band

H zone

Z line

Collagen

Nucleus

10 μ

Human, Zenker's fluid, Verhoeff & Van Gieson stain, 1416 x.

**I band:** Isotropic band determined by polarization microscopy. Note the darker Z line bisecting the I band. Electron microscopy has shown that the I band contains thin filaments 50 Å in diameter and approximately 2 $\mu$ in length. The contractile protein actin is found in the thin I band filaments.

**A band:** Anisotropic band determined by polarization microscopy is bisected by the lighter H zone. The A band contains filaments of the protein myosin which are 100 Å in diameter and 1.6 $\mu$ in length, as well as thin (actin) filaments extending from the I band into the A band. The A band filaments are composed of myosin molecules, which through enzymatic activity (adenosine triphosphatase) release energy essential for the contractile process.

**Z line:** Bisects the I band. Z from the German word Zwischenscheibe or in-between line.

**H zone:** Variable in width, it bisects the A band and vanishes in contraction as the thin I band filaments are drawn further into and through the middle of the A band. When seen, it contains only thick filaments. H for the German word Hell (bright) and also for the zone's discoverer, Henson.

**Sarcomere:** The contractile substance between two Z lines constitutes a convenient structural unit but not the precise functional or primary contractile unit of muscle fibers. See Plate 66.

**Nucleus:** Elongated and located beneath the sarcolemma. The sarcolemma is seen in Plate 62.

**Collagen:** Bundles of this connective tissue separate individual muscle fibers (endomysium), bind fascicles, or bundles, of muscle fibers (perimysium), and invest the entire muscle (epimysium). Through this tough and inelastic connective tissue contractile forces are transmitted to bone and skin.

# STRIATED MUSCLE
## Relaxed and contracted muscle fibers

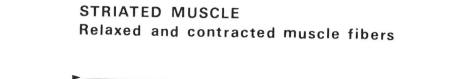

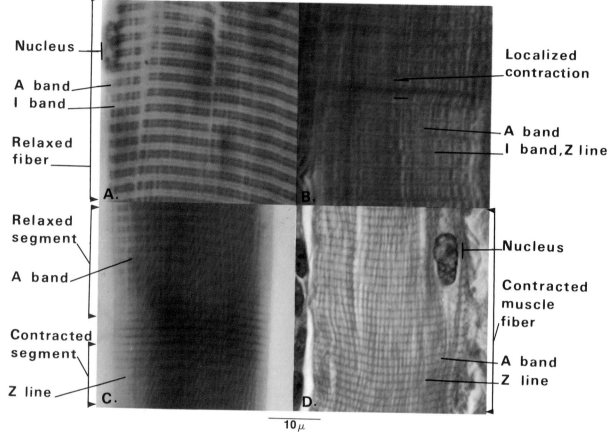

Nucleus

A band
I band

Relaxed fiber

A.

B.

Localized contraction

A band
I band, Z line

Relaxed segment

A band

Contracted segment

Z line

C.

D.

Nucleus

Contracted muscle fiber

A band
Z line

$10\mu$

Human; Helly's fluid; A.,C., Phosphotungstic acid hematoxylin, B. Mallory-azan, D. H. & E.; 1416x.

In this plate, the structural basis of skeletal muscle fiber contraction is shown.

**A:** Relaxed fiber showing distinct cross striations, the darker staining A band and the lighter staining I band. Note that the I band is bisected by a thin but deeply staining line (Z line), while the A band is bisected by a lightly staining line (H zone).

**B:** A fiber seen in the relaxed state except for a small segment of localized contraction. Note the change in the band pattern in this segment. Two adjacent A bands are in contact, and the I band has disappeared.

**C:** A fiber shown with both a relaxed and contracted segment. The A and I bands are clearly outlined in the relaxed segment but not in the contracted segment. In contraction, the I band becomes narrower and disappears. The A band does not normally become shorter except in extreme contraction. Contraction bands appear as a result of an increase in density and staining of the Z line.

**D:** A portion of a fully contracted muscle fiber is shown. The changes here are similar to those described in C for a contracted segment except that the normal distance between the thickened Z lines (contraction bands) is reduced, denoting extreme contraction.

## STRIATED MUSCLE
### Lateral rectus
### cross section

Epimysium

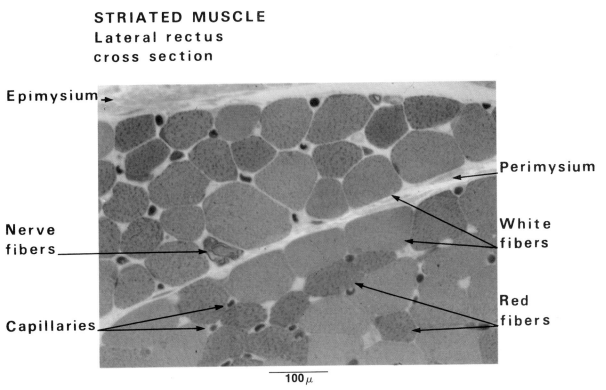

Perimysium

White
fibers

Nerve
fibers

Red
fibers

Capillaries

$\overline{100\,\mu}$

## Cat, Glutaraldehyde – osmium fixation, Toluidine blue stain, 162 x.

**Epimysium:**  Envelope primarily composed of collagenous connective tissue wrapping the entire muscle.

**Perimysium:**  Connective tissue partitions between bundles, or fascicles, of muscle fibers.

**White fibers (A fibers):**  Also known in the human as Type II fibers. These large fibers demonstrate pronounced myofibrillar ATPase activity and glycogen stores. These fibers are fast contracting.

**Red fibers (B fibers):**  Also known in the human as Type I fibers. Characteristically smaller than white fibers, they contain numerous mitochondria and lipid stores. These fibers are slow contracting. See Plate 9.

Note variation in fiber diameter. Normally, skeletal muscle fibers vary from 10 to 100 $\mu$ in diameter, depending on muscle and species.

**Nerve fibers:**  Somatic motor nerve fibers are distributed in the connective tissue septa of the muscle. These terminate on individual muscle fibers (see Plates 105, 106 and 107).

**Capillaries:**  Widely distributed in the connective tissue septa (endomysium) between and around individual muscle fibers. Blood cells are seen within some capillaries.

## STRIATED MUSCLE
Cremaster muscle
myofibrils

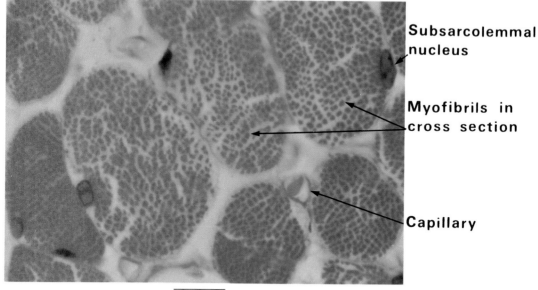

Subsarcolemmal
nucleus

Myofibrils in
cross section

Capillary

10 μ

## Human, 10% Formalin, H. & E., 1416 x.

**Myofibrils:**  Subunits of each muscle fiber. Each myofibril is composed of myofilaments. Myofibrils vary in size, depending on the number of myofilaments they contain. Myofilaments cannot be resolved by the light microscope.

**Nucleus with nucleolus:**  The nucleus shown in this mature muscle fiber is characteristically located near the sarcolemma. In some skeletal muscles, particularly those which are slow contracting (Type I, Type B or red), the nuclei may be found more centrally located within the muscle fiber.

A capillary containing a red blood cell is seen between muscle fibers. Muscle fibers are provided with a rich capillary network which supplies essential nutrients and oxygen and removes metabolic wastes.

## STRIATED MUSCLE
### Semitendinosus, cross section
### Mitochondria; succinic dehydrogenase localization

Red muscle fiber 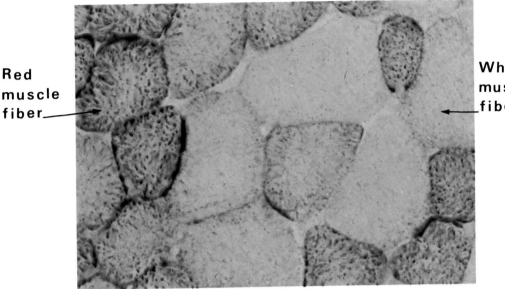 White muscle fiber

20 μ

### Rat, Frozen section, Tetrazolium method, 612 x.

**Red muscle fiber (B fiber):**   Rich in mitochondria and lipids, this type of fiber is slow contracting. Known in the human as Type I muscle fiber.

**White muscle fiber (A fiber):**   Relatively poor in mitochondria and lipid, but rich in myofibrillar ATPase activity and glycogen, these fibers are fast contracting. Known in the human as Type II muscle fiber.

Histochemical methods similar to the one used here have been instrumental in distinguishing muscle fiber types in health and disease.

# MOTOR END PLATE, SUBNEURAL APPARATUS
## Intercostal muscle

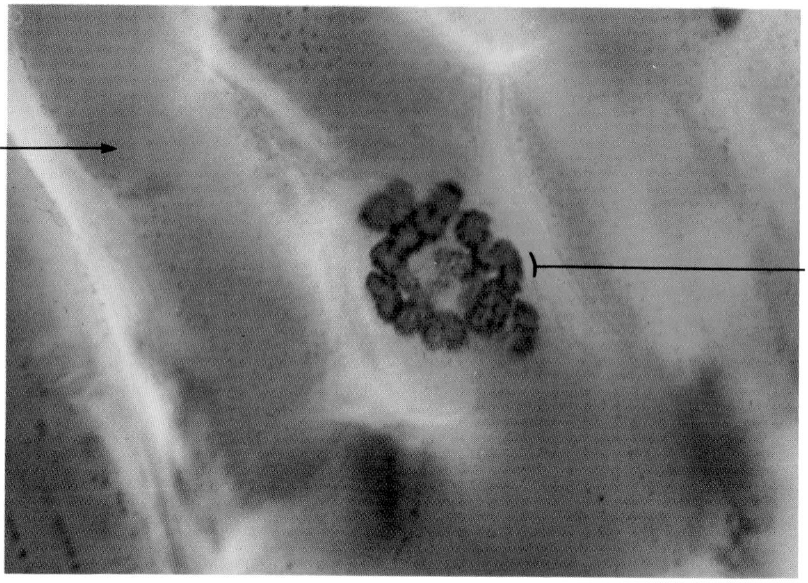

Muscle
fiber

Enzyme
location

20 μ

## Rat, Seligman acetylcholinesterase method, 612x.

**Enzyme location:**  The muscle sarcolemma which forms the primary and secondary clefts of the subneural apparatus is rich in acetylcholinesterase activity. Axon terminals (not seen in this preparation) lie within the primary synaptic cleft (refer to Plates 105 and 106).

## NEUROMUSCULAR SPINDLE
Cross section
A. tongue    B. sartorious

Capsule

Intrafusal
muscle
fibers

Nerve
fibers

Extrafusal
muscle
fibers

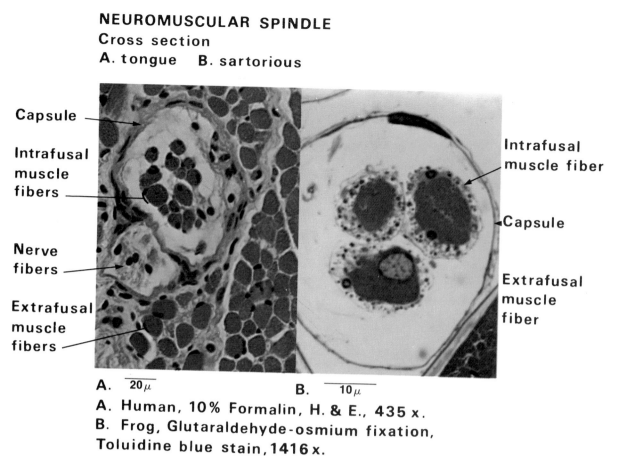

Intrafusal
muscle fiber

Capsule

Extrafusal
muscle
fiber

A. $\overline{20\mu}$    B. $\overline{10\mu}$

A. Human, 10% Formalin, H. & E., 435 x.
B. Frog, Glutaraldehyde-osmium fixation,
Toluidine blue stain, 1416 x.

This plate shows some of the histologic features of neuromuscular spindles as seen in the human tongue (A) and frog sartorius (B). Note that the neuromuscular spindle is surrounded by skeletal muscle fibers (extrafusal fibers). Each spindle contains several small muscle fibers (the intrafusal fibers), myelinated nerve fibers enclosed within a connective tissue capsule which is pierced by the nerve fibers reaching the spindle. Nerve fibers of the spindle are both sensory and motor. Information conveyed from and to the muscle spindle is not consciously received but is important in reflex regulation of muscle tone. Intrafusal muscle fibers of the spindle receive axons of the gamma motor neurons in the spinal cord while the extrafusal muscle fibers receive axons of the larger alpha motor neurons. See Plates 108 and 109.

## CARDIAC MUSCLE

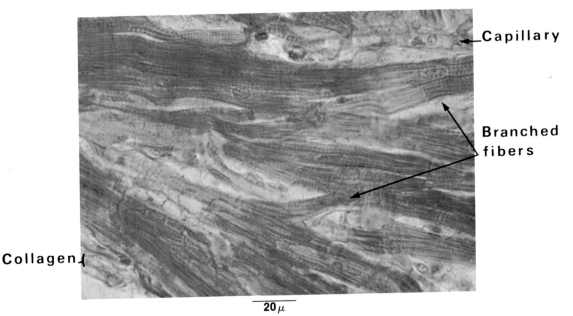

Capillary

Branched fibers

Collagen

20 μ

**Human, Helly's fluid, Mallory's stain, 612x.**

The characteristically branched cardiac muscle fibers are separated by collagenous connective tissue. The differentiation of collagenous connective tissue and cardiac muscle is clearly seen with this stain. Note the capillary containing red cells. Compare capillary diameter (approximately 8μ) with that of the cardiac muscle fiber.

## CARDIAC MUSCLE
### Longitudinal section

Intercalated disc

Muscle fibers

Branching fibers

Striations

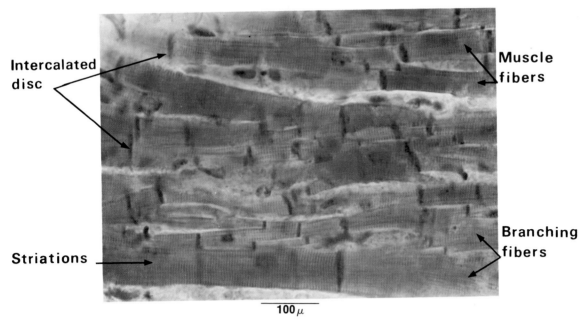

100 μ

### Human, Zenker's fluid, Phosphotungstic acid hematoxylin stain, 162 x.

**Muscle fibers:** Each 9 to 22 $\mu$ in diameter, serially arranged in columns with short branches contacting adjacent fibers.

**Branching fibers:** Characteristic of cardiac muscle fibers. Each branching fiber limited by an intercalated disc constitutes a single muscle fiber.

**Striations:** A and I bands. A bands are usually inconspicuous. Z lines are particularly prominent. Contractile apparatus and cross striations, although not usually stained well in cardiac muscle, are similar to those found in skeletal muscle (Plates 63, 64 and 65).

**Intercalated disc:** Site of termination and junction of adjacent cardiac muscle fibers. Consists of snugly fit projections and indentations of adjacent cell membranes. Intercalated discs are the sites of transmission of excitatory impulses from cell to cell and provide firm attachment for contiguous fibers. The stain used in this preparation is particularly useful for demonstrating intercalated discs.

## CARDIAC MUSCLE
### Relaxed and contracted muscle fibers

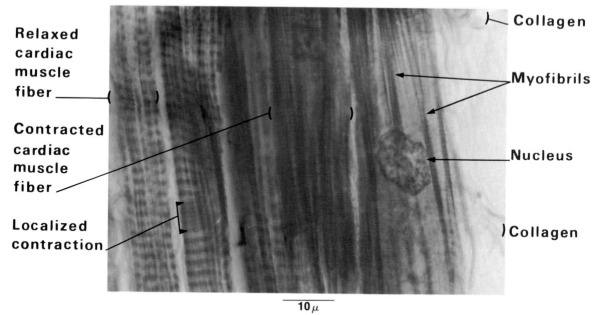

Relaxed
cardiac
muscle
fiber

Contracted
cardiac
muscle
fiber

Localized
contraction

Collagen

Myofibrils

Nucleus

Collagen

10 μ

### Human, Helly's fluid, Mallory-azan stain, 1416 x.

This is a longitudinal section of cardiac muscle stained with Mallory-azan, which differentiates muscular tissue (red-brown) from collagenous connective tissue (blue).

Several muscle fibers are seen. A vesicular nucleus is seen in one. The muscle fibers are separated by narrow spaces containing delicate strands of collagen fibers. Each muscle fiber is formed of subunits, the myofibrils. To the extreme left of the figure is shown a muscle fiber in the relaxed state. Note the distinct striations. Adjacent to this fiber is another relaxed fiber except for a small area of localized contraction. Note that the muscle striations are less distinct in the contracted area. In the middle of the plate is a contracted fiber in which the striation pattern is indistinct, although the Z lines are evident.

## PURKINJE FIBERS

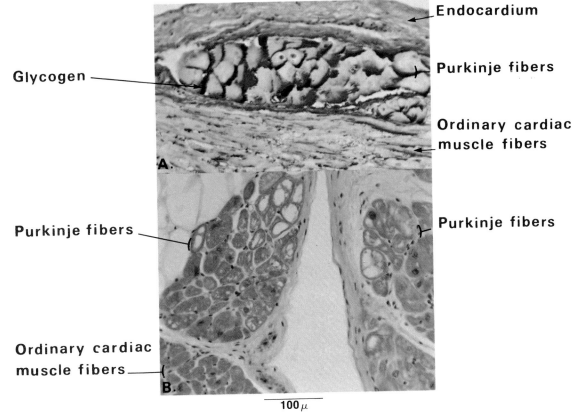

Endocardium

Glycogen

Purkinje fibers

Ordinary cardiac muscle fibers

Purkinje fibers

Purkinje fibers

Ordinary cardiac muscle fibers

100 µ

A. Sheep, Rossman's fixative, Periodic acid-Schiff and hematoxylin stains, 162 x.

B. Human, 10 % Formalin, H. & E., 162 x.

In this figure, the contrast between ordinary cardiac muscle fibers and their specialized variety, the Purkinje fibers, is evident. Purkinje fibers are larger than ordinary cardiac muscle fibers and stain less intensely. Note the clear areas in the cytoplasm of Purkinje fibers in B. These represent areas from which glycogen was lost during the preparation of the tissue. By contrast, in the Purkinje fibers seen in A, the glycogen is preserved by the fixation method used. Note the subendocardial location of Purkinje fibers.

## CARDIAC MUSCLE
Purkinje fibers
cross section

Cardiac
muscle
fibers

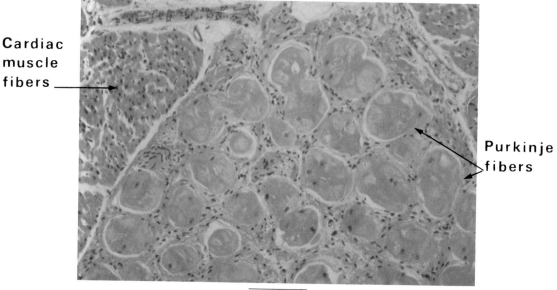

Purkinje
fibers

100 μ

Sheep, Bouin's fluid, H. & E., 162 x.

**Purkinje fibers:**  Larger and paler than ordinary cardiac muscle fibers. Areas of clear sarcoplasm represent regions which normally contain glycogen as well as areas devoid of myofibrils. These fibers contain irregularly arranged small myofibrils and nuclei.

## CARDIAC MUSCLE
### Lipochrome pigment

Cross
striations

Nuclei

Lipochrome
pigment

Lipochrome
pigment

Nucleus

Nucleolus

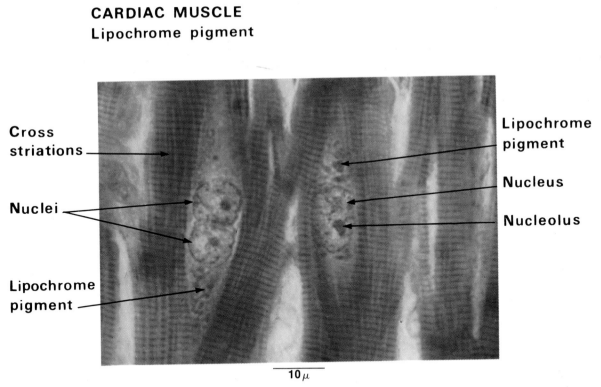

10 μ

## Human, Helly's fluid, Mallory's stain, 1416 x.

Several cardiac muscle fibers are seen in this plate. Note the transverse striations characteristic of cardiac and skeletal muscle fibers. Two ovoid nuclei are seen in one fiber. Nuclei are oriented in the long axis of the fiber and contain prominent nucleoli. Binucleate fibers are seen only occasionally in cardiac muscle. Adjacent to the nuclei, note the yellowish granules of lipochrome pigment. This pigment increases with age and is thought to be a product of normal metabolic activity.

## SMOOTH MUSCLE
Duodenum
longitudinal section

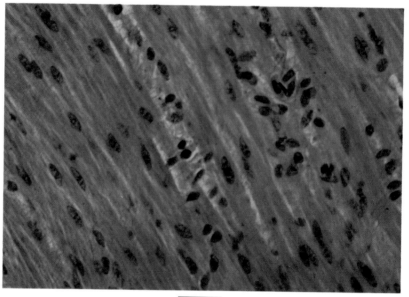

20 μ

**Human, Helly's fluid, H. & E., 612 x.**

Outer longitudinal layer of smooth muscle in the tunica muscularis of the duodenum. Muscle fibers are divided by connective tissue septa into bundles. Each muscle cell has a central nucleus and abundant sarcoplasm. The muscle fibers are long, slender and spindle-shaped. Note that differentiation between smooth muscle cells and connective tissue fibers is difficult in this preparation because of the staining method used (H. & E.). Differentiation of smooth muscle from connective tissue using specific stains is shown in Plates 34, 37, 138 and 139.

## SMOOTH MUSCLE
Duodenum
cross section

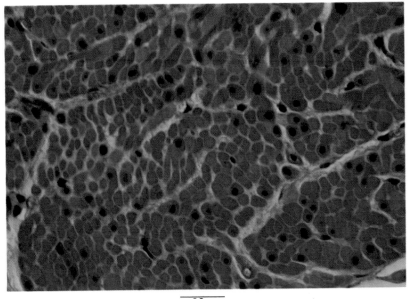

20 μ

Human, Helly's fluid, H. & E., 612 x.

Bundles of smooth muscle fibers separated by connective tissue septa. Each fiber is characterized by abundant sarcoplasm and central nucleus. Myofibrils are not seen in smooth muscle. Note variation in cross-sectional diameter which can be accounted for on the basis of their spindle shape (as seen in longitudinal section).

## SMOOTH MUSCLE
### A. Longitudinal and circular (jejunum)
### B. Small fascicle (skin)

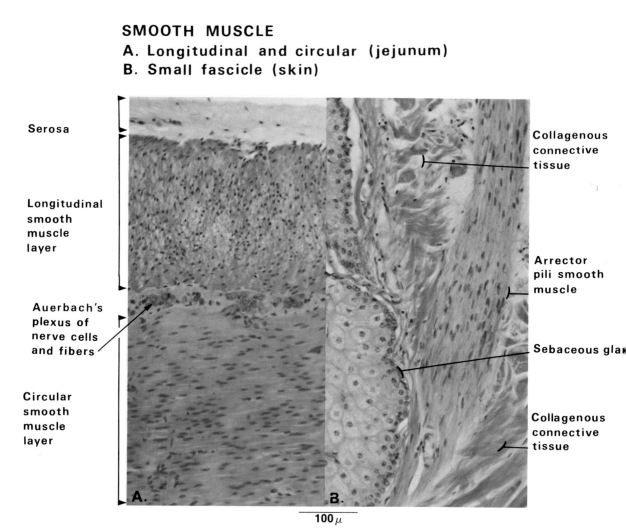

Serosa

Longitudinal
smooth
muscle
layer

Auerbach's
plexus of
nerve cells
and fibers

Circular
smooth
muscle
layer

Collagenous
connective
tissue

Arrector
pili smooth
muscle

Sebaceous gland

Collagenous
connective
tissue

100 μ

A.   B.

**Human, 10% Formalin, H. & E., 162x.**

This plate shows smooth muscle fibers from two locations. In *A*, they are seen distributed as an outer longitudinal and an inner circular layer in the wall of the jejunum. These two layers are separated by connective tissue and by neurons and fibers of Auerbach's autonomic plexus. In *B*, a smooth muscle fiber bundle of the arrector pili muscle is seen between bundles of connective tissue in the skin. Note the elongated nuclei and homogeneous cytoplasm. Arrector pili muscles originate in the papillary connective tissue and insert on hair follicles. Their contraction erects hairs in animals and produces "goose-flesh" in man. Note the proximity of the arrector pili muscle to a sebaceous gland.

# Nervous Tissue

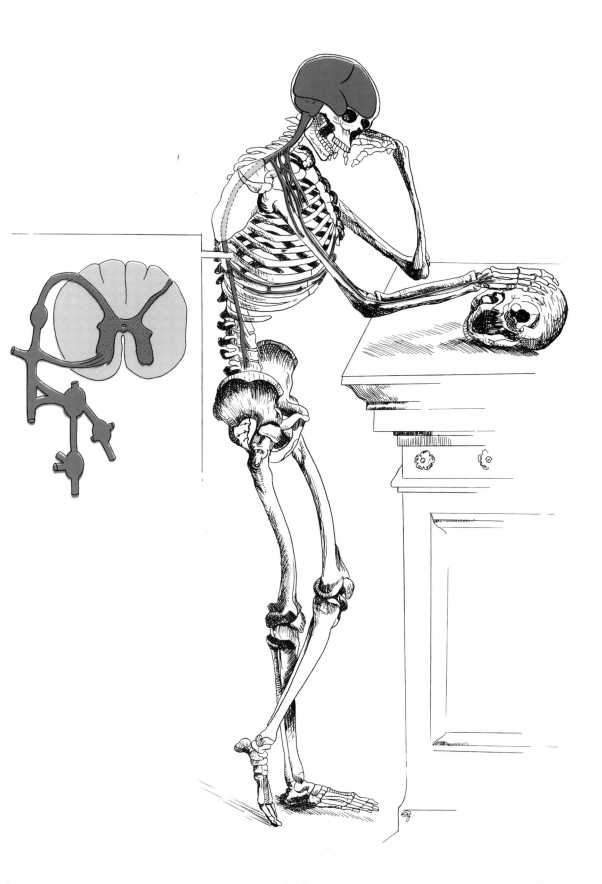

# Nervous Tissue

The nervous system is developed entirely from ectoderm. It manifests optimally the two properties of protoplasm, irritability and conductivity, and is the most highly differentiated tissue in the body.

Neural tissue is made up of cells and their processes. Cells of the nervous system fall into two general categories: (1) nerve cells or neurons and (2) supporting cells and satellite cells. In addition, neural tissue contains blood vessels and a protective covering (meninges).

To study neural tissue several stains are utilized. None of them alone is capable of revealing all the desired details of structure. Because of the affinity of nerve cells and their processes for silver solutions (argyrophilia), silver impregnation methods are frequently used.

The Golgi silver methods selectively impregnate relatively few cells, but accomplish this most completely. These methods are good for outlining the external shape of nerve cells and their processes, but do not reveal details of internal cell structure such as neurofibrils and Nissl bodies.

The Cajal and Bielschowsky silver methods are later developments of the silver impregnation methods. They are utilized to demonstrate axons, neurofibrils and nerve endings including synapses. Originally used on blocks of tissues, they have been modified for use on mounted sections. The most useful modification is that of Bodian in which activated protargol (silver proteinate) is employed (Plates 101 and 293).

The Nissl substance (cytoplasmic ribonucleoprotein) of nerve cells is revealed, using basic aniline dyes, such as cresyl violet, gallocyanin and toluidine blue (Plates 1 and 86).

For the myelin sheath a variety of methods are used, such as the osmium tetroxide, Pal-Weigert, Weil and Marchi techniques. The Marchi method is used to demonstrate degenerating myelin (Plates 272 and 273), while the Pal-Weigert and Weil methods stain normal myelin (Plates 265, 267 and 290).

A neuron (nerve cell) consists of the cell body (perikaryon) and all its processes. Neurons, with a range of 4 to 135 $\mu$ in diameter, are generally larger in size than other cells in the body. The shape of neurons varies with the number and arrangement of their processes. In general, three types of neurons are recognized. (1) Unipolar or pseudounipolar neurons are spherical cell bodies with single processes that later bifurcate. Such cells are found in the dorsal root ganglia (Plates 95 and 97). (2) Bipolar neurons are spindle-shaped, with one process at each end. Such neurons are found in peripheral ganglia, such as in the acoustic and olfactory systems (Plates 96 and 246). (3) Multipolar neurons have polygonal cell bodies and many processes. Such neurons are encountered in the autonomic ganglia (Plate 98) and central nervous system (Plates 10 and 85).

Nuclei of neurons are usually large, rounded and centrally located and are characterized by well defined, strongly RNA-positive nucleoli (Plate 86). Bi- and trinucleated neurons are rarely found in some autonomic ganglia (Plate 99).

The cytoplasm of neurons is rich in Nissl bodies, which are particularly coarse in the somatic motor neurons (Plates 1 and 86). Electron microscopy has shown the Nissl substance to be composed of ribonucleoprotein bound to membrane (granular endoplasmic reticulum). Nissl material extends into the proximal portions of dendrites but is absent in the axons and axon hillocks. Nissl substance, because of its RNA content, is stained by basic aniline dyes. Nissl substance undergoes definite changes in response to axonal injury. In addition to the Nissl substance, neuronal cytoplasm is rich in mitochondria and contains a prominent perinuclear Golgi apparatus (Plate 7). Neurofibrils are seen in the cytoplasm of neurons and their processes (Plate 10). They are made up of subunits (neurofilaments) which are beyond the limit of resolution of the light microscope. The argyrophilic neurofibrils are unique to nerve cells. In addition to the above cell organelles, neuronal cytoplasm may contain lipid droplets, glycogen, pigment granules (Plate 12) and secretory products (hormones) (Plate 104).

Neurons in the central nervous system have a variety of shapes. They may be stellate in the anterior horn of the spinal cord (Plate 85) or flask-shaped, as in the Purkinje cells of the cerebellum (Plate 89). Neurons in the peripheral ganglia are surrounded by satellite cells forming a capsule around the neuron. Those located in sensory ganglia are unipolar, whereas those in autonomic ganglia are multipolar.

The cell body of a neuron is its trophic center. Separation of a process from the cell body results in the death of that process. Neuronal processes are extensions of the cell body and serve to initiate or conduct nerve impulses. Dendrites generally receive and then conduct impulses toward the cell body, while axons conduct them away from the cell body. In unipolar (pseudounipolar) neurons, in which the single process bifurcates into a peripheral and a central branch, both branches are structurally axon-like. In bipolar neurons, the effector and receptor portions of the neuron are found at the extreme ends of the two processes, and the entire intermediate portion is conductive. Multipolar neurons have several dendrites arising from the cell body (Plate 87) and one axon that arises from the cell body or from the base of a dendrite (Plate 85). Dendrites branch repeatedly and their surfaces are studded with spines or gemmules (Plate 84), thus expanding the receptive cell surface. It is estimated that some neurons receive as many as 100,000 axon terminals on their dendritic expansion. A striking example of the vast dendritic expansion is seen in Golgi preparations of the Purkinje cell of the cerebellum (Plate 91).

Axons are more slender than dendrites (Plate 83) and more uniform in diameter. The point of origin of the axon from a nerve cell is termed the axon hillock and is devoid of Nissl substance. It is the most excitable part of the neuron and the site at which the nerve impulse is initiated. Distally, each axon breaks up into simple or complex arborizations, the telodendria, which end on other neurons, glands or muscle (Plates 87, 105, 106 and 107). Axons invariably acquire sheaths along their course. The axon and its sheath are referred to as a nerve fiber. Nerve fibers that run together in a bundle and share a common origin and destination in the central nervous system constitute a tract (Plates 267 and 273). A nerve fiber bundle in the peripheral nervous system constitutes a nerve (Plate 103). Nerve fibers may be myelinated or unmyelinated. Myelin sheaths are elaborated and maintained by oligodendroglia in the central nervous system, and by Schwann cells in the peripheral nervous system. Unmyelinated and myelinated peripheral nerve fibers are in intimate contact with Schwann cell cytoplasm and nucleus and the plasma membrane is covered by a basement membrane (the neurolemmal sheath or sheath of Schwann). The relationship of such nerve fibers to oligodendroglia in the central nervous system is not quite so intimate. The myelin sheath around an axon is interrupted at regular intervals to form the nodes of Ranvier (Plate 95). The flow of an electrical impulse along the nerve fiber skips from one node of Ranvier to the next. Myelin sheaths serve to insulate axons and to speed up conduction of the nerve impulse (saltatory conduction). Myelin is made up of a lipid-protein complex. Some of the lipid is usually lost during tissue preparation, leaving behind a resistant proteo-lipid, neurokeratin (Plate 102), unless special methods are used to preserve it (Plate 103).

In addition to the myelin sheath and the sheath of Schwann, peripheral nerve fibers are surrounded by connective tissue, the endoneurium. The endoneurium is continuous with the more abundant connective tissue perineurium which envelops bundles of nerve fibers. The nerve trunk is ensheathed in turn by the epineurium.

Nerve fibers, both axons and myelin sheaths, vary in size. The size of the nerve fiber (axon and its myelin coat) bears a direct relationship to its rate of impulse conduction. Large and heavily myelinated fibers conduct faster than small, unmyelinated ones.

Axons which branch at their termination to establish synapses on other neurons (dendrites, perikarya or other axons) or muscle (Plates 87, 105 and 106) come in close proximity but not in contact with the postsynaptic components of the synapse. Synaptic junctions vary in configuration, from the bouton-type (end bulb) of synapse (Plate 87), to the side-to-side contact seen in the climbing fiber system of the cerebellum (Plate 294), to the basket-type seen in the cerebellum (Plates 293 and 295).

Supporting cells of the nervous system include the capsule or satellite cells of peripheral ganglia, ependyma, neuroglia and Schwann cells.

Satellite cells surround neurons of peripheral ganglia, forming a capsule one cell layer thick (Plate 94). They are derived from neural crest elements and are continuous with the neurolemmal (Schwann) sheath or neural processes.

Ependymal cells line the cavities of the brain and spinal cord (Plate 117). A specialized form of ependymal cell is seen in some areas of the nervous system (subcommissural organ).

Neuroglia are the "supporting elements" of the central nervous system. Three cell types are found: (1) astrocytes with their two varieties, protoplasmic and fibrous, (2) oligodendroglia and (3) microglia.

The astrocytes, as their name implies, are star-shaped cells with relatively lightly staining nuclei and processes closely applied to blood vessels. Two varieties are distinguished on the basis of the morphology of their processes. The protoplasmic variety, found mostly in gray matter, have plump and abundant cell processes which branch repeatedly (Plate 114). The fibrous variety, found mostly in white matter, have more slender but well defined and fewer cell processes. They are longer and straighter than those of the protoplasmic variety (Plate 115). Both varieties of astrocyte play a role in metabolite transfer within the central nervous system. The fibrous astrocytes, in addition, play a role in healing and scar formation in the nervous system.

Oligodendroglia are smaller than astrocytes and have a denser nucleus and cytoplasm. As their name indicates, they have few delicate processes (Plate 116). These glial cells are seen adjacent to myelinated nerve fibers in the white matter or forming satellite cells to the neurons in the gray matter. Oligodendroglia elaborate central nervous system myelin.

Microglia are the smallest of the neuroglia and, unlike the ectodermally derived macroglia (astrocytes and oligodendroglia), they are formed from the mesoderm. They are dense cells with deeply staining nuclei (Plate 114) and are frequently seen in gray matter in close proximity to neurons. The perikaryon of a microglial cell is irregular in shape and, if elongated, the few processes emanate from both of its poles. Microglia are believed to be the scavenger cells of the central nervous system.

The central nervous system is covered by three protective coats (meninges). (1) The outermost layer is the dura mater, made up of a vascular dense fibrous connective tissue. (2) The middle layer is the arachnoid, a non-vascular delicate connective tissue coat. (3) The innermost layer is the pia mater, a delicate vascular layer adherent to the surface of the brain and spinal cord. Between the pia and arachnoid membranes is the subarachnoid space in which the cerebrospinal fluid circulates. The small arteries and capillaries of the pia mater in certain regions of the ventricular system form tufts which invaginate into the ventricular cavity (choroid plexus). The invaginated tufts are lined by cuboidal epithelium. The choroid plexus elaborates cerebrospinal fluid.

Peripherally located receptors constantly feed information into the central nervous system. These receptors may convey general sensation such as touch, pain, thermal sense, pressure, position and movement, or specialized sensations such as vision, audition, taste and smell. The latter variety are dealt with in the section on special senses. Illustrations of most of the former are seen in this section. Such receptors are found as (1) free nerve endings in epithelia or connective tissue or as (2) encapsulated endings in which the neural component of the receptor is surrounded by a connective tissue sheath of varying thickness. The sheath is continuous with the endoneurium and perineurium of the nerve fiber. Examples of such encapsulated endings are Meissner's (Plates 111 and 124), Krause's (Plate 113), and Pacinian corpuscles (Plate 112), the neuromuscular spindle (Plate 108) and the Golgi tendon organ (Plate 110).

Stimulation of any of these receptors results in the initiation of a nerve impulse which travels to the central nervous system. The translation of this impulse into a conscious sensation is a function of the brain.

Although doubt has been cast upon the functional specificity of the different varieties of receptors, it is still generally believed that free nerve endings convey sensations of pain, and possibly touch and thermal sense; Meissner's corpuscles convey touch sensations whereas Pacinian corpuscles convey pressure sensibility. Krause's end bulb and Ruffini receptors are believed to be cold and warmth receptors, respectively. The receptors in muscle and tendon are concerned with movement and posture. They respond to stretch and tension resulting from muscular contraction or passive stretch of muscles.

# CEREBRAL CORTEX
## Motor area, Precentral region

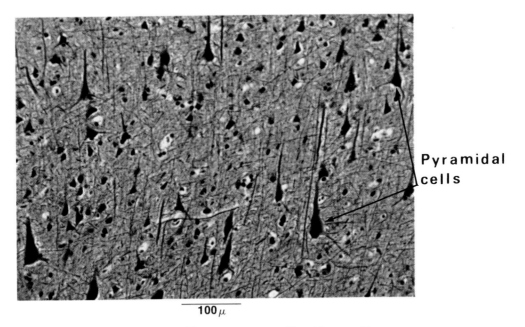

Pyramidal cells

100 μ

## Rhesus monkey, 10% Formalin, Bodian silver, 162x.

**Pyramidal cells:** Characteristic of cerebral cortex. The apex of the cell directed toward the surface of the cortex is termed the apical dendrite. Horizontally oriented basal dendrites also arise from the cell body. Note the variation in size of pyramidal cells (10 to 100 μ). The pyramidal cells located in the motor cortex are the largest of their kind and are known as Betz cells. The unstained region between pyramidal and glial cells is termed the neuropil and is filled with glial cell processes and axonal and dendritic processes of nerve cells.

## CEREBRAL CORTEX
### Betz cell

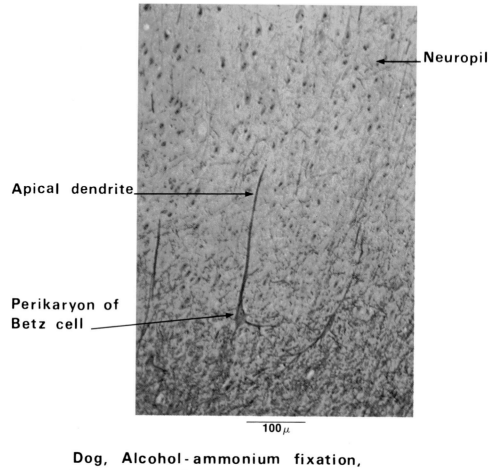

Neuropil

Apical dendrite

Perikaryon of
Betz cell

100μ

Dog, Alcohol-ammonium fixation,
Ranson's method, 162x.

This is a section from the cerebral motor cortex (Area 4), where the pyramidal cells of Betz are found. Note the large multipolar cell body (perikaryon) and the apical dendrite directed toward the surface of the cortex. Surrounding these nerve cell bodies are processes of neural and glial origin (neuropil). In the neuropil, innumerable synaptic contacts occur between nerve cells and their processes.

## CEREBRAL CORTEX
### Pyramidal cells

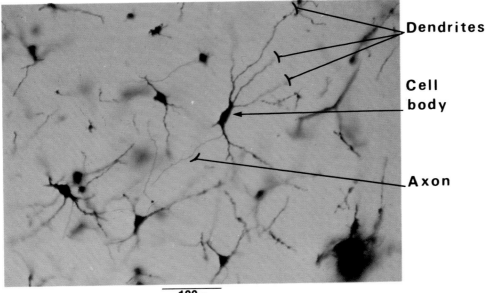

Dendrites

Cell body

Axon

100 μ

**Mouse , Golgi – Cox method , 162 x.**

**Cell body:** Pyramidal in shape.

**Dendrites:** Each cell possesses several large tapering processes containing cytoplasmic organelles similar to those found in the cell body. Some dendrites possess spine-like side processes called gemmules which are seen at higher magnification in Plate 84.

**Axon:** This process arises in this particular cell from the proximal part of the dendrite. It is slender and of uniform diameter, but variable in length depending on location. The axon of a motor neuron may exceed 1 meter in length.

# CEREBRAL CORTEX
## Pyramidal cell

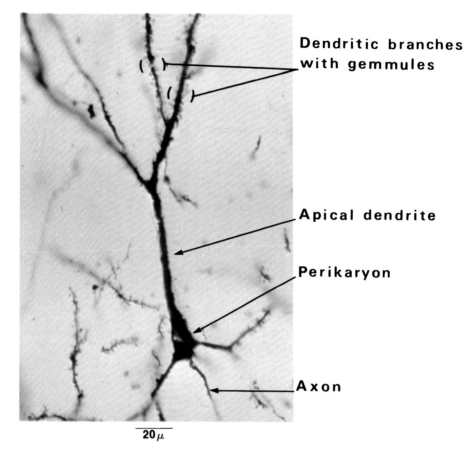

Dendritic branches
with gemmules

Apical dendrite

Perikaryon

Axon

20 μ

## Cat, Golgi preparation, 500 x.

**Perikaryon:** Pyramid-shaped cell body impregnated with silver. Details of inner structure of nerve cells are not revealed by this method.

**Apical dendrite:** Stout tapering process. Directed toward surface of brain. Highly branched (Greek, *dendron*, tree).

**Dendritic branches with gemmules:** Dendritic branches increase the neuron surface for reception of many axon terminals or synapses. Dendritic branches are studded with spiny processes which increase greatly the surface area of the dendrite. It is estimated that this elaboration of surface area allows large neurons to receive as many as 100,000 separate axon terminals or synapses.

**Axon:** Arise from the nerve cell body (as in this figure) or from the proximal part of a dendrite (see Plate 83). Slender extensions with a smoother contour than dendrites and uniform in diameter. The method used in this preparation is the only one capable of revealing the whole neuron (perikaryon and its processes).

## LOWER MOTOR NEURON
### Spinal cord ventral horn

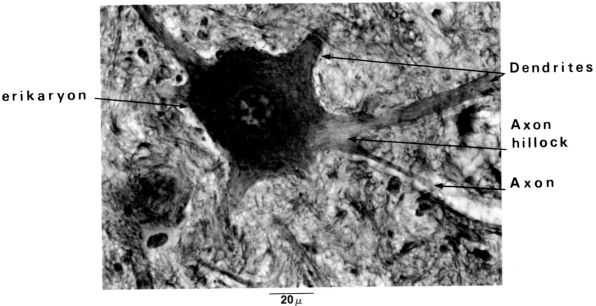

erikaryon

Dendrites

Axon
hillock

Axon

20 μ

### Rhesus monkey, 10% Formalin, Glees' method, 612 x.

**Perikaryon:**  Multipolar (*i.e.*, possesses a single axon and several dendrites). Central prominent nucleus. Cytoplasm rich in Nissl bodies except at the axon hillock (lighter area of cell body from which axon arises). Nissl bodies can be seen in Plates 1 and 86.

**Dendrites:**  Stout tapering processes similar in structure to the perikaryon.

**Axon:**  Arising from axon hillock. Slender process of uniform diameter and great length. The myelin sheath is not seen around the axon in this preparation because it is not preserved by the fixation method employed.

## NISSL BODIES
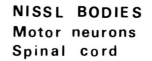
Motor neurons
Spinal cord

Perikaryon

Nucleus

Nucleolus

Dendrite

Neuropil

Nissl bodies

Axon hillock

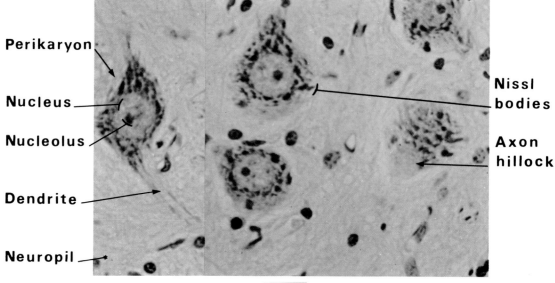

20 μ

Rhesus monkey, 10% Formalin, Gallocyanin, 612 x.

**Perikaryon:** Cell body, multipolar and large.

**Nucleus:** Spherical, pale, centrally placed with widely dispersed chromatin.

**Nucleolus:** Prominent in the pale background of the nucleus.

**Dendrite:** A process of the neuron that allows an expansion of the neuron surface for reception of stimuli. Nissl material is restricted to the proximal region of the dendrite.

**Neuropil:** Region between neurons. Composed of neuronal and glial processes.

**Nissl bodies:** Named after the German histologist Nissl, who first described them. They are one of the major characteristics of the neurons. Found in perikarya and in the proximal part of the dendrite. Electron microscopy reveals Nissl substance to be composed of ribosomes bound to the endoplasmic reticulum. Nissl bodies undergo a distinctive change (chromatolysis) in response to axon section or injury.

**Axon hillock:** The region in the neuronal cell body that marks the emerging axon. Devoid of Nissl bodies.

## THE SYNAPSE
### Spinal cord, Lower motor neuron

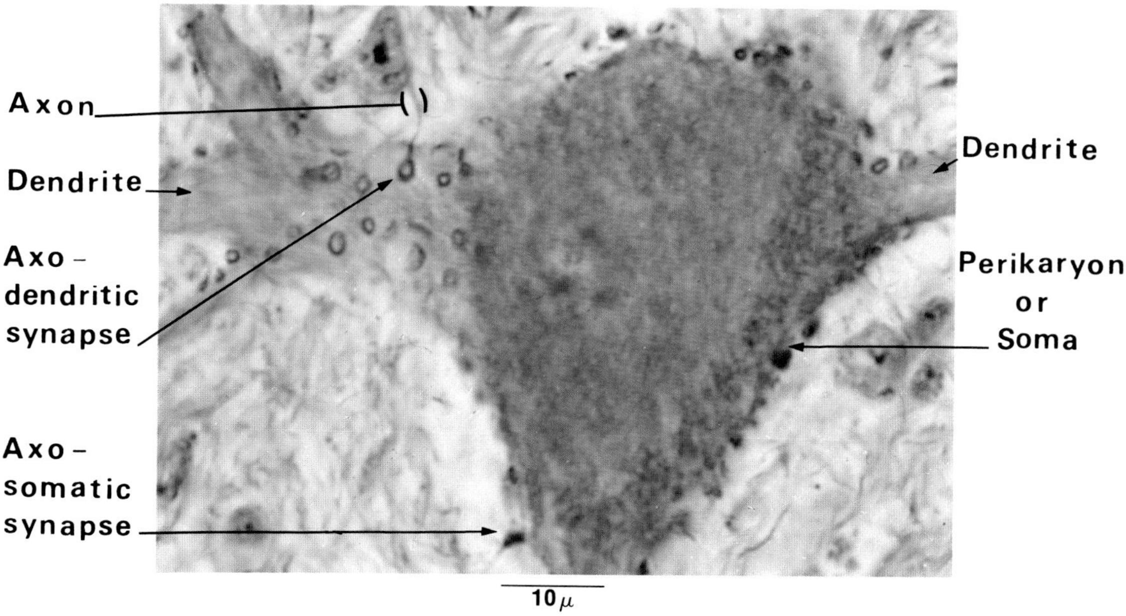

Axon

Dendrite

Axo-
dendritic
synapse

Axo-
somatic
synapse

Dendrite

Perikaryon
or
Soma

10 μ

### Rhesus monkey, 10% Formalin, Glees' method, 1416 x.

**Axon:** Preterminal portion before establishing contact.

**Dendrite:** Stout branching process.

**Axodendritic synapse:** Synaptic knob arising from an axon which is in contact with a dendritic process.

**Axosomatic synapse:** Axon terminal knob in contact with the cell body or perikaryon of the motor neuron.

**Perikaryon or soma:** Multipolar. Studded with terminal knobs. Variation of fine focus in such preparations will reveal the richness of synaptic terminals. The synaptic knobs seen in this photomicrograph represent only a minute fraction of the total synaptic terminals. It has been estimated that as many as 1200 to 1800 synaptic knobs may establish contact with one spinal motor neuron.

## CEREBELLUM

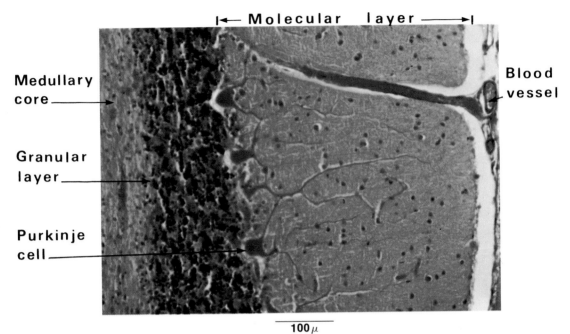

Human, 10% Formalin, Hematoxylin and carmine stains, 162x.

**Medullary core:** The white matter of the cerebellum contains nerve fibers which carry the afferent input and efferent output of the cerebellum.

**Granular layer:** Closely packed with the nuclei of small neurons (granule cells). Receives the major input to the cerebellum (the mossy fiber input).

**Purkinje cell:** Single row of large flask-shaped neurons. Dendrites arborize richly in the molecular layer. Axons exit in the medullary core.

**Molecular layer:** Most superficial layer. Sparsely cellular. Primarily composed of unmyelinated fibers, the dendrites of Purkinje cells, stellate and basket cells.

**Blood vessel:** Located in the subarachnoid space, blood vessels penetrate deeply into folds of the cerebellum to nourish and remove metabolic waste products from the nerve cells and neuroglia.

## CEREBELLUM

**Molecular layer**

**Stellate cell**

**Purkinje cell dendrite**

**Molecular layer**

**Purkinje layer**

**Purkinje cell**

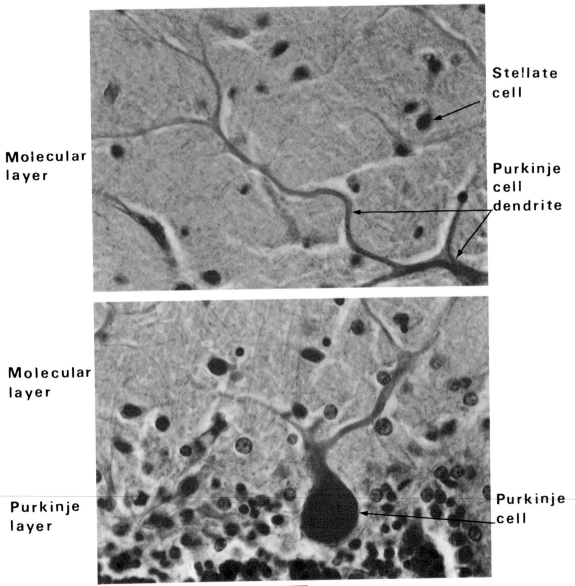

20 μ

## Human, Müller's fluid, Carmine stain, 612 x.

**Molecular layer:** Most superficial layer of the cerebellum. Sparsely cellular. Primarily composed of unmyelinated fibers and dendrites of Purkinje cells.

**Stellate cells:** Sparsely scattered in the molecular layer. Usually small cells with short dendrites and fine unmyelinated axons that run horizontally. Larger stellate cells in the vicinity of Purkinje cells are known as basket cells.

**Purkinje layer:** Single row of large flask-like cell bodies situated between the molecular and granule cell layer.

**Purkinje cell:** Flask-shaped. Each cell gives off two or three main dendrites which arborize richly in the molecular layer. Their axons pass through the granule layer and enter the medullary core to leave the cerebellum.

# CEREBELLUM

Molecular
layer

Golgi
type II

Granule
cell layer

Molecular
layer
Basket cell

Purkinje
cell

Granule
cell layer

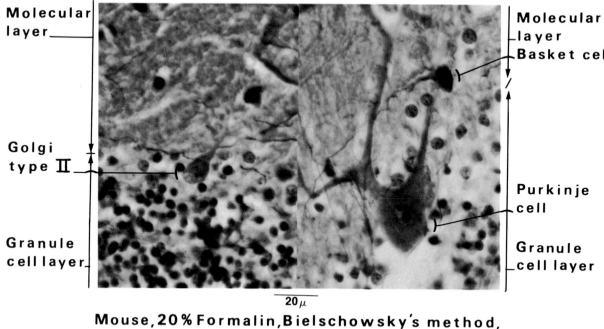

20μ

Mouse, 20% Formalin, Bielschowsky's method,
612 x.

**Molecular layer:**  Most superficial layer of the cerebellar cortex. Sparsely cellular. Primarily composed of nonmyelinated fibers. Dendrites of Purkinje cells arborize in this layer.

**Basket cell:**  A large variety of stellate cells deep in the molecular layer in the vicinity of Purkinje cells. Axons run transversely in the molecular layer and send collaterals that arborize around the perikarya of Purkinje cells like a basket.

**Purkinje cell:**  Single row of large, flask-shaped cells. Form a distinct layer bordering the molecular and granule cell layers. Dendrites arborize richly in the molecular layer. These cells are named after Johannes Purkinje, a Bohemian physiologist, who described them in 1837.

**Granule cell layer:**  Closely packed with chromatic nuclei of small granule cell neurons. Major input to the cerebellum projects into this layer.

**Golgi Type II:**  This type of cerebellar neuron is found in the upper part of the granule cell layer close to the Purkinje cell layer. Larger than the granule cell neuron. Dendrites extend to the molecular layer. Axons establish synapses with dendrites of granule cells in the glomeruli of the granule cell layer. It is estimated that there is one Golgi Type II cell for every ten Purkinje cells.

# CEREBELLUM
## Purkinje cell

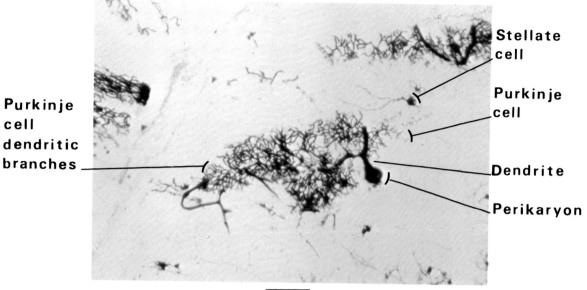

Stellate cell

Purkinje cell

Purkinje cell dendritic branches

Dendrite

Perikaryon

$\overline{100\,\mu}$

## Cat, Golgi preparation, 123x.

**Purkinje cell:** Single row of large cell bodies in the Purkinje cell layer of the cerebellum. Only one complete cell is seen in this figure.

**Perikaryon:** Flask-shaped Purkinje cell body impregnated with silver. Details of inner structure are not revealed by this method.

**Dendrite:** Directed toward surface of cerebellum. Each Purkinje cell possesses several main dendrites which enter the molecular layer.

**Purkinje cell dendritic branches:** Purkinje cell dendrites arborize richly in the molecular layer. The arborization is fan-shaped and extends at right angles to the cerebellar folia.

**Stellate cell:** Located in molecular layer. Small cell body with short, thin dendrites ramifying near the cell body, and fine unmyelinated axon extending transversely to the folia, which establishes synaptic contact with Purkinje cell dendrites.

PLATE 92

# DORSAL ROOT GANGLION
## Sensory neurons

Cell
bodies

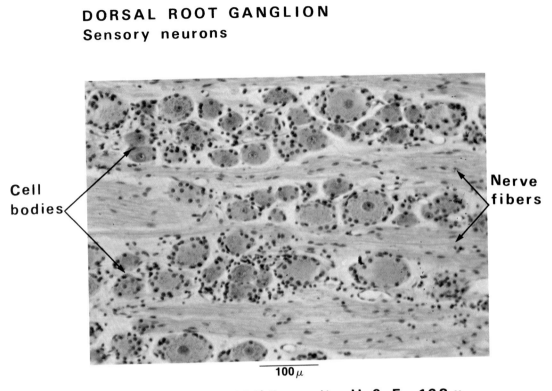

Nerve
fibers

100 μ

**Rhesus monkey, 10% Formalin, H. & E., 162 x.**

**Cell bodies:** Unipolar and ovoid or spherical in shape. Note the variation in size and density of staining of the large "clear" cells and the more numerous, small, densely staining "obscure" cells. See also Plates 93 and 94. Each ganglion cell is surrounded by deeply stained nuclei of the capsule cells (satellite cells).

**Nerve fibers:** These are shown separating groups of nerve cells. Constitute central and peripheral axons of ganglion cells.

## DORSAL ROOT GANGLION

Nerve
fibers

Ganglion
cell bodies

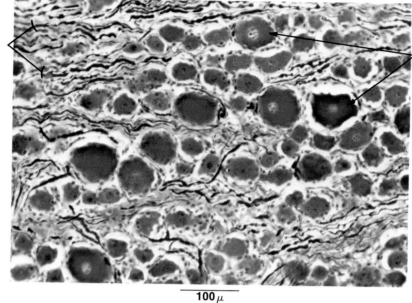

100 μ

### Rhesus monkey, Glees' method, 162 x.

**Ganglion cell bodies:**   Unipolar cells of variable size.

**Nerve fibers:**   Myelinated fibers separate cell bodies. Constitute the afferent and efferent nerve fibers. In this preparation the axons, but not the myelin sheaths, are stained. The myelin sheath can be seen in Plate 95.

# DORSAL ROOT GANGLION
## Cell bodies

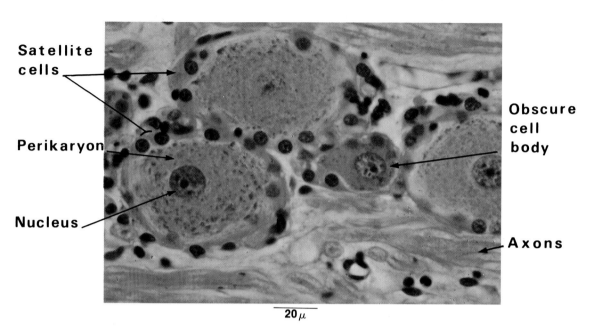

Satellite cells

Perikaryon

Nucleus

Obscure cell body

Axons

20 μ

**Rhesus monkey, 10% Formalin, H. & E., 612 x.**

**Satellite cells:** Of neural crest origin and concentrically arranged around ganglion cells. Also called capsule cells. Rounded or elongated nuclei are darker than nuclei of adjacent ganglion cells.

**Perikaryon:** Dorsal root ganglion cell body of neural crest origin. Ovoid or spherical in shape. Finely scattered cytoplasmic ribonucleoprotein (Nissl substance). Prominent central nucleus with a well defined nucleolus. Indentations of the surface margin are caused by satellite cells.

**Obscure cell body:** Smaller and darker variety of ganglion cells. The nature and functional significance of obscure cells are uncertain.

**Axons:** Processes of ganglion cells. See Plate 95.

# DORSAL ROOT GANGLION
## Sensory neurons

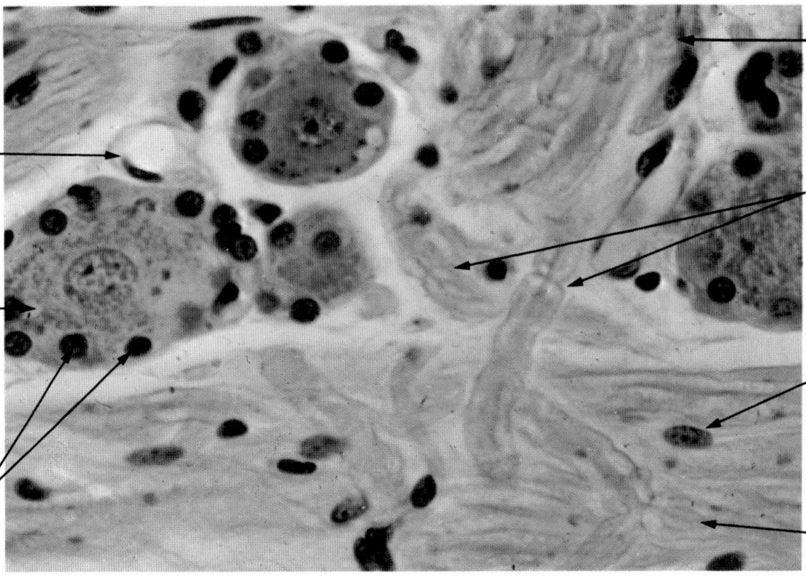

Capillary

Ganglion
cell body

Satellite
cells

Axons

Nodes of
Ranvier

Schwann
cell
nucleus

T—bifur-
cation

20 μ

## Rhesus monkey, 10% Formalin, H. & E., 612 x.

**Ganglion cell body:**  Ovoid or spherical. Note variation in size and intensity of staining. Nucleus central.

**Satellite cells:**  Concentrically arranged around the ganglion cells.

**Capillary:**  With endothelial cell nucleus. Located in the connective tissue stroma between ganglion cells. Absence of blood cells from the capillary lumen is due to vascular perfusion fixation.

**Axons:**  Processes of ganglion cells. Intricate coiling and winding denote its proximity to the cell of origin.

**Nodes of Ranvier:**  Site of termination of myelin sheath segments.

**Schwann cell nucleus:**  Flat to oval in shape. Close proximity to myelinated fibers. Schwann cells elaborate myelin sheaths.

**T-bifurcation:**  Ganglion cell axon bifurcates to form peripheral and central processes. Hence dorsal root ganglion cells are termed pseudounipolar.

## SPIRAL GANGLION CELLS
Cochlear nerve

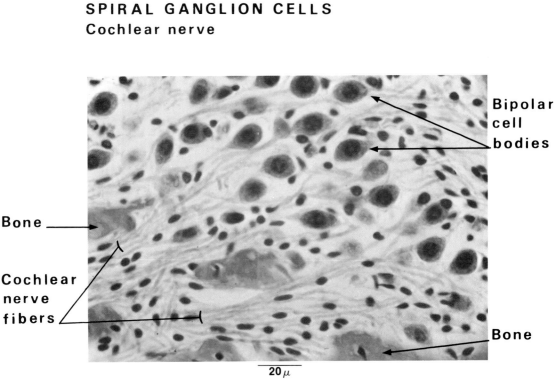

Bipolar
cell
bodies

Bone

Cochlear
nerve
fibers

Bone

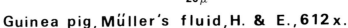

20 μ

Guinea pig, Müller's fluid, H. & E., 612 x.

**Bone:**   Modiolus or central conical pillar of spongy bone of the osseous cochlea.

**Cochlear nerve fibers:**   Central processes of the bipolar ganglion cells.

**Bipolar cell bodies:**   Spiral ganglion. Peripheral processes of sensory hair cells located in the organ of Corti. Central processes from the spiral ganglion cells form the cochlear nerve (auditory part of the eighth cranial nerve).

See Plate 259.

## SENSORY GANGLION (GASSERIAN)
### Pseudounipolar neurons

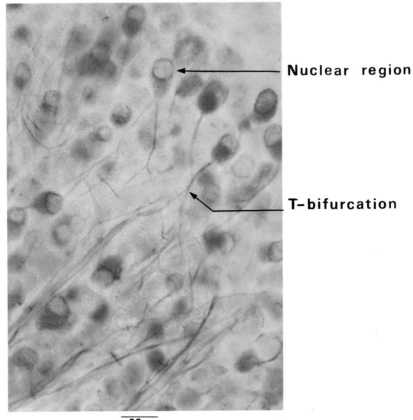

Nuclear region

T-bifurcation

$\overline{20\,\mu}$

### Cat, Alcohol-ammonium fixation, Ranson's method, 500 x.

This figure is taken from an embryonic Gasserian or trigeminal ganglion (fifth cranial nerve) and shows pseudounipolar sensory neurons. Nuclei of neurons are seen as negative images. These neural processes characteristically bifurcate into central and peripheral extensions.

# SYMPATHETIC GANGLION CELLS

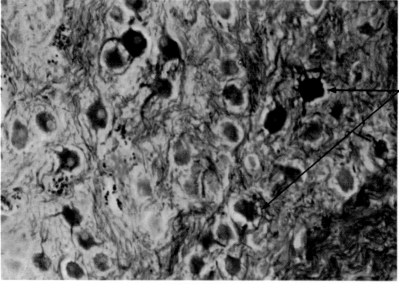

Multipolar ganglion cell bodies

100 μ

**Human, Glees' method, 162 x.**

**Multipolar ganglion cell bodies:** Numerous dendrites, eccentric pale nucleus. Compare the multipolar ganglion cells of sympathetic ganglia with the unipolar ganglion cells of dorsal root ganglia (Plate 93) and with the bipolar cells of sensory ganglia (Plate 96).

# PARASYMPATHETIC GANGLION
## Seminal vesicle

Venule

Ganglion
cell
body

Nerve
fibers

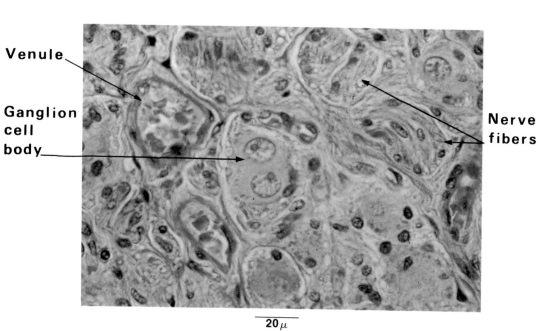

20μ

## Human, Helly's fluid, H. & E., 612x.

**Ganglion cell body:**   Multipolar neurons. Large, eccentrically placed nucleus. Binucleate cells are commonly found in pelvic ganglia and occasionally in the heart. Note the dark nuclei of satellite or capsule cells surrounding the neuron.

**Nerve fibers:**   Myelinated preganglionic and unmyelinated postganglionic fibers of the parasympathetic nervous system.

**Venule:**   A venule is seen in the connective tissue stroma between ganglion cells. Blood is carried away in venules from the capillary bed supplying the ganglion cells and other tissue.

PLATE 100

NERVOUS TISSUE

# PARASYMPATHETIC GANGLION CELLS
## Pancreas

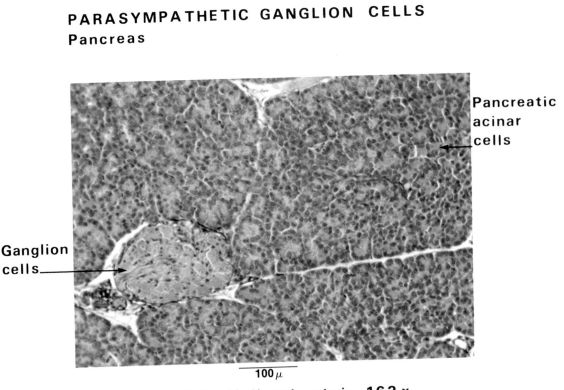

Pancreatic
acinar
cells

Ganglion
cells

$\overline{100\,\mu}$

## Cat, Helly's fluid, Mallory's stain, 162 x.

**Ganglion cells:** Aggregates of parasympathetic ganglion cells enclosed in a thin connective tissue sheath between pancreatic lobules. Afferent input to these cells is from the vagus nerve.

**Pancreatic acinar cells:** Irregular clusters of pancreatic exocrine secretory cells arranged in lobules separated by thin connective tissue septa.

Pancreatic secretion is under neural and hormonal control. The chyme (semifluid mass of partially digested food mixed with gastric enzymes and hydrochloric acid) arriving in the intestine and contacting the intestinal epithelium results in pancreatic secretion. When hydrochloric acid and products of partial protein digestion (proteoses and peptones) contact the intestinal mucous membrane two hormones are released and carried in the blood to the pancreas. The hormone secretin promotes the secretion of water and salts while the hormone pancreozymin depletes zymogen granules (digestive enzymes) from the pancreatic acinar cells. Zymogen granules are also secreted from acinar cells by vagal (parasympathetic) and splanchnic nerve (sympathetic) stimulation.

Secretin was discovered by Bayliss and Starling in 1902. They correctly suggested that secretin was the first example of a whole group of chemical regulators (as yet to be discovered) produced in the body that could be designated as hormones.

## NERVE FIBERS
### White matter, Spinal cord
### cross section

Axon 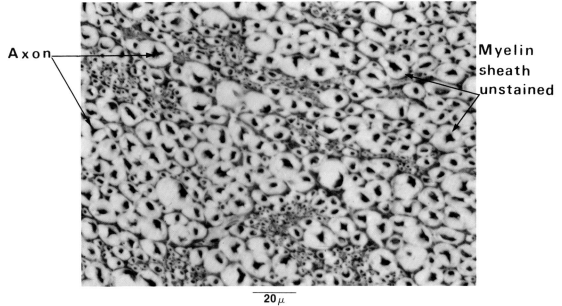 Myelin
sheath
unstained

20 μ

### Rhesus monkey, 10% Formalin, Bodian silver, 612 x.

**Axon:** Shrunken axis cylinder appears black because of silver impregnation. Note the variation in axon diameter. The diameter of a nerve fiber is directly related to the speed of nerve impulse transmission; larger fibers carry electrical impulses faster than smaller fibers.

**Myelin sheath:** Unstained, surrounds axis cylinder.

## SPINAL ROOT NERVE FIBERS
### A) Dorsal root
### B) Ventral root

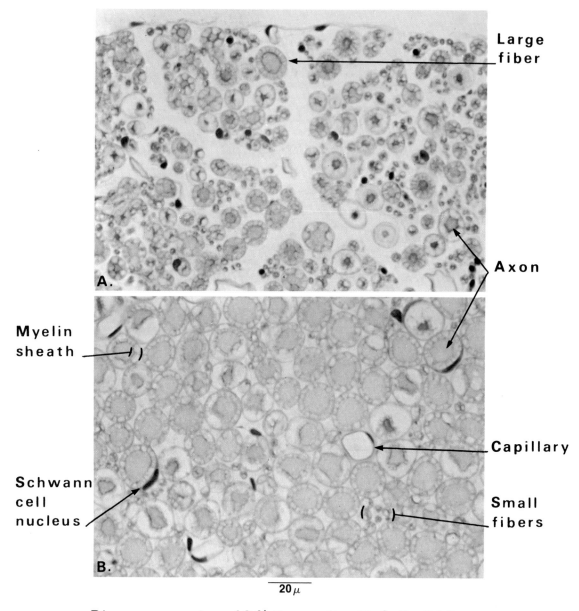

Large fiber

Axon

Myelin sheath

Capillary

Schwann cell nucleus

Small fibers

20 μ

**Rhesus monkey, 10% Formalin, H. & E., 612x.**

The method used here demonstrates axons but not myelin, hence the clear areas around the centrally placed axons represent unstained myelin. The partitions in the clear areas are artifacts of fixation.

Note that nerve fibers in the ventral root (B) are, on the whole, larger than those in the dorsal root (A). Note also the variation in fiber size within both the dorsal and ventral roots. Very small fibers seen in B are unmyelinated. The capillary seen in B shows a crescent-shaped dark endothelial cell nucleus and clear lumen (perfusion fixation). A large, dark, crescent-like Schwann cell nucleus is also seen in B. Schwann cells elaborate the myelin sheath.

## PERIPHERAL NERVE
### Sciatic nerve
### cross section

**Axons
unstained**

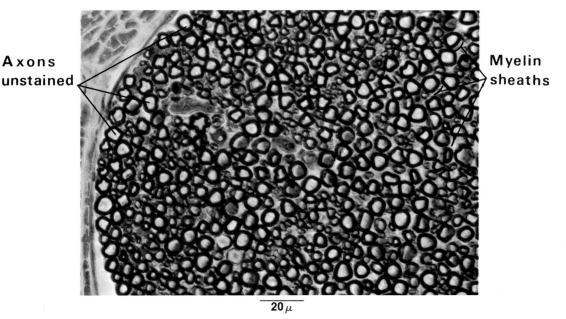

**Myelin
sheaths**

20 μ

### Rhesus monkey, Osmium tetroxide, 612 x.

**Axons unstained:**  Note variation in size.

**Myelin sheath:**  Dense sleeve around axons. Myelin sheaths in the peripheral nervous system are elaborated by Schwann cells.

Compare this preparation with that of Plate 101, in which axons only are stained.

## NEUROHYPOPHYSIS
### Axon terminations of hypothalamic secretory neurons

Nerve fibers

Nerve terminals around a capillary

Neurosecretory substance

Capillaries

Neurosecretory substance

A. $\overline{20\,\mu}$     B. $\overline{100\,\mu}$

A. Pig, 10% Formalin, Ranson's method, 500 x.
B. Rat, Helly's fluid, Gomori's chrom alum hematoxylin and phloxine stains, 162 x.

The posterior lobe of the hypophysis, the neurohypophysis, is composed of nerve fibers which arise in the hypothalamus. Their cell bodies lie in the supraoptic and paraventricular nuclei. In *A*, nerve fibers and their pericapillary terminations are shown. In *B*, the method employed selectively demonstrates neurosecretory material located in the axons. Note the abundance of blood vessels and the stained neurosecretory material surrounding the pericapillary spaces. It is believed that the nerve terminals release oxytocin and vasopressin into the blood stream. These two hormones are polypeptides. Oxytocin causes the smooth muscle fibers of the uterus to contract, a function essential for parturition, and can be used clinically to induce labor. Oxytocin also causes the myoepithelial cells of the mammary gland to contract, bringing about the flow of milk from the gland.

Vasopressin or antidiuretic hormone (ADH) raises blood pressure by acting on arterial blood vessels, stimulates the adrenal cortex, and increases the permeability of the distal and collecting tubules of the kidneys. This increases water reabsorption from the glomerular filtrate, inhibiting an abnormally large flow of urine (diuresis) and resulting in the formation of a urine hypertonic with respect to blood plasma.

## MOTOR END PLATE
Lateral rectus muscle
cross section

Muscle
fiber

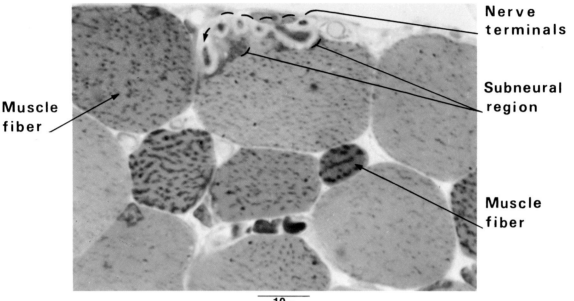

Nerve
terminals

Subneural
region

Muscle
fiber

10μ

## Cat, Glutaraldehyde – osmium fixation, Toluidine blue stain, 1416 x.

**Nerve terminals:** Nonmyelinated, dip into specialized sarcolemmal folds or gutters in the muscle fiber.

**Subneural region:** Specialized synaptic region of the muscle fiber. Multiple sarcolemmal folds.

**Muscle fiber:** Note the variation in size of fibers and in staining pattern. Compare with Plates 106 and 107.

# NEUROMUSCULAR JUNCTION
## Intercostal muscle

Nerve fibers

Muscle fiber

Axon

Motor end plate

Muscle striations

20μ

## Rat, 10% Formalin, Bodian silver, 612x.

**Nerve fibers:** Myelinated somatic motor nerve fibers branch extensively within and between the muscle fibers. Axons (but not their myelin sheaths) are stained in this preparation.

**Axon:** Although not shown, nerve fibers lose their myelin sheaths as they approach the motor end plate region. These nonmyelinated axons branch extensively on the surface of the muscle fiber.

**Motor end plate:** A well defined junction of axon terminals on the muscle fiber surface. It is at this place that the electrical nerve impulse is chemically (acetylcholine) transferred to the muscle fiber. A muscle action potential is generated and the electrical impulse is conducted over the fiber surface, resulting in muscular contraction.

**Muscle striations:** Note that the striated myofibrils do not extend inside the motor end plate region.

**Muscle fiber:** The number of muscle fibers supplied by a single motor nerve fiber varies greatly. The ratio is low (about 1:3) for muscles which perform delicate functions, such as the extrinsic eye muscles. In limb muscles the ratio may be 1:80 or greater.

# MOTOR END PLATE
## Intercostal muscle

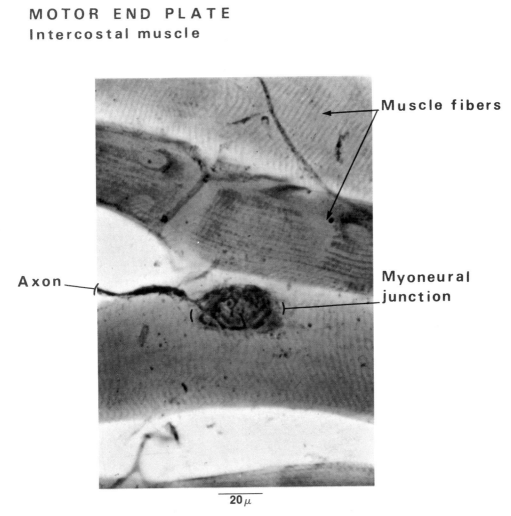

Muscle fibers

Axon

Myoneural junction

20 μ

### Rabbit, Ranvier's Gold chloride method, 612x.

**Muscle fibers:**  A small portion of three cross striated muscle fibers is seen in this preparation.

**Axon:**  A myelinated nerve fiber, upon reaching the muscle surface, loses its myelin sheath and branches extensively in a well defined region called the motor end plate or myoneural junction.

**Myoneural junction:**  The specialized region between the axon terminals and muscle fiber surface at which the nerve impulse is transmitted to the sarcolemma, resulting in muscular contraction.

The method used in this preparation is a classical technique for staining nerve endings (see also Plate 110).

## MUSCLE SPINDLE
### Neural components

Annulo-
spiral
ending

Nuclear
bag
muscle
fiber

Motor
end
plates

Intra-
fusal
muscle fiber

Nerve
fiber

Sheath

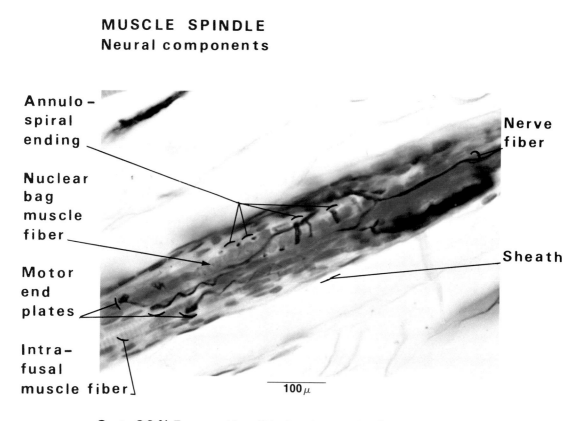

100 μ

### Cat, 20% Formalin, Bielschowsky's method, 162 x.

Muscle spindles are found within skeletal muscles. Each spindle is formed of two to ten small muscle fibers, the intrafusal fibers, enclosed within a sheath of connective tissue which is pierced by nerve fibers.

**Nerve fibers:**  Leaving and entering the muscle spindle, they may carry the sensory signals (output) or the motor signals (input).

**Sheath:**  Connective tissue capsule that surrounds the intrafusal muscle fibers of the spindle.

**Annulospiral endings:**  Also known as primary or nuclear bag endings. Large axon with many branches and terminal enlargements. Arborization of this type of ending occurs around the nuclear bag variety of intrafusal muscle fibers. These endings have a low threshold to stretch. They discharge when the intrafusal muscle fibers are stretched. The receptors are silent when the extrafusal (ordinary) muscle fibers contract and the intrafusal fibers are relaxed. Central processes of the annulospiral endings in the spinal cord participate in the monosynaptic (myotatic) reflex.

**Nuclear bag muscle fibers:**  Larger variety of intrafusal muscle fibers. Have an enlarged equatorial region to accommodate numerous small nuclei (Plate 109). It is here that annulospiral endings arborize.

**Motor end plates:**  The smaller nerve fibers within the spindle are axons of gamma neurons in the spinal cord. The axons terminate as typical motor end plates on intrafusal muscle fibers.

**Intrafusal muscle fibers:**  Small striated muscle fibers rich in sarcoplasm and arranged parallel to the extrafusal skeletal muscle fibers. Two to ten fibers enclosed in a connective tissue capsule form the muscle spindle.

## MUSCLE SPINDLE
### Gastrocnemius muscle

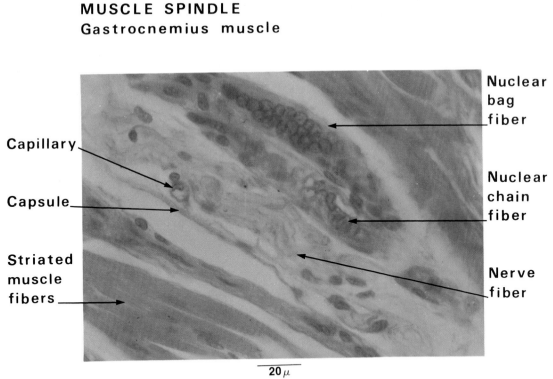

Capillary

Capsule

Striated
muscle
fibers

Nuclear
bag
fiber

Nuclear
chain
fiber

Nerve
fiber

20 μ

### Human, Zenker's fluid, H. & E., 612 x.

**Striated muscle fiber:** Extrafusal (ordinary) skeletal muscle fiber oriented parallel to the intrafusal (en-capsulated) fibers.

**Capsule:** Thin connective tissue sheath which surrounds the muscle spindle.

**Nerve fiber:** Myelinated axon. One of several nerve fibers related to the sensory and motor function of the muscle spindle.

**Nuclear chain fiber:** Smaller variety of intrafusal muscle fibers (10 to 12 μ in diameter and 3 to 4 mm in length). Has a single row or chain of central nuclei.

**Nuclear bag fiber:** Larger variety of intrafusal muscle fibers. Enlarged equatorial region accommodates numerous small nuclei.

This specimen was obtained from a patient with a rhabdomyosarcoma, a very uncommon, highly malignant tumor of striated muscle. The tumor cells are not seen in this section.

## GOLGI TENDON ORGAN
### Tendon of Achilles

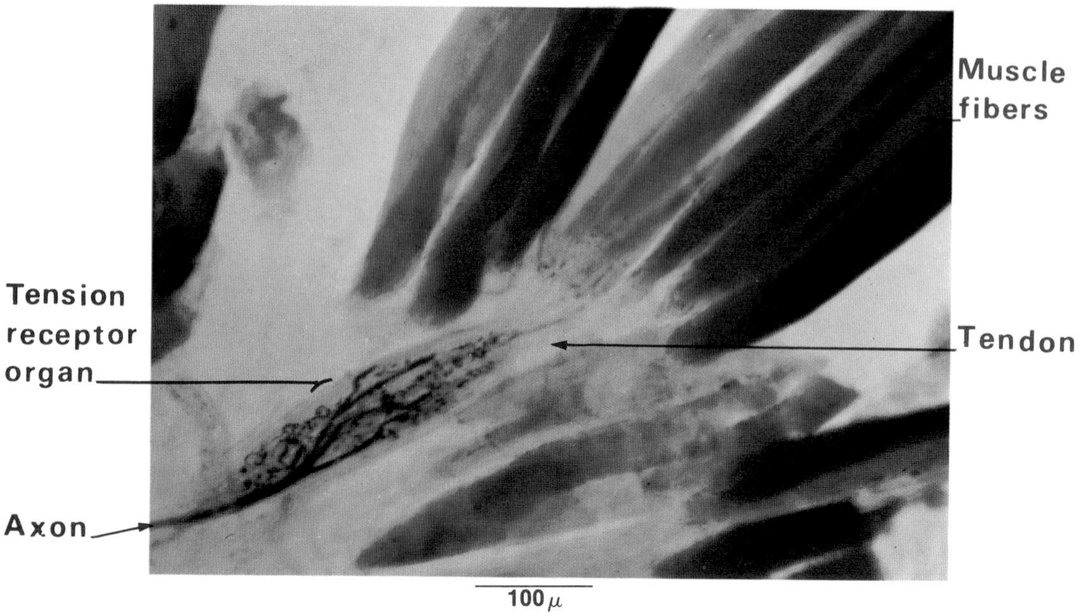

Muscle fibers

Tension receptor organ

Tendon

Axon

100 μ

**Rabbit, Formic acid – gold chloride, 162 x.**

**Axon:** Myelinated axons break into primary, secondary and tertiary branches. Unmyelinated branches from these axons wind around and in between tendon fascicles.

**Tendon:** Collagenous connective tissue bundle joined to several muscle fibers.

**Muscle fibers:** Skeletal (striated) muscle fibers.

**Tension receptor organ:** Discharges electrical impulses in response to tension on the tendon produced by muscular contraction. Provides information about state of muscle tension which determines in part the response of the central nervous system in the appropriate use of the muscle or muscles for precise motor function.

# MEISSNER'S TACTILE CORPUSCLE
Finger tip

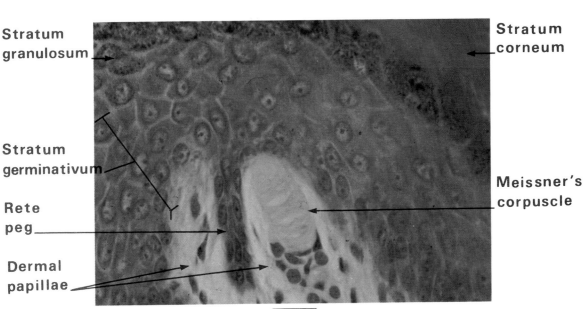

Stratum granulosum

Stratum corneum

Stratum germinativum

Rete peg

Meissner's corpuscle

Dermal papillae

20 μ

Rhesus monkey, Helly's fluid, H. & E., 612 x.

**Meissner's corpuscle:** Contained within a dermal papilla. Surrounded by a thin connective tissue sheath. Common in hairless (glabrous) portions of skin. Most numerous in fingertips, palms and soles. Nerve terminals within Meissner's corpuscle are not seen with this method. See also Plate 124.

**Stratum corneum:** Consists mainly of sheets of dead keratinized squamous cells.

**Stratum granulosum:** One to three layers of cells that contain keratohyalin granules.

**Stratum Malpighii:** Few layers of irregular polyhedral cells with intercellular bridges (see Plate 123).

**Rete peg:** Peg like projections of epidermis into dermis forming dermal papillae.

**Dermal papillae:** Superficial portion of dermis between epidermal pegs. Contains free nerve endings and Meissner's corpuscles or blood vessels.

# CORPUSCLE OF VATER – PACINI
# (PACINIAN CORPUSCLE)
## Pancreas

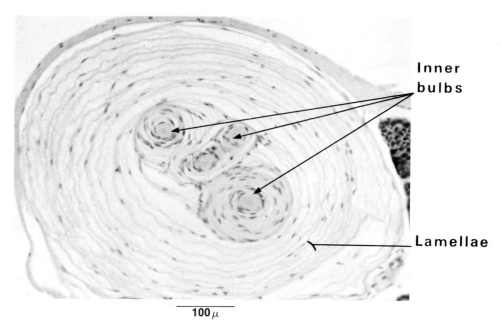

Inner
bulbs

Lamellae

$\overline{100\,\mu}$

## Cat, Helly's fluid, H. & E., 162 x.

**Inner bulbs:**   Transverse section of branches of terminal unmyelinated nerve endings.

**Lamellae:**   Concentric layers of collagenous connective tissue and flattened fibroblasts.

Pacinian corpuscles are found in the pancreas of cats but not man. In man and other animals they are readily seen in sections of the dermis from the fingers and palm of the hand, the conjunctiva, near joints, in the mesenteries, branching blood vessels, penis, urethra, clitoris, parietal peritoneum and loose connective tissue.

The Pacinian corpuscle is a pressure receptor. Since the corpuscle is fluid-filled it is essentially incompressible. The corpuscle transmits mechanical stimuli, through the connective tissue lamellae and fluid, to excite the nonmyelinated receptor axon in its core.

Pacinian corpuscles vary in size but many are large enough to be easily dissected without magnifying lenses in the fingers of man.

## END BULB OF KRAUSE
### Tongue
### lamina propria

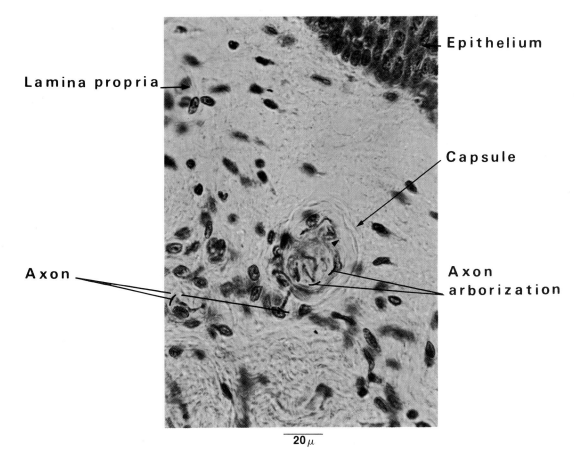

Epithelium

Lamina propria

Capsule

Axon

Axon
arborization

20μ

**Rhesus monkey,10% Formalin,Bodian silver,550x.**

**Axon:**  Sensory axon leading to the central nervous system.

**Axon arborization:**  Encapsulated receptor branches of the sensory axon.

**Sheath:**  Collagenous connective tissue spherical sheath or capsule enclosing the axon arborizations.

**Connective tissue:**  Collagenous connective tissue of the lamina propria.

The end bulbs of Krause are believed to be cold temperature receptors.

## NEUROGLIA
## Protoplasmic astrocytes
## Microglia

Protoplasmic
astrocytes

Microglia
cell

Nuclear
region

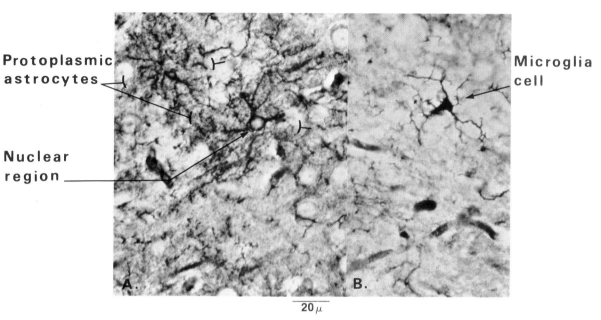

20 μ

**Human, 10 % Formalin, Silver diammine hydroxide, 500 x.**

**Protoplasmic astrocyte:** Stellate in shape, with many cytoplasmic processes. Found chiefly in gray matter of brain and spinal cord. Important in metabolite transport.

**Nuclear region:** Nucleus unstained. Large, rounded or ovoid.

**Microglia cell:** Small, dark cell. Processes fewer than those of the astrocyte, spiny and much more delicate.

# NEUROGLIA
## Fibrous astrocytes

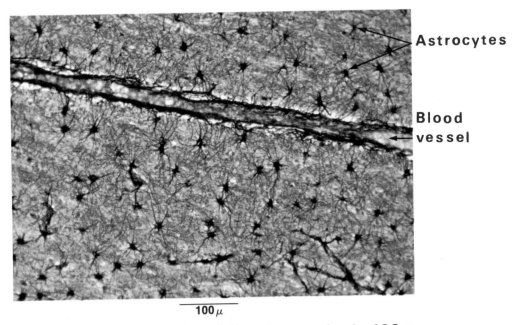

Human, Cajal's gold sublimate method, 162 x.

**Astrocytes:** Stellate cells. Processes fewer, straighter and much longer than those of protoplasmic astrocytes (Plate 114). Note the relationship to blood vessels. Astrocyte processes with end feet are applied to the walls of blood vessels forming a continuous glial membrane surrounding blood vessels and capillaries. This important component of the so-called blood-brain barrier modifies the diffusion of substances from the blood to the extracellular fluid.

## NEUROGLIA
### Oligodendroglia

Neuropil 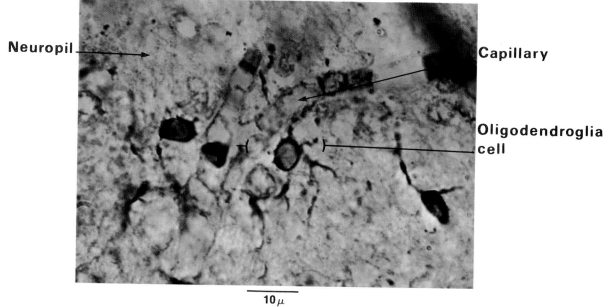 Capillary

Oligodendroglia
cell

10 μ

Rabbit, 10% Formalin, Nassar-Shanklin method,
1376x.

**Oligodendroglia cell:** Rounded nucleus, scanty cytoplasm and a few delicate processes that extend for a short distance. Oligodendroglia are found in gray and white matter. They are usually seen in relation to neuronal cell bodies or between myelinated fibers. A cell of this type has also been described in juxtaposition to blood vessels. Oligodendroglia are believed to elaborate central nervous system myelin.

**Neuropil:** The region between neuronal and glial cells packed with neuronal and glial cell processes.

## EPENDYMA
### Spinal cord

Ependymal cells

Central canal

Ependymal cells

Central canal

Anterior white commissure

Obliterated central canal

Posterior funiculus

Blood vessel

Anterior white commissure

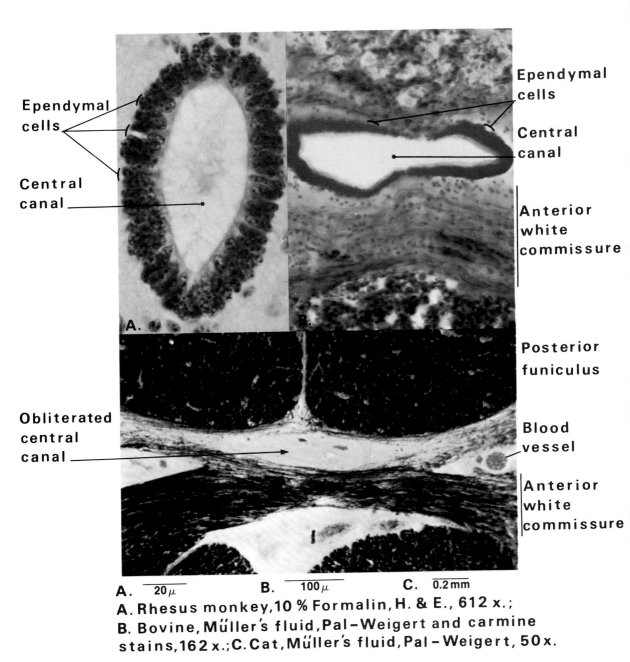

A. ‾20 μ‾   B. ‾100 μ‾   C. ‾0.2 mm‾
A. Rhesus monkey, 10 % Formalin, H. & E., 612 x.;
B. Bovine, Müller's fluid, Pal−Weigert and carmine
   stains, 162 x.; C. Cat, Müller's fluid, Pal−Weigert, 50 x.

The ependymal lining of the central canal of the spinal cord is shown in this plate. In *A*, note that the ependymal cells are columnar in shape and are closely packed with their long axes perpendicular to the central canal. Their nuclei are elongated. Ependymal cells line the cavities of the spinal cord and brain (central canal and ventricles). Although the central canals seen (*A* and *B*) are patent, in adult humans and some animals the canal is usually obliterated (*C*). In *B*, note the anterior white commissure passing anterior (ventral) to the central canal. In *C*, in addition, note the posterior funiculus located posterior (dorsal) to the central canal.

## CHOROID PLEXUS

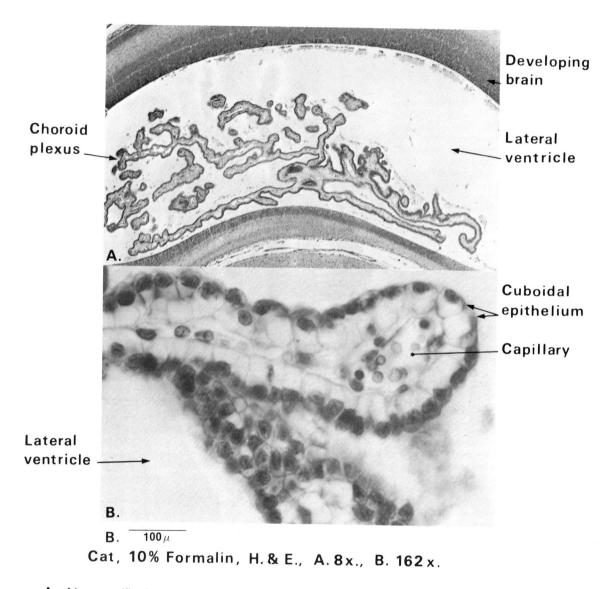

Developing brain

Choroid plexus

Lateral ventricle

Cuboidal epithelium

Capillary

Lateral ventricle

A.

B.

B. ‾‾‾‾‾ 100 μ

**Cat, 10% Formalin, H. & E., A. 8x., B. 162x.**

**A:**  A low magnification plate showing the branched projections of the choroid plexus within the cavity of the lateral ventricle in a developing cat brain.

**B:**  A high magnification plate showing the histology of the choroid plexus. Note the single layer of cuboidal epithelium with large spherical nuclei. Beneath the epithelium is a connective tissue core containing vascular channels. The choroid plexus is a major site for production of cerebrospinal fluid.

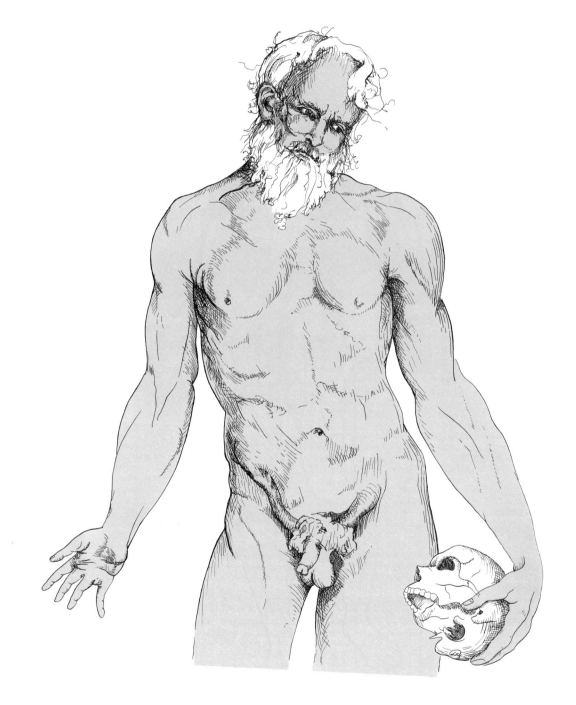

# The Integument

The integument is composed of the skin, which covers the entire body, in addition to accessory organs derived from the skin. The accessory organs include the nails, hair and glands of various kinds.

Skin serves many important functions. (1) It is an impervious barrier which excludes harmful substances and prevents desiccation; (2) plays a role in the regulation of body temperature; (3) readily repairs itself; (4) receives sensory stimuli (touch, pressure, temperature and pain); (5) sweat glands excrete waste products; and (6) sebaceous and mammary glands secrete sebum and milk, respectively.

Skin consists of the epidermis (keratinized stratified squamous epithelium) and the dermis (corium) which is composed of connective tissue (Plate 121). Beneath the dermis is the hypodermis or subcutaneous superficial fascia, a loose connective tissue which in some places is composed primarily of fat cells (panniculus adiposus), a stored energy reserve.

### The Epidermis

This epithelium varies in thickness in different regions of the body but is usually 0.1 mm thick. In the skin of the palms and soles it may be 0.8 to 1.4 mm in thickness. The epidermis of the palm and sole can be divided into five distinct layers. From the deepest layer outward they are: (1) stratum basale, (2) stratum spinosum, (3) stratum granulosum, (4) stratum lucidum and (5) stratum corneum. The strata basale and spinosum are also referred to as the Malpighian layer. The cells of stratum basale comprise a single layer of columnar or cuboidal cells in contact with the underlying basement membrane and connective tissue of the dermis. The stratum basale is often referred to as the stratum germinativum. Melanin pigment granules are richly concentrated in the basal layer but may be found throughout the stratum Malpighii (Plate 11). Above the basal layer is the stratum spinosum composed of polyhedral cells, the so-called prickle cells (Plate 123). The stratum granulosum is composed of a layer of three to five cells which contain keratohyalin granules of irregular shape that stain with basic dyes. The stratum lucidum consists of a tightly packed layer of cells without nuclei containing a refractile substance called eleidin. This layer is strongly eosinophilic. The most superficial layer, the stratum corneum, is composed of many dead cells without nuclei which are filled with keratin. The surface cells of this layer are continually desquamated.

Over most of the body the epidermis is much thinner and simpler in composition. The strata Malpighii and corneum are always present and the stratum granulosum, consisting of two or three layers of cells, can usually be seen. The stratum lucidum is rarely seen in the thinner epidermis. The epidermis is devoid of blood vessels but is nourished by diffusion from the capillaries in the underlying dermis (Plates 124 and 140).

### The Dermis

The dermis or corium underlying the epidermis is 0.3 to 4.0 mm in thickness and may be divided into two layers, papillary and reticular. The papillary layer includes the ridges and papillae which protrude between the epidermal pegs. Some papillae contain tactile corpuscles of Meissner, while other papillae contain only small blood vessels (Plate 124). The papillary connective tissue is composed primarily of collagenous and elastic fibers. The reticular layer is composed primarily of coarse interlacing collagenous fibers and an elastic network. Hair follicles and smooth muscle (arrector pili), sweat and sebaceous glands, and Pacinian corpuscles are located in the reticular layer (Plates 128, 129, 130 and 131). In the face and neck, striated muscle fibers (the muscles of facial expression) terminate in the dermis.

## Subcutaneous Layer

This layer, not a part of the skin, is also called the superficial fascia and is a loose network of connective tissue bundles and septa which blends indistinctly with the dermis. The arrangement of the connective tissue of the superficial fascia permits the movement of skin except on the palm of the hand and sole of the foot. In some regions, particularly the abdomen, lobules of fat are abundant, and the layer is then called the panniculus adiposus.

## Epidermal Derivatives

The epidermal derivatives include the nails, hair and glands. The fingernails, found only in man and other primates, are convex rectangular specializations of the epidermis called the nail plates. Underlying the nail plate is the nail bed consisting of the germinative layer of the epidermis.

Hair is a characteristic of mammals. These elastic, horny filaments may grow to a length of five or more feet and vary in thickness from 0.005 to 0.2 mm. Hair is found on all parts of the skin except the palm and sole, and the oral, anal and urogenital orifices. Hair consists of a free shaft and a root located in the dermis. The hair is surrounded by a tubular epithelial follicle. Associated with the follicle are a sebaceous gland and the arrector pili smooth muscle fiber bundle (Plates 80, 129 and 131).

The cutaneous glands include the sebaceous, sweat, lacrimal and mammary glands. The sebaceous glands produce sebum, which is an oily substance formed by the degeneration of cells rich in lipid droplets and cellular remnants. The glands discharge their contents by the contraction of the arrector pili muscle and by any pressure applied to the gland. Sweat glands are coiled tubular glands which are widely distributed and vary regionally. On the palm and sole they number about 100 per $cm^3$. The merocrine sweat gland consists of a duct and a coiled secretory tubule. At the periphery of the coiled secretory tubule, and enclosed by a basement membrane, spindle-shaped myoepithelial cells wind in longitudinal spirals around the tubule. Myoepithelial cells resemble smooth muscle fibers, and it is believed that their contraction empties the contents of the gland onto the surface of the skin (Plate 127).

Another variety of sweat gland is the apocrine gland, which is less widely distributed. These glands are large, branched and less coiled than the ordinary merocrine glands. The lumen of the secretory tubule is wide, the cells are larger with distinctive projections from their surfaces and the myoepithelial cells are larger and more numerous than in ordinary sweat glands. The axillary apocrine glands develop their large size at puberty (Plate 126).

The lacrimal gland is a compound tubuloalveolar serous gland and is an outgrowth of the upper lateral margin of the conjunctiva. The secretion is a clear, salty liquid (tears) that flushes and moistens the conjunctiva and cornea (Plates 248 and 258).

The mammary glands are specialized cutaneous glands that develop rapidly but incompletely in the female at puberty. Additional differentiation begins during pregnancy, and functional activity begins after childbirth. Marked regression of the glandular tissue occurs when nursing ceases. The gland comprises 15 to 20 lobes, each with its own duct system surrounded by interlobar connective tissue and abundant fat cells. The glandular epithelium resembles that seen in apocrine glands. See Plate 222.

## SKIN
### Shoulder

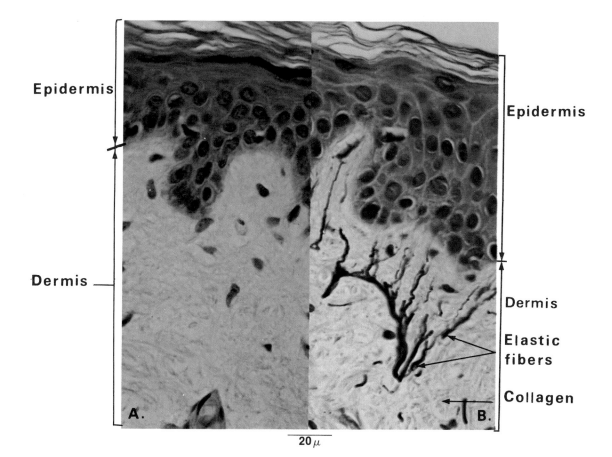

Epidermis

Dermis

Epidermis

Dermis

Elastic fibers

Collagen

A.

B.

$\overline{20\,\mu}$

A. Human, 10% Formalin, H. & E., 612 x.
B. Human, 10% Formalin, Pinkus' Acid
   Orcein - Giemsa method, 612 x.

This figure illustrates the value of special staining techniques in histology. In *A*, the routine H. & E. method shows clearly the epidermis and dermis. The special technique used in *B* differentiates elastic fibers from collagen fibers, both of which are important components of the dermis. The H. & E. stain does not specifically reveal elastic fibers. While the elastic tissue stain provides contrasting colors in collagen and elastic fibers, the essential point is that the orcein stain specifically discriminates and delineates elastic fibers from collagen and other tissue components and is therefore an important research tool. In addition, this method provides useful information about tissue and organ structures which the H. & E. fails to provide. The H. & E. stain is a good general method, with marked limitations, which should be appreciated if more than a superficial understanding of microscopic structure and function is to be obtained.

## SKIN, EPIDERMIS
### Stratified squamous epithelium
### shoulder

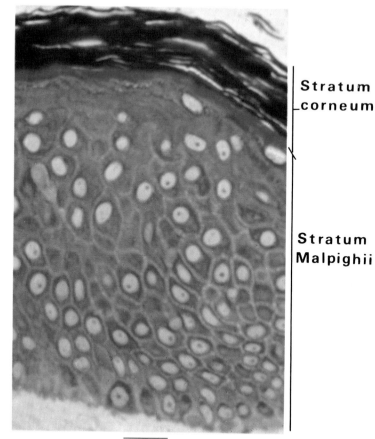

Stratum
corneum

Stratum
Malpighii

20 μ

### Human, Glutaraldehyde – osmium fixation,
### Toluidine blue stain, 612 x.

**Stratum corneum:** Flattened nonviable epithelial cells containing keratin. Superficial layers desquamate continuously.

**Stratum Malpighii:** Mitotic cell division occurs in this layer. Desmosomes join adjacent cells. Prominent nuclei with small dark nucleoli. Nuclear staining characteristics indicate that these nuclei are functionally active.

## EPIDERMIS
## A. Shoulder, B. Scalp, and C. Palm.

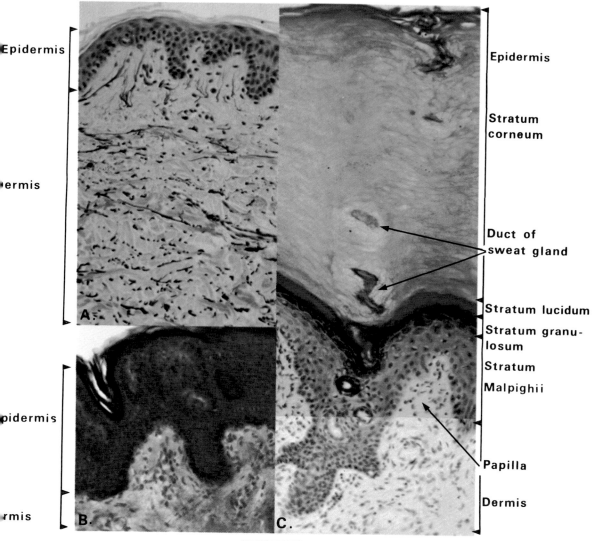

Human, 10% Formalin, A. Pinkus' acid Orcein-Giemsa
method, B. and C. H. & E., 162 x.

This plate shows the structural variation of the epidermis in different parts of the body.

The epidermis in all three areas is keratinized stratified squamous epithelium. The thickness varies from one site to the other. Note the marked thickness of the epidermis in *C* (palm). The epidermis of palms of the hands and soles of the feet is the thickest in the body. In these regions four layers of the epidermis are well delineated.

**Stratum Malpighii:** Named for Marcello Malpighi, the Italian anatomist who described this layer. This layer is responsible for the proliferative activity of the epidermis. Cells in this layer are connected by intercellular bridges. See Plate 123.

*Text continued on following page.*

**Stratum granulosum:** Cells in this layer are deeply stained and rather flattened. This stratum is thin in most parts of the body. Nuclei are pyknotic (inactive), and cytoplasm contains keratohyalin granules.

**Stratum lucidum:** Usually seen only in thick epidermis of palms and soles. It appears as a homogeneous translucent layer in which cellular outlines are indistinct and nuclei are not seen.

**Stratum corneum:** A layer of cornified cells which are closely packed, flat and anucleate. They contain keratin. Thickness of this layer varies in different regions of the body and is thickest in the palms and soles. Superficial layer is shed continuously.

**Dermis:** A layer of dense connective tissue underlying the epidermis. Varies in thickness in different body regions. Note the thick dermis in the shoulder skin (*A*).

**Papilla:** A projection of dermis between epidermal pegs. Particularly abundant in the soles and palms.

**Duct of sweat gland:** Seen spiraling through the stratum corneum of the epidermis to open at its free surface.

## KERATINIZATION
### Filiform papilla
### tongue

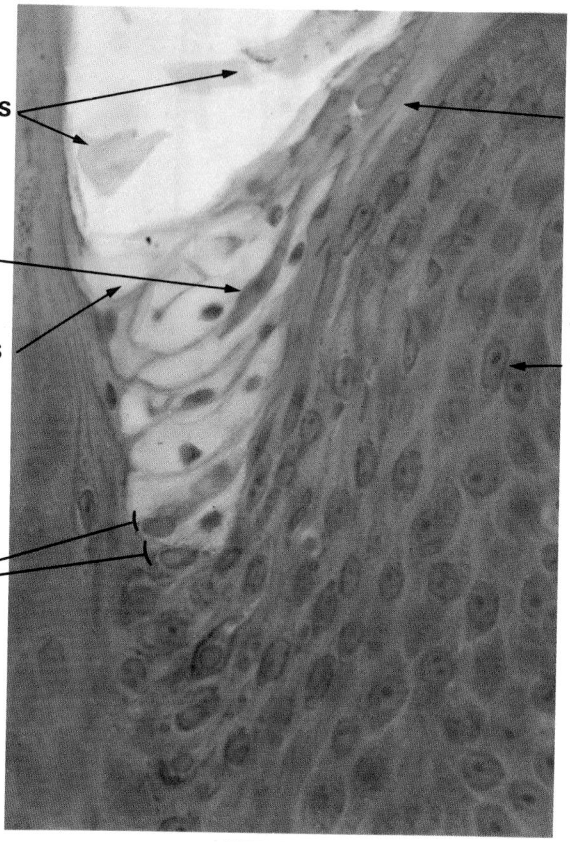

Desquamated superficial cells

Keratinized epithelium

Keratinized cell

Desquamating superficial cells

Stratified squamous epithelium

Keratohyalin granules

100 μ

**Rhesus monkey, 10% Formalin, H. & E., 162 x.**

This plate shows the cellular changes in the process of keratinization. The stratified squamous epithelium covering a filiform papilla is seen. Note the keratohyalin granules in cells of the zona granulosa. In the more superficial zona pellucida, the cells lose their keratohyalin granules, become flattened and elongated and some lose their nuclei. The cytoplasm of these cells appears homogeneous. In the most superficial zone the cells become clear and flattened.

The structural changes in keratinization involve aggregation and arrangement of filaments, formation of keratohyalin granules and loss of cell organelles as a result of the accumulation of these granules. Desquamated cells are continually replaced by new cells which are formed in the germinative basal layer and move toward the surface during the process of keratinization.

PLATE 123

# STRATIFIED SQUAMOUS EPITHELIUM
## Prickle cells

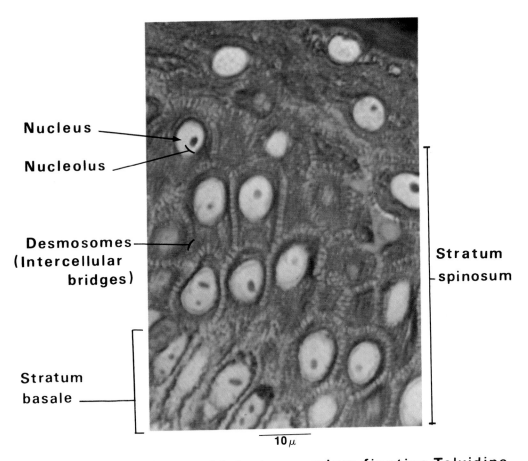

Nucleus

Nucleolus

Desmosomes
(Intercellular
bridges)

Stratum
spinosum

Stratum
basale

10 μ

**Human, Glutaraldehyde – osmium fixation, Toluidine blue stain, 1416 x.**

**Stratum basale:** Single cell layer which underlies the prickle cell layer (stratum spinosum). Cell division most active in this layer.

**Desmosomes (intercellular bridges):** Found between cells in the stratum spinosum overlying the stratum basale. Represent sites of firm attachment between adjacent cells. Cells in this layer are also characterized by a large nucleus and a prominent nucleolus.

# DERMAL PAPILLAE
## Finger tip

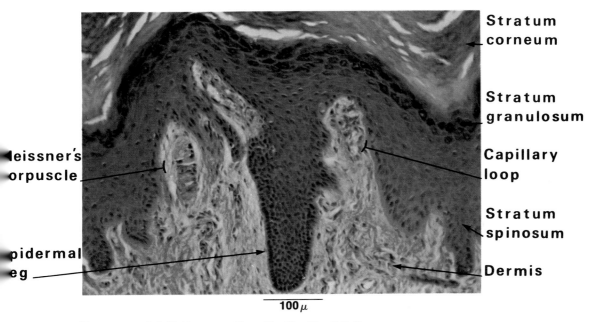

Stratum corneum

Stratum granulosum

Capillary loop

Stratum spinosum

Meissner's corpuscle

Epidermal peg

Dermis

100μ

**Human, 10% Formalin, H. & E., 162 x.**

Skin of the fingertip is characterized by a thick cornified epithelium, an absence of hair and an abundance of tactile corpuscles of Meissner in the dermis.

Note the thick stratum corneum; the stratum granulosum, containing keratohyalin granules; and the stratum spinosum, overlying the stratum basale. An epidermal peg is seen dividing a primary dermal papilla into secondary papillae. Note the Meissner's corpuscle in the dermal papilla. This is an oval, encapsulated touch receptor composed of flattened connective tissue stacked horizontally and a sensory nerve fiber. The sensory nerve fiber leaves the corpuscle and enters the spinal cord with the dorsal root fibers. Another component of dermal papillae is a capillary loop which supplies the overlying epithelium with nutrients and oxygen and removes metabolic waste.

## SWEAT GLAND
### Finger

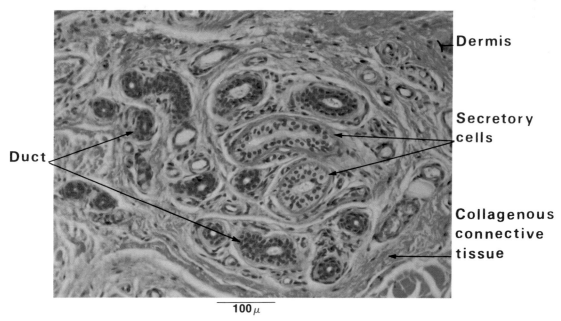

Duct

Dermis

Secretory cells

Collagenous connective tissue

100 μ

**Human, 10% Formalin, H. & E., 162x.**

Most sweat glands are of the eccrine variety, in which the secretory cells remain intact. They play an important role in temperature regulation in man and are widely distributed. Sweat glands are innervated by cholinergic nerves of the sympathetic nervous system. They secrete only when stimulated and, in a hot environment or during strenuous exercise, over 1 liter per hour can be secreted by an average individual. However, the sweat glands of the palms of the hands and soles of the feet appear to respond to emotional states (anxiety and mental stress) rather than to increase in external temperature.

Sweat glands are located deep in the dermis of the skin and are surrounded by fat cells and the collagenous connective tissue septa of the dermis.

**Secretory cells:**   The secretory portion of sweat glands is made up of tubules lined by a single layer of simple cuboidal or columnar cells, with faintly staining cytoplasm and a prominent round nucleus located in the middle of the cell. A distinct basement membrane and myoepithelial cells surround the secretory cells.

**Secretory ducts:**   Spiral course to the free surface of the skin. Lined by two layers of darkly staining cuboidal cells surrounded by a distinct basement membrane.

## AXILLARY SWEAT GLAND
### Apocrine type

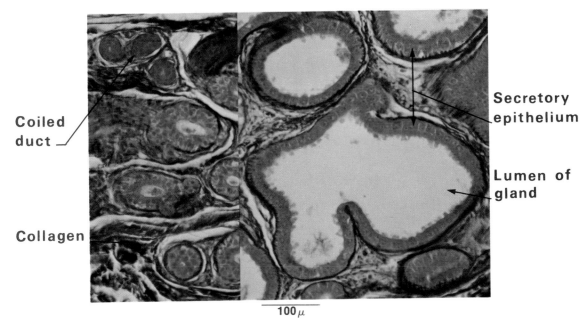

Coiled duct

Collagen

Secretory epithelium

Lumen of gland

100μ

**Human, Zenker's fluid, Mallory-azan stain, 162 x.**

While most sweat glands are of the merocrine or eccrine variety (*i.e.*, they do not lose cytoplasmic components in any appreciable amount during the secretory process), a specialized variety of sweat gland in the axilla has been considered by some investigators to be of the apocrine variety, in which the apices of the gland cells apparently break off and are lost with the secretory product. These sweat glands are characterized by their large size and large lumen and are less coiled than ordinary sweat glands. (See Plate 125.)

The epithelial lining is columnar or high cuboidal and varies with secretory activity. Nuclei stain deeply and lumina are wide. Collagenous connective tissue separates individual glands and ducts.

The apocrine glands are found in the axillary and pubic regions of the body and begin their functional activity at puberty. The secretory product is rich in organic matter which, when acted upon by bacteria, produces an objectionable odor. The apocrine glands are activated by adrenergic nerves and the secretion of these glands can be increased by emotional stress. The secretory activity of the adrenal medulla plays a role in this increased secretion.

Recent phase and electron microscopic studies have questioned the apocrine mechanism of secretion by the axillary sweat glands.

# AXILLARY SWEAT GLAND
## Myoepithelium

Lumen of gland

Secretory epithelium

Myoepithelial cell

Myoepithelial cells

Capillary

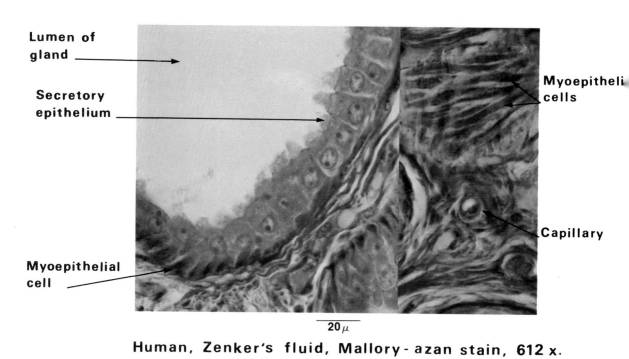

20 μ

## Human, Zenker's fluid, Mallory-azan stain, 612 x.

**Secretory epithelium:** Simple columnar or high cuboidal in type. The nuclei of these gland cells are round. In mucous glands the nuclei are flattened against the basal cell membrane, and in sebaceous glands the nuclei degenerate and form part of the secretory product. In glands which produce a watery secretion (*e.g.*, parotid gland and sweat glands) spherical nuclei are characteristically found.

**Myoepithelial cells:** Spindle-shaped contractile cells found between the secretory epithelium and the underlying basement membrane. They lie with their long axes tangential to the secretory epithelium. Nuclei are elongated. Their contractile activity forces secretions into the excretory duct of the gland. Electron micrographs reveal myoepithelial cells to be similar to smooth muscle fibers and to contain myofilaments. These contractile cells are particularly well developed in the large apocrine glands found in the axilla and perianal region.

## HYPODERMIS
### Finger tip

Pacinian
corpuscle —

Dense
irregular
connective
tissue

Fat cells

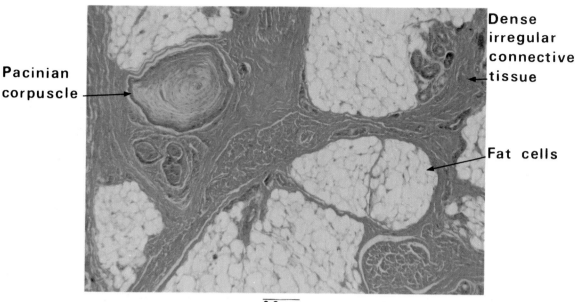

0.2 mm

**Human, 10% Formalin, H. & E., 50x.**

The hypodermis is a layer of subcutaneous connective tissue beneath the dermis. It is composed of connective tissue fibers disposed in all directions and continuous with those of the dermis. The density of the connective tissue elements varies in different locations, being less dense in "loose" skin (*e.g.*, arm) and more compact where the skin is firmly attached (*e.g.*, fingers). Groups of fat cells are also found in the hypodermis. The concentration of fat is regionally variable. In addition, the hypodermis is rich in nerve fibers and sensory receptors (Pacinian corpuscles) as well as blood vessels.

## SCALP

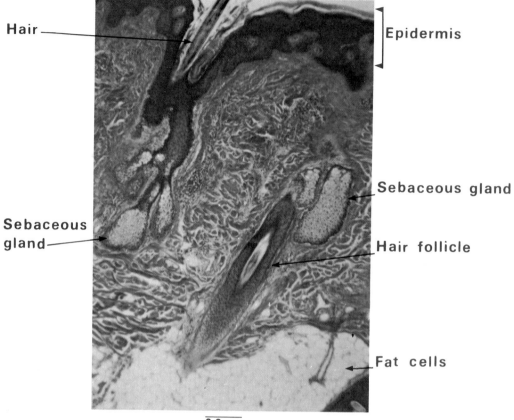

Hair

Epidermis

Sebaceous gland

Sebaceous gland

Hair follicle

Fat cells

0.2 mm

**Human, 10 % Formalin, H. & E., 50 x.**

The structure of skin varies in different regions of the body. For comparison of scalp skin with other sites examine Plates 121 and 124.

**Epidermis:** Stratified squamous keratinized epithelium.

**Hair:** The free end of the hair shaft is seen projecting from the skin.

**Sebaceous gland:** Holocrine variety of glands, in which cells are lost along with their secretion product. Closely applied to hair follicles into which they drain. The ducts are composed of a stratified squamous epithelium. Some sebaceous glands around the mouth and in the genital region are not associated with hair and their ducts open directly onto the surface of the skin.

**Hair follicle:** Surrounds the hair shaft. Composed of an inner epidermal layer and outer connective tissue sheath.

**Fat cells:** Located in the dermis.

## SCALP
## Cross section

Sweat
gland

Connective
tissue

Hair
follicles

Sweat
gland
duct

Sebaceous
glands

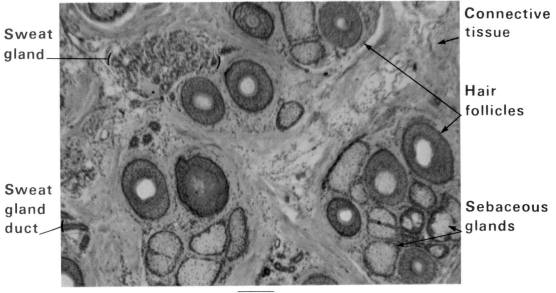

0.2 mm

Human, 10% Formalin, H. & E., 50 x.

This is a section of skin from the scalp showing the abundance of hair follicles. Note the proximity of sebaceous glands to hair follicles. Sweat glands and their ducts are scattered in the connective tissue stroma.

## SEBACEOUS GLAND
### Hairy skin
### dorsum of arm

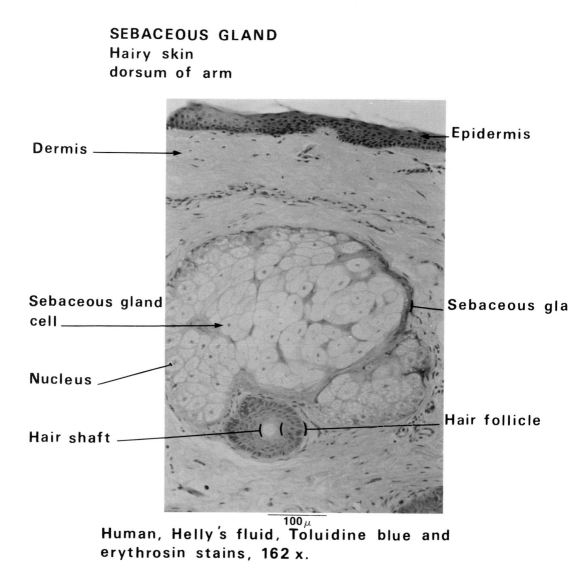

Dermis —————→

Epidermis

Sebaceous gland
cell —————→

Sebaceous gla

Nucleus —————→

Hair follicle

Hair shaft —————→

100 μ

### Human, Helly's fluid, Toluidine blue and erythrosin stains, 162 x.

**Epidermis:**  Stratified squamous cornified epithelium of the skin.

**Dermis:**  Connective tissue layer beneath the epidermis. Thickness varies in different parts of the body. Rich in collagenous and elastic fibers. The part of the dermis underlying the epithelium is called the papillary layer. The deeper part is the reticular layer, in which sebaceous glands are found. In addition, hair follicles, sweat glands and Pacinian corpuscles occur in this layer. In the face, the striated muscles of facial expression terminate in the dermis.

**Sebaceous gland:**  Holocrine variety of gland in which the entire cell is lost along with the secretory products. Intimately associated with hair follicles into which they drain. Composed of a group of saclike alveoli ensheathed by a thin layer of connective tissue. The alveoli are composed of stratified cuboidal or polyhedral epithelial cells that fill the sac. The secretion of the sebaceous gland is an oily substance (sebum) which lubricates the epidermis and hair.

**Sebaceous gland cell:**   Note the peripheral, small cuboidal cells and the more central, larger polyhedral or spheroidal cells. Oily droplets increase with an increase in size of the cells. See Plate 80.

**Nucleus:**   Nuclei of peripheral cells are rounded. Nuclei of centrally located cells are either shrunken or absent. This nuclear change is part of the degenerative process by which the entire cell is lost, along with its secretion product.

**Hair follicle:**   Surrounds the hair shaft and is composed of inner epidermal epithelial elements and outer dermal connective tissue elements.

**Hair shaft:**   Located within the follicle. The free end of the hair projects from the surface of the skin.

# Section 8

# The Cardiovascular System

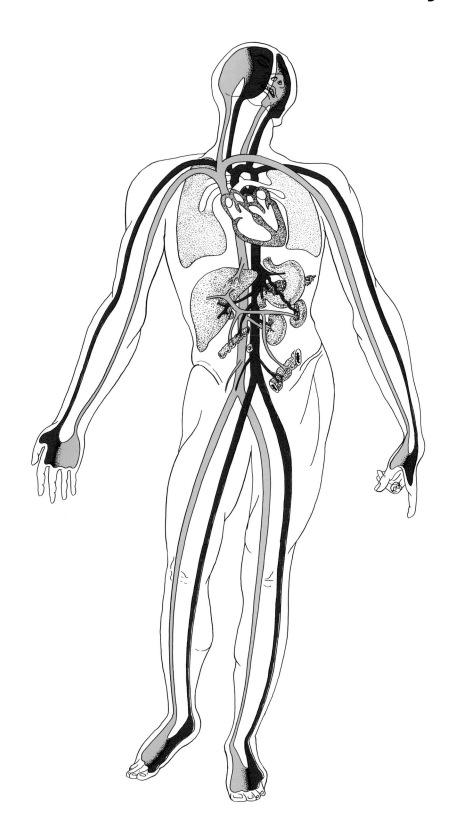

# The Cardiovascular System

The heart and the blood vessels comprise the cardiovascular system. The heart wall can be divided into three layers: (1) the endocardium, which is an endothelial cell-lined layer continuous with the tunica intima of the blood vessel wall; (2) the myocardium, composed of cardiac muscle, corresponds to the tunica media of the blood vessel wall; and (3) the epicardium, covered by a reflection of the mesothelium-lined serous membrane (visceral pericardium), contains blood vessels (coronary vessels) and nerves and corresponds to the tunica adventitia of the blood vessel wall (Plates 133 and 135).

The mammalian heart has four chambers, two thin walled atria and two thicker walled ventricles. The central supporting structure is the "cardiac skeleton," composed of dense white fibrous (collagenous) tissue into which the cardiac muscle fibers of the two atria and two ventricles insert and to which the heart valves are attached. The orifices of the four chambers are guarded by the heart valves, which are endocardial folds supported by an internal plate of dense collagenous and elastic connective tissue continuous with the cardiac skeleton. The right atrioventricular valve has three cusps and is called the tricuspid valve. The left atrioventricular valve has two cusps and is called the bicuspid, or mitral, valve. Two semilunar valves at the ventricular entrance to the aorta and pulmonary arteries have three cusps each. The valves are arranged to direct the appropriate movement of blood and to prevent retrograde blood flow. The heart is a four-chambered pump which moves the blood throughout the vascular system. We will begin the sequence of events with the two atria. Blood enters the right atrium from the great veins (superior and inferior vena cavae) and coronary veins, which carry blood poor in oxygen and rich in carbon dioxide from the entire body. Blood rich in oxygen and devoid of carbon dioxide enters the left atrium from the lungs via the pulmonary veins. Contraction of the right and left atria forces the blood past the right tricuspid and left bicuspid valves into the right and left ventricles, respectively. At the end of their contraction, the right and left atria begin to fill once again with blood. Contraction of the right and left ventricles forces the oxygen-poor blood from the right ventricle past the right semilunar valve into the pulmonary artery, and the oxygen-rich blood past the left semilunar valve into the aorta to supply the entire body and into the coronary arteries, which supply the heart itself. A red blood corpuscle, for example, moves through the heart in the following way: right atrium, right ventricle, pulmonary artery, lung, pulmonary vein, left atrium and left ventricle, and leaves the heart to enter the aorta and the systemic or coronary arteries. The contractile force required to move the blood through the pulmonary system is less than that required to force the blood throughout the entire body. This fact is reflected in the thickness of the myocardium of the right and left ventricles (see Plates 132 and 133).

The mammalian heart possesses a special system of cardiac fibers which function to coordinate the heart beat. These modified cardiac fibers lie beneath the endocardium. Two specialized pacemakers which determine the rate of the heart beat are recognized: (1) the sinoatrial node (SA node) fibers, in continuity with atrial cardiac fibers, lie at the junction of the superior vena cava and right atrium and (2) the atrioventricular node (AV node), a mass of irregularly arranged, highly branched specialized cardiac fibers located in the floor of the right ventricle near the termination of the coronary sinus. Extending from the AV node is a bundle of small, unbranched cardiac muscle fibers called the atrioventricular bundle, which passes to the midline of the heart to branch and form two bundles beneath the endocardium on either side of the interventricular septum. These fibers are continuous with a system of Purkinje fibers and, through them, with ordinary cardiac fibers (Plates 75, 76 and 134).

The blood vessels which originate from the right and left ventricles are designated as arteries and possess a distinctive structure. The wall of an artery has three tunics: (1) the innermost layer or tunica intima, consisting of an endothelial cell layer exposed to the blood, a delicate subendothelial connective tissue layer and an elastic tissue layer, the internal elastic membrane; (2) the middle coat, or tunica media, consisting of smooth muscle fibers and variable amounts of elastic and collagenous tissues; and (3) the outer coat, or tunica adventitia, composed primarily of collagenous connective tissue (Plates 135 and 136).

The exact structure and relative thickness of the three coats vary with the size of the artery. The changes that occur are gradual but, in general, three different types of arterial vessels may be distinguished: (1) large elastic (conducting) arteries leaving the heart, (2) medium and small muscular arteries, and (3) arterioles which are continuous with the capillary vessels. From the structural-functional point of view elastic tissue is the most important component in the larger vessels while smooth muscle is the most important in the smaller vessels. Blood is ejected from the heart in a pulsatile manner (systole of the heart), and the aorta and pulmonary arteries must expand to receive the output of the right and left ventricles. The passive elastic recoil between systoles (diastolic period) maintains the blood pressure and smooths the flow of blood while the ventricles are filling from the atria. Muscular arteries (Plate 140) regulate the blood flow to different parts of the body depending on need. These vessels are also termed distributing arteries. Arterioles (Plates 137 and 138) are small arteries about 0.04 to 0.3 mm in diameter with one to five layers of smooth muscle fibers. Arterioles have a relatively thick wall in comparison to their lumen and determine the local blood flow with precapillary sphincters at the beginning of the capillary beds (Plate 141). The blood pressure falls sharply and blood flow slows in arteriole vessels. Capillaries (Plates 140 and 142) are endothelial cell tubes whose walls appear as thin lines with bulging nuclei. Capillaries, because of their intimate relationship with the cells of the body and their special permeability characteristics, are functionally the most interesting of the blood vessels. Their thin walls and slow blood flow favor exchange of nutrients and oxygen for metabolic wastes and carbon dioxide. In addition, hormones from endocrine glands enter and leave the vascular system through regionally specialized capillaries. The submicroscopic structure and function of capillaries, as revealed by electron microscopy, can be found in comprehensive textbooks of histology and physiology.

As with the arterial system the veins can be divided into three groups according to size: venules, small and medium sized veins, and large veins. Venules can be recognized as such when they are about 20 $\mu$ in diameter and possess an endothelial lining, a thin layer of collagenous fibers and some fibroblasts. They have neither muscle fibers nor elastic fibers. With increasing size (about 45 $\mu$), some elastic fibers appear in the tunica intima along with collagenous fibers, and smooth muscle begins to appear between the endothelium and the outer fibrous coats. With still greater increases in caliber a distinct intima, media and adventitia become recognizable. The largest veins possess some longitudinal smooth muscle and a delicate internal elastic membrane in the tunica intima, a thin smooth muscle coat (which may be absent) forms the tunica media, and prominent bundles of smooth muscle separated by collagenous fibers appear in the thickest of the three coats, the tunica adventitia (Plates 140 and 143).

Many small and medium sized veins contain valves which prevent retrograde blood flow. They are especially frequent in the limbs. The erect posture of man, in particular, necessitates this structural specialization in veins. Valves are paired folds of the intima which are commonly located just distal to the entry of a communicating vein. Blood flow against gravity and toward the heart in the thin walled veins is aided by the contraction of skeletal muscle and the system of valves. Blood pressure in the venous system is less than one-tenth of that in the aorta, and the blood travels slowly and smoothly through relatively large thin walled vessels. In spite of the differences in blood pressure and velocity of flow the venous return to the heart must equal the ventricular output. The vascular system contains about 5 liters of blood which is pumped and circulated throughout the body about 3200 times daily.

## HEART CHAMBERS
### Aorta

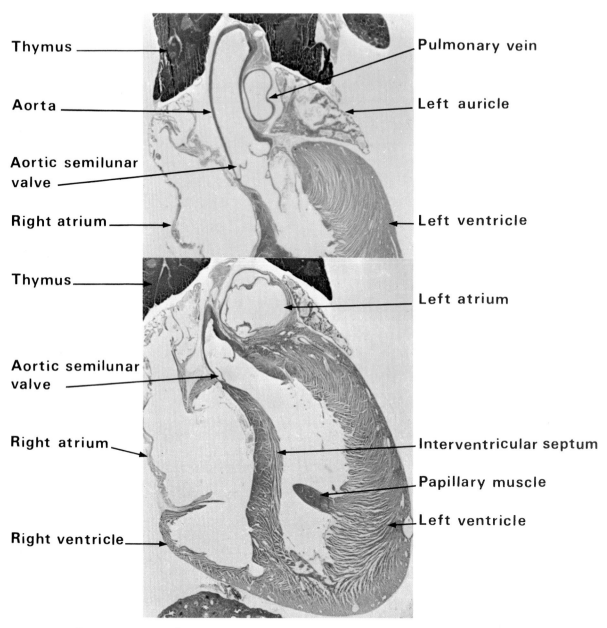

Thymus

Aorta

Aortic semilunar valve

Right atrium

Thymus

Aortic semilunar valve

Right atrium

Right ventricle

Pulmonary vein

Left auricle

Left ventricle

Left atrium

Interventricular septum

Papillary muscle

Left ventricle

### Rat, Helly's fluid, H. & E., 6x.

This plate, in two parts, shows the four cardiac chambers and adjoining large vessels. In the upper part of the plate the left auricle, the left ventricle and the right atrium are seen, along with the aorta and pulmonary vein. Note the thicker muscular wall of the ventricle and the aortic semilunar valve that closes the aortic orifice. The pulmonary vein wall is thinner than the wall of the aorta. It brings oxygenated blood from the lung into the left atrium. The lower part of the plate shows both atria and ventricles as well as the aortic outlet. Note that the left ventricular wall is thicker than the right ventricular wall. This is essential for the movement of blood throughout the entire body, the systemic circulation. The interventricular septum separates the right and left ventricles and contains the conductive tissue of the heart. In the wall of the left ventricle note the papillary muscle. This muscle is continuous with the wall of the ventricle and projects into the cavity, where it gives origin to the chordae tendinae which are attached to the segments of the tricuspid valve.

The thymus is seen here molded over the aortic arch. The thymus is well developed in early life and involutes after puberty. It plays a fundamental role in the development of the immune mechanism of the body.

## HEART
### Ventricular wall

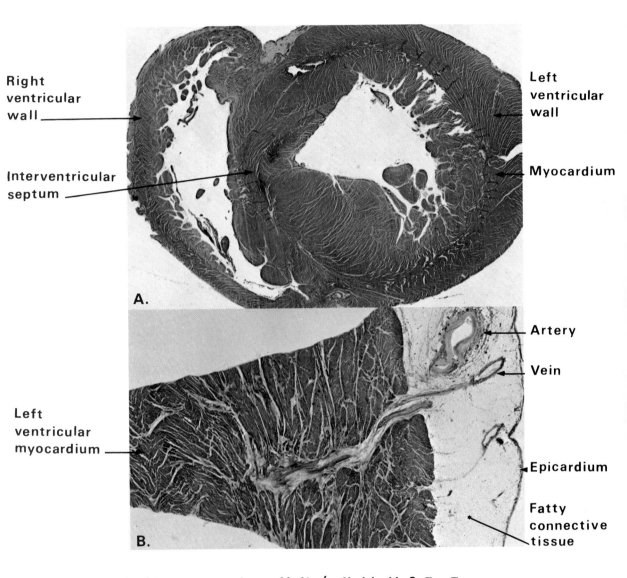

Right ventricular wall

Interventricular septum

Left ventricular wall

Myocardium

Left ventricular myocardium

Artery

Vein

Epicardium

Fatty connective tissue

A.

B.

A. Rhesus monkey, Helly's fluid, H. & E., 5 x.
B. Human, Helly's fluid, Phosphotungstic acid, hematoxylin stain, 7 x.

In *A*, the right and left ventricular cavities are shown in cross section. Note the thick wall of the left ventricle and the muscular interventricular septum separating the two cavities. In this septum courses the impulse-conducting tissue, *i.e.,* the Purkinje fibers. Note the different orientation of muscle bundles in the myocardium.

In *B*, the thick left ventricular myocardium is shown separated from the epicardium by the subepicardial space filled with blood vessels and connective tissue containing fat. The epicardium is the visceral layer of the pericardial sac in which the heart is located. It is covered by a single layer of mesothelial cells.

## ATRIOVENTRICULAR NODE AND BUNDLE
Specialized cardiac muscle fibers

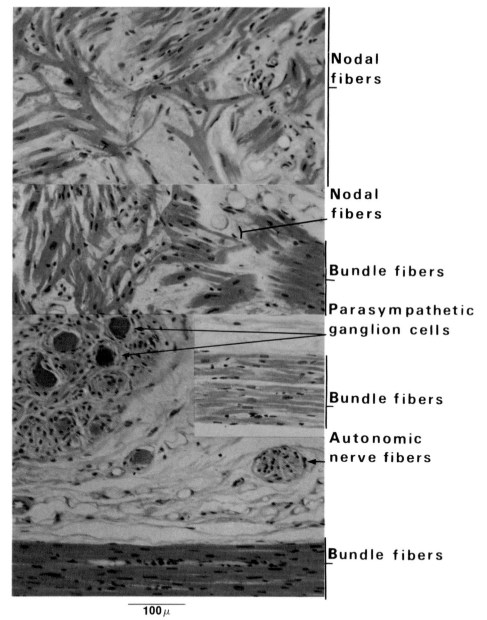

Nodal fibers

Nodal fibers

Bundle fibers

Parasympathetic ganglion cells

Bundle fibers

Autonomic nerve fibers

Bundle fibers

100 μ

Human, 10% Formalin, H. & E., 162 x.

*See text on following page.*

The atrioventricular (AV) node and bundle are composed of cardiac muscle fibers specialized for impulse conduction. The atrioventricular node (node of Tawara) is found in the subendocardium of the right atrium, close to the termination of the coronary sinus. Note the irregularly arranged branching fibers (nodal fibers) that form the AV node. Note also how the AV nodal fibers become continuous with the small unbranched fibers of the AV bundle (bundle of His). The latter originate in the AV node, continue into the interventricular septum and divide into two trunks composed of Purkinje fibers, which pass to the right and left ventricular wall, where they become continuous with ordinary cardiac muscle fibers. Stimuli for cardiac contraction are initiated in the sinoatrial (SA) node, reach the AV node and spread to the myocardium via the AV bundle. Injury to the bundle results in dissociation of atrial and ventricular rhythms.

Note the parasympathetic ganglion cells and the autonomic nerve fibers in the wall of the heart. The parasympathetic ganglia receive vagal fibers which slow the heart rate while the sympathetic postganglionic fibers carry impulses which increase the heart rate. The autonomic fibers include sympathetic postganglionic and parasympathetic preganglionic fibers.

## AORTA

Tunica intima

Elastic fibers

Smooth muscle

Tunica adventitia

Erythrocytes

Tunica media

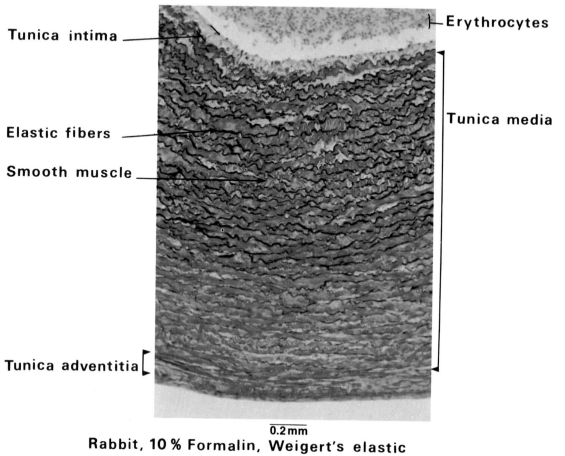

0.2 mm

Rabbit, 10 % Formalin, Weigert's elastic
tissue and phloxine stains, 50x.

The aorta is an example of an elastic artery. The wall of the aorta has three tunicae: intima, media and adventitia. The transition from one tunica to the other is indistinct. The tunica intima is small and merges with the much thicker tunica media. The latter is composed mainly of concentrically arranged laminae of elastic tissue. The spaces between the elastic tissues are filled with smooth muscle fibers and fibroelastic tissue. Adjacent circles of elastic fibers connect by slanting bands to form complex elastic nets.

The adventitia is small and is made up of collagenous connective tissue. The richness of elastic tissue in the aorta permits distensibility and maintenance of a uniform blood flow. The collagenous fibrous tissue of the adventitia prevents overdistension of the vessel. The lumen of the aorta is seen filled with erythrocytes.

# AORTA

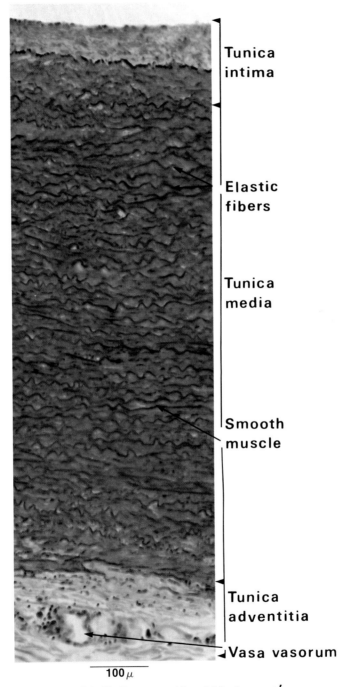

Tunica
intima

Elastic
fibers

Tunica
media

Smooth
muscle

Tunica
adventitia

Vasa vasorum

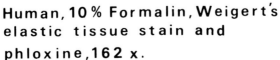

100 μ

Human, 10 % Formalin, Weigert's
elastic tissue stain and
phloxine, 162 x.

*See text on following page.*

The aorta is an elastic artery. The intima is a small tunica and consists of collagenous and elastic fibers. Small bundles of smooth muscle fibers and concentrically arranged elastic fibers are found in deeper layers of the intima.

The media is the thickest tunica and consists mainly of concentrically arranged laminae of elastic tissue which are connected with each other to form a complex elastic net. Between these elastic fibers are found smooth muscle fibers and connective tissue.

The adventitia is small and not well organized. It is composed of fibroelastic tissue containing blood vessels (vasa vasora).

The abundant elastic tissue in the wall of the aorta helps to make the wall easily distensible and helps maintain a constant blood flow.

## ARTERIOLE AND VENULE
### Peripheral nerve

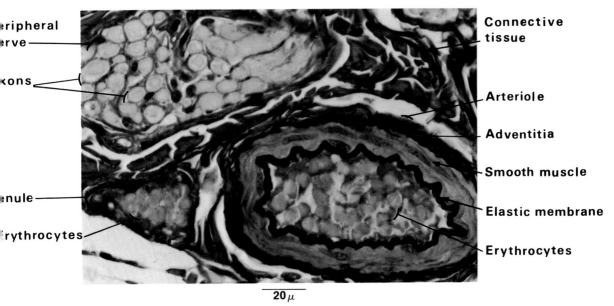

Peripheral nerve —

Axons

Venule —

Erythrocytes

Connective tissue

Arteriole

Adventitia

Smooth muscle

Elastic membrane

Erythrocytes

20 μ

### Rhesus monkey, Helly's fluid, Modified aldehyde fuchsin stain, 612 x.

This figure shows a commonly seen triad; a peripheral nerve, an arteriole and a venule. The peripheral nerve is enclosed in a connective tissue sheath and is formed by a number of nerve fibers. Each nerve fiber is made up of an axon and its myelin sheath. The latter is unstained in this preparation. Surrounding each nerve fiber is a delicate connective tissue sheath, the endoneurium.

The arteriole shows the component layers. These are the adventitia (a connective tissue sheath) and the smooth muscle coat (tunica media) which is the thickest and most prominent coat of the arteriolar wall. Note the well defined internal elastic membrane internal to the smooth muscle coat. The intima is an extremely thin layer. Erythrocytes fill the lumen of the arteriole.

The venule seen here is smaller than the adjacent arteriole. Typically, venules are larger than arterioles. Note that the bulk of the wall is made up of connective tissue adventitia, the other coats being thin and inconspicuous.

The stain used in this preparation is useful to differentiate muscular and connective tissue elements.

## ARTERIOLE

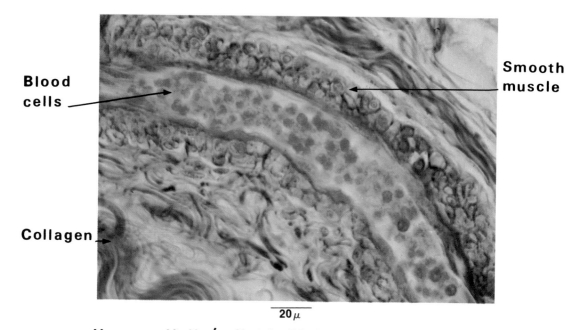

Blood cells

Smooth muscle

Collagen

20μ

**Human, Helly's fluid, Mallory-azan stain, 612 x.**

    This is a longitudinal section of an arteriole. The stain used in this preparation provides good differentiation between collagenous connective tissue, which stains blue, and muscular elements in the wall of the arteriole, which stain reddish brown. Note the centrally placed nuclei in the smooth muscle cells which are seen in cross section. The lumen of the artery is filled with blood cells.

# ARTERIOLE

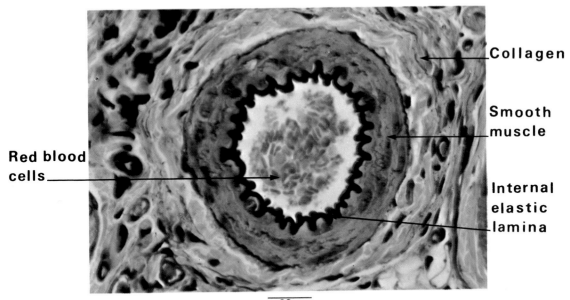

Human, Zenker's fluid, Phosphotungstic acid hematoxylin, 612 x.

**Red blood cells:** Abnormally clumped together in the lumen of the arteriole as a result of the fixation of the tissue.

**Internal elastic lamina:** Corrugated band due to the contraction of the circular smooth muscle. Prominent diagnostic structure found between intima and media.

**Smooth muscle:** Circularly arranged in the media. Note the presence of delicate elastic fibers in this layer. Although not shown, collagenous and reticular connective tissue fibers are also found in this layer.

**Collagen:** In the thick adventitia. Note the thin layer of slightly corrugated elastic fibers between the adventitia and media.

# MUSCULAR ARTERIES, VEINS AND CAPILLARY BLOCK VESSELS

Artery

Artery

Vein

Ovary
zona vasculos

Seminal
vesicle
epithelium

Stratified
squamous
epithelium

Venule

Arteriole

Capillary

B.

C.

A. $\overline{\quad 100\mu \quad}$          B. & C. $\overline{\quad 20\mu \quad}$
Human, 10% Formalin, H. & E., A. 162 x., B. 612 x.
Human, Glutaraldehyde-osmium fixation,
Toluidine blue stain, C. 612 x.

This plate compares the histology of arteries, veins and capillaries.

In *A*, a muscular artery and a vein from a human ovary are seen. Note, in the artery, the thick tunica media composed of many concentric layers of smooth muscle. The intima of such arteries is small and the adventitia is either equal to or smaller than the thick media. The internal and external elastic membranes between the intima-media and the media-adventitia are not seen in this type of preparation. Compare the predominantly muscular tunica media of muscular arteries with that seen in elastic arteries such as the aorta (Plate 135). The adjoining vein by contrast has a much thinner wall. Scattered smooth muscle fibers and fibroelastic connective tissue form this thin wall. Compare the sizes of the arterial and venous lumina.

In *B*, a venule and an arteriole are shown. Arterioles are not visible to the naked eye. Their walls are thick in comparison to the lumina. The tunica intima is thin and is composed almost exclusively of the endothelial lining. The tunica media is muscular and is the thickest coat. The tunica adventitia is smaller than the tunica media. Note the pseudostratified epithelium of the seminal vesicle.

In *C*, a capillary is seen in a section of human skin. Note the extremely thin wall and the bulging endothelial cell nuclei. Capillaries are tiny endothelial tubes between terminal arterioles and venules through which gases, nutrients and metabolic wastes are transferred. The endothelium is continuous throughout the vascular system and heart.

## BLOOD VESSELS
### Mesentery

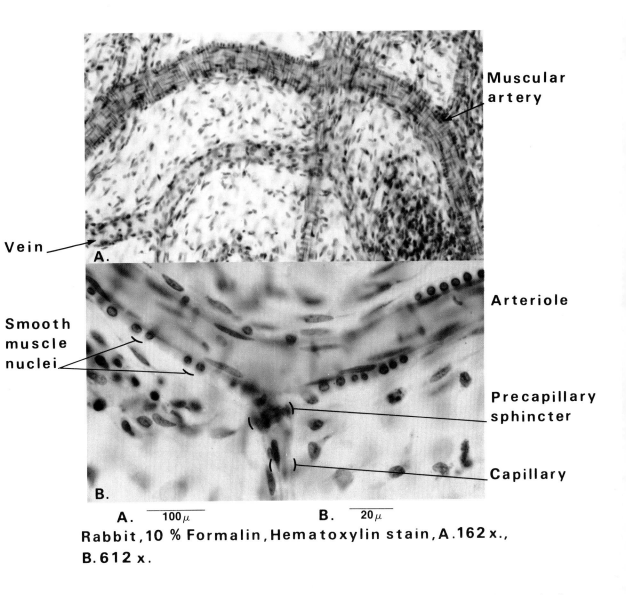

**A.** $\overline{\quad 100\,\mu \quad}$       **B.** $\overline{\quad 20\,\mu \quad}$
Rabbit,10 % Formalin,Hematoxylin stain,A.162x.,
B.612 x.

This plate is taken of a thin spread of mesentery showing the configuration of blood vessels. Compare the size of the muscular artery and vein in *A*. Note the thicker wall of the artery and the circular bands of smooth muscles in the wall. In *B*, a row of smooth muscle nuclei is seen, circumferentially arranged in the wall of the arteriole. Their elongated form is not seen because they are shown here in only two dimensions. Note the precapillary sphincter at the junction of an arteriole and capillary. The precapillaries are larger than ordinary capillaries and contain smooth muscle fibers that encircle the vessel and act as sphincters to control blood flow in the capillary bed. Note the absence of smooth muscle nuclei from the capillary. The nuclei oriented along the long axis of the capillary belong to the endothelial cells.

# CAPILLARY BASEMENT MEMBRANE
## Gastrocnemius muscle, Myasthenia gravis

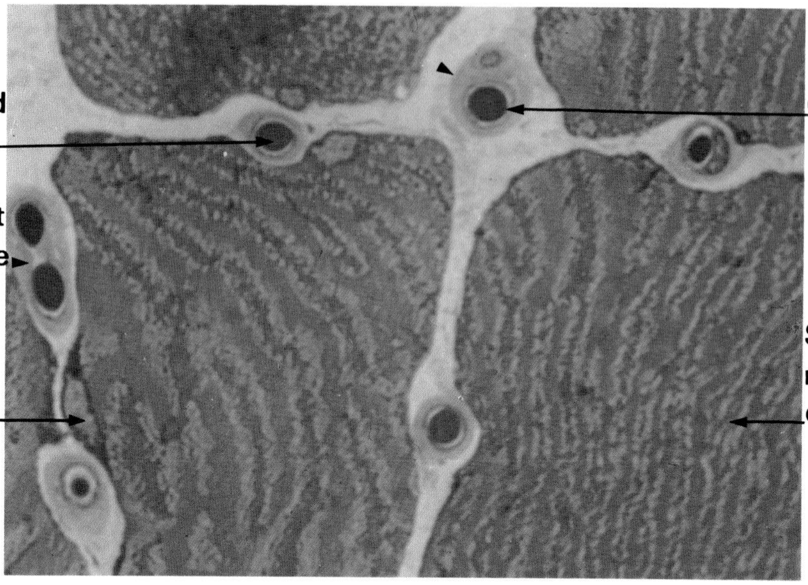

Red blood cell

Basement membrane

Muscle nucleus

Capillary

Striated muscle, cross sect.

10 μ

Human, Glutaraldehyde – osmium fixation, Toluidine blue stain, 1416 x.

**Capillary:** Extensive network, one red blood cell in diameter, found between the muscle fibers. A single red blood corpuscle fills the lumen. Arrowheads point to thickened basement membranes.

**Striated muscle, cross section:** Distinct A and I bands. Further details of skeletal muscle structure are seen in Plates 64, 65 and 68.

**Muscle nucleus:** Characteristic subsarcolemmal location in skeletal muscle.

**Basement membrane:** Usually quite thin and difficult to visualize in normal tissue, it is shown here abnormally thickened around capillaries. Composed of protein polysaccharides. Thickening of the capillary basement membrane has been described in this and other muscle disorders, in diabetes mellitus and in some kidney diseases.

**Red blood cell:** Fills the lumen of a capillary and is a useful, but rough, internal micron marker. In man, the red blood corpuscle is approximately 7.0 to 8.0 μ in diameter. The diameter of blood cells varies markedly due to species differences, disease states and methods of preparation. It is important to remember, therefore, that the red cell gives an "order of magnitude" only if used as an internal measure.

## VENA CAVA

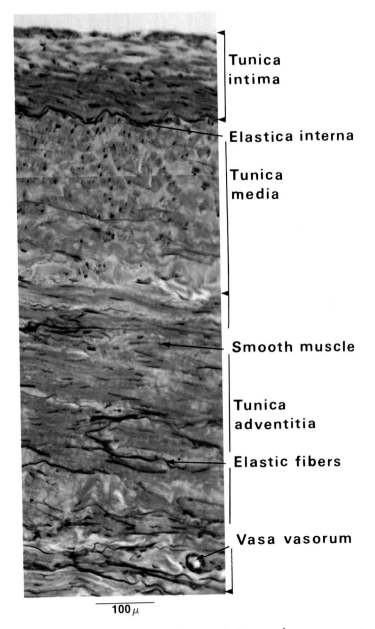

Tunica intima

Elastica interna

Tunica media

Smooth muscle

Tunica adventitia

Elastic fibers

Vasa vasorum

100 μ

Human, 10 % Formalin, Weigert's
elastic tissue stain and
phloxine, 162 x.

The superior and inferior vena cavae are examples of large veins. The walls of large veins have three tunicae: intima, media and adventitia.

The tunica intima is thick compared to that of other veins. A delicate internal elastic membrane may be seen in it.

In the tunica media, smooth muscle fibers are lacking or markedly reduced. This tunica is relatively small.

The tunica adventitia is the thickest of all tunicae. It consists of loose connective tissue and contains longitudinally arranged bundles of smooth muscle as well as thick elastic fibers. The vasa vasora (blood vessels of blood vessels) that nourish the wall of the vein are found in this tunica and may penetrate into the media or even the intima.

# Section 9     The Lymphatic System

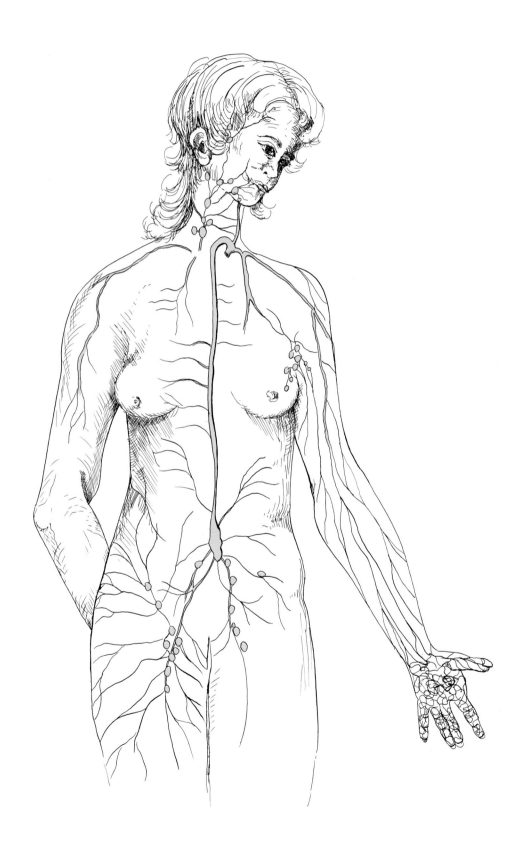

# The Lymphatic System

Lymphoid tissue consists of reticular cells and fibers supporting masses of lymphocytes. Lymphoid tissue is remarkably variable and may appear as a diffuse infiltration into the lamina propria of mucous membranes or as well defined organs, such as the thymus. One classification of lymphoid tissue based upon increasing complexity is: (1) diffuse lymphoid tissue; (2) lymph nodules; (3) tonsils; (4) lymph nodes; (5) the thymus; and (6) the spleen. The simplest form, diffuse lymphoid tissue, is found throughout the body, but in particular in the alimentary and respiratory tracts. Located in the lamina propria, it underlies the surface epithelium, surrounds mucosal glands and their ducts and is characterized by a loosely organized mass of lymphocytes. The diffuse form of lymphatic tissue grades into a more dense form, termed lymph nodules, circumscribed masses of densely packed lymphocytes which may be considered the basic structural unit of lymphoid tissue. Each nodule may contain a light staining central area, termed the germinal center, the presence of which indicates a site of active lymphocyte proliferation. These "primary" nodules or lymph follicles are found in large numbers in the mucosa of the intestinal tract.

Groups of lymph nodules may be partially encapsulated as small organs with a definite lymphatic and blood vascular supply. Such is the case in the tonsils, found in the pharynx. The three distinct tonsillar masses include the palatine, lingual and pharyngeal (clinically the adenoids), which form an incomplete ring around the entrance to the throat. The palatine and lingual tonsils are covered with a stratified squamous epithelium, while the pharyngeal tonsil is covered with a pseudostratified columnar ciliated epithelium, with some goblet cells characteristic of the nasopharynx. In adults the pharyngeal tonsil is covered by a stratified squamous epithelium. The palatine and lingual tonsils have numerous epithelium-lined pits, referred to as crypts, which may bifurcate. Surrounding the crypts is a single layer of lymph nodules with germinal centers. The pharyngeal tonsil does not possess true crypts but rather widened ducts of underlying glands. The epithelium covering the tonsils is extensively infiltrated by lymphocytes, plasma cells and polymorphonuclear leucocytes.

Lymph nodes are completely encapsulated ovoid structures, in contrast to the lymphatic tissue described above. The capsule admits afferent lymphatic vessels containing valves to the subcapsular sinus. The lymph circulates through sinuses located in the cortex (containing the lymph nodules) and the medulla (containing lymphatic cords), and leaves the node via larger but fewer efferent lymphatic vessels. These also contain valves and emerge from a specific region of the node, the hilus. The lymph nodes, which vary in diameter from 1 to 25 mm, receive their blood supply only at the hilus of the node. The arterial vessels enter both the trabeculae formed from the capsular connective tissue and the medullary cords and they regionally supply the node by giving off capillaries; they continue to the cortex, where an arterial branch penetrates each cortical lymph nodule and forms a capillary plexus around the germinal center. From the capillary beds blood is carried by veins, which follow a pathway similar to the arteries, leaving the node at the hilum along with the efferent lymphatic vessels.

The thymus varies in size and undergoes structural alterations with age. It undergoes rapid growth until the end of the second year, after which time the rate of growth slows until approximately the fourteenth year. After this the thymus begins to involute or decrease in size, and gradually the lymphatic tissue is replaced by fat and connective tissue. In old age very little thymic tissue may be present. The thymus consists of two lobes joined by connective tissue. Each lobe contains many lobules which are 0.5 to 2 mm in diameter and which are incompletely separated from each other. A lobule is composed of a cortex and a medulla, which sends a projection to join with the medullae of adjacent lobules. The cortex consists of lymphocytes which are densely and uniformly packed, obscuring the sparse reticular framework. The cortex lacks lymph nodules. The medulla stains less intensely due to a thinning of the concentration of lymphocytes, and it is here that reticular cells can be recognized. Hassall's thymic corpuscles located in the medulla are diagnostic for the identification of the thymus. The diameter of Hassall's corpuscles varies from 20 to 150 $\mu$.

Arteries supplying the thymus follow the connective tissue septa and give off branches which enter the lobular cortex and break up into capillaries which supply the cortex and medulla. The medulla is more richly supplied than the cortex. The capillaries terminate in thin walled veins which pass into the connective tissue septa along with the arteries. Lymphatic vessels arise within the thymic lobule and join to form larger vessels which accompany the arteries and veins in the connective tissue septa. In contrast to lymph nodes, the thymus contains no lymph sinuses or afferent lymphatic vessels.

The spleen is the largest lymphatic organ in the body. Like the thymus, it has no afferent lymphatic vessels and no lymph sinuses. Splenic vessels enter and leave the spleen at the hilum and are located in thick trabeculae which extend inward from the capsule. The capsule and trabeculae are composed of collagen and elastic fibers and some smooth muscle fibers. A reticular fiber network and lymphocytes are between the trabeculae. Sections of fresh spleen reveal two different regions, the red pulp and the white pulp. The red pulp is traversed by a plexus of venous sinuses separated by lymphatic splenic cords. The venous sinuses contain tightly packed red blood corpuscles when they perform a storage function. The white pulp is composed of compact lymphoid tissue arranged in spherical or ovoid aggregations around arterioles (central arterioles). These aggregations are called splenic or Malpighian corpuscles and bear a resemblance to lymph nodes. The vascular supply is critical for an understanding of the spleen. The arteries enter at the hilus and are carried in and branch with the trabeculae. Arterioles emerge from the trabeculae and pass into the splenic parenchyma, where the adventitia of the arterioles is infiltrated by lymphocytes to form the splenic corpuscles. These arterioles supply the capillaries for the white pulp and continue their course, lose their lymphatic investment and enter the red pulp, where they subdivide into several branches called penicilli. These branches become smaller and are differentiated into three distinct regions: pulp arterioles, sheathed arterioles and terminal capillaries. The nature of the termination of these capillaries and their ultimate union with the venous sinuses is controversial. A discussion of this can be found in comprehensive histology textbooks. The venous sinuses are lined not by endothelium but by specialized reticular cells which are fixed macrophages. The reticular cells are encircled by reticular fibers. The venous sinuses unite to form pulp veins which are lined by endothelial cells. The pulp, or collecting, veins enter the trabeculae and leave the spleen at the hilum. Lymphocytes and monocytes are formed in both the red and white pulp, the primary source being, however, the white pulp. They migrate to the red pulp to gain access to the venous sinuses. Although the spleen is not essential for life it carries out several important functions which include: (1) filtering the blood by removing from the circulation foreign particles and aging and damaged red blood corpuscles and leucocytes; (2) conservation and temporary storage of iron recovered from hemoglobin; (3) storage of normal red blood corpuscles with the splenic sinuses; (4) an important role in antibody formation; and (5) the generation of lymphocytes and monocytes which enter the general circulation.

## PALATINE TONSIL

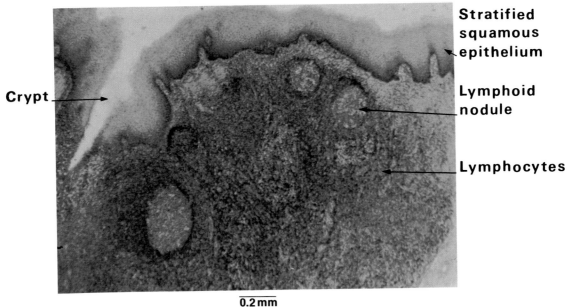

0.2 mm

**Human, 10% Formalin, H. & E., 50 x.**

**Crypt:** Epithelial invaginations into the tonsillar substance lined by surface epithelium.

**Stratified squamous epithelium:** Covers the free surface of the tonsil and lines the crypts.

**Lymphoid nodule:** Compact aggregate of lymphocytes in the midst of a diffuse sheet of lymphatic tissue. Occurs close to the epithelium. May contain germinal centers.

**Lymphocytes:** Predominant cell type in the palatine tonsil.

## LYMPH NODES
Mesenteric

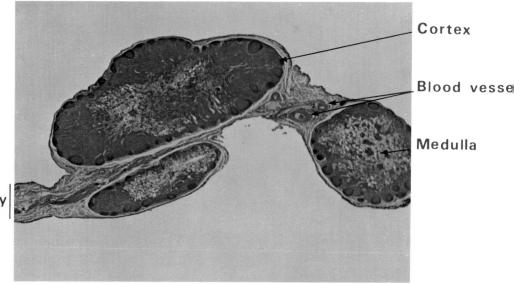

Cortex

Blood vesse

Medulla

Mesentery

Rhesus monkey, Helly's fluid, H. & E., 8.5 x.

The mesentery is composed of loose connective tissue covered by peritoneum. Three lymph nodes are seen within the mesentery. The division of each into cortex and medulla is well defined. Note the poor development of trabeculae in these nodes. This is often observed in lymph nodes situated deep in the body. The abundance of medullary substance noted in two of the nodes is also characteristic of abdominal nodes.

PLATE 146

## LYMPH NODE

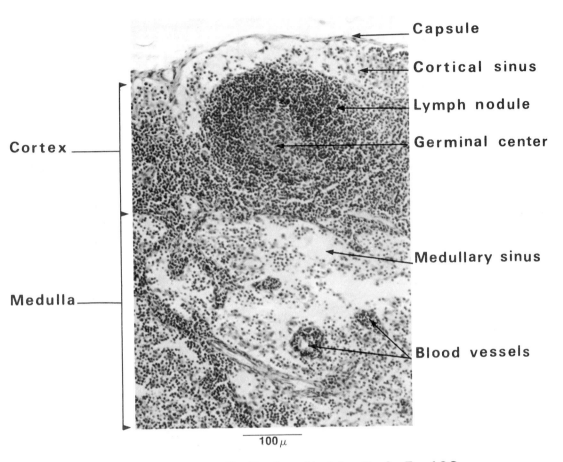

Capsule

Cortical sinus

Lymph nodule

Germinal center

Cortex

Medullary sinus

Medulla

Blood vessels

100 μ

Rhesus monkey, Helly's fluid, H. & E., 162 x.

**Cortex:** Underneath the capsule. Formed of a series of closely packed regularly arranged lymph nodules.

**Medulla:** Formed of anastomosing cords of lymphocytes separated by the abundant lymphatic sinuses.

**Capsule:** Well defined connective tissue cover from which septa or trabeculae penetrate the substance of the lymph node.

**Cortical sinus:** Lymphatic sinus separates cortical nodules from the capsule. Lymph from the afferent lymphatic vessels enters the node via the cortical sinus.

**Lymph nodule:** Closely packed aggregate of lymphocytes in the cortex of the node. Also known as cortical follicles or primary nodules. Lymphatic nodules are temporary structures which may develop, disappear and redevelop. The size and number of nodules vary widely.

**Germinal center:** Also known as secondary nodule or reaction center. The lighter-staining area in the center of the lymph nodule. Vary in size with age, being best developed in childhood. They are believed to be cytogenic or lymphocytopoietic centers. They are temporary structures like lymph nodules.

**Blood vessels:** Branches of the artery that enter at the hilus of the node.

# LYMPHOCYTES
## Lymph node

Lymphocyte nuclei

Mitotic cell division; anaphase

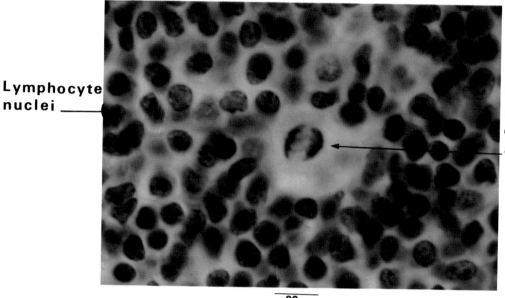

20μ

## Human, Helly's fluid, H. & E., 612 x.

**Lymphocyte nuclei:**   Densely staining, they fill most of the cell. The cytoplasm is not seen at this magnification but can be seen in Plate 51.

**Mitotic cell division:**   Anaphase. Medium and large lymphocytes are capable of multiplication by mitosis. Anaphase is a period in the continuous process of cell division in which the replicated chromosomes separate and are drawn toward the spindle poles prior to cytoplasmic division. For an illustration of the complete mitotic cycle and human chromosomes at high magnification see Plates 3 and 4.

## LYMPHATIC VESSEL

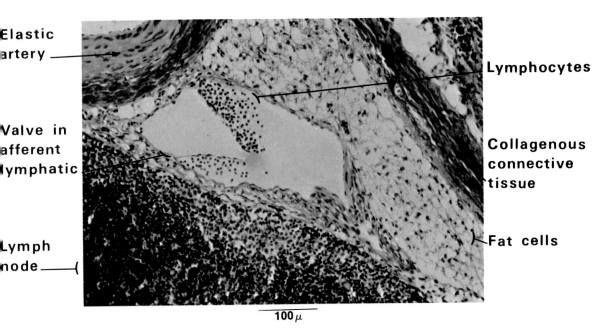

Elastic artery

Lymphocytes

Valve in afferent lymphatic

Collagenous connective tissue

Lymph node

Fat cells

100 μ

### Rat, Helly's fluid, Mallory's stain, 162 x.

This plate shows an afferent lymphatic vessel near a lymph node. The lymph vessel is lined with endothelium and has a valve which opens toward the node. The valve is a fold of that part of the vessel wall known as the intima (Plates 135 and 143). Valves, by preventing retrograde flow, are essential for the movement of lymph to major lymphatic trunks. Lymph is formed in part from materials and fluid which leave the capillaries and venules of the blood vascular system. This extracellular fluid contains small molecular weight substances, neutral fat, protein and metabolic products from cells which enter lymphatic capillaries and are carried by a system of lymphatic vessels to and from lymph nodes to the thoracic duct where the lymph enters the blood vascular system. Lymphatic vessels also have a primary role in the transport of absorbed fats and fat-soluble substances from the digestive tract. The total volume of lymph carried by lymphatic vessels which passes into the blood is estimated to be about 1.5 to 2.2 liters per day.

Collagenous connective tissue forming the capsule of the lymph node, as well as fat cells and an artery, is seen adjacent to the afferent lymph vessel.

Lymphatic vessels and the fluid they carry (lymph) were discovered in 1627 by Gasparo Aselli, the Professor of Anatomy at the University of Pavia.

## THYMUS

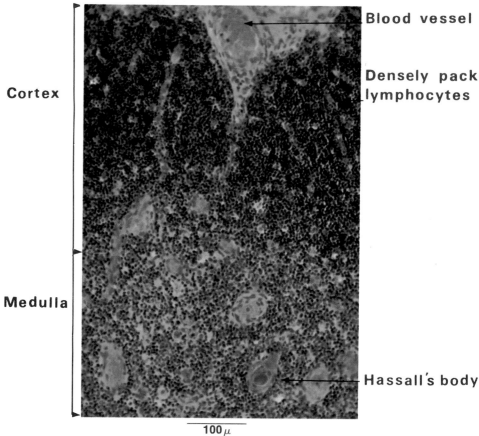

Human, 10% Formalin, H.& E., 162x

**Cortex:** Denser staining than the medulla. Consists of densely packed lymphocytes of all sizes.

**Medulla:** Less densely staining and less compact than cortex. Made up of lymphocytes and epithelial reticular elements.

**Hassall's corpuscle:** A diagnostic structure found in the medulla. Composed of epithelioid cells arranged in layers. Dense hyalinized core surrounded by flattened cells. Increase in size and number with age. Origin is epithelial reticular cells.

**Blood vessel:** Located in the connective tissue capsule.

The thymus is an organ which produces lymphocytes, plasma cells and, in embryonic life, myelocytes. This organ is most highly developed in the embryo and child until puberty, after which it involutes gradually throughout life. The principal cell types in this organ are lymphocytes and reticular cells. The lymphocytes produced by the thymus in the embryo populate the spleen and lymph nodes, where they reproduce themselves. The thymus plays an early and essential role in the development of immunological competence by the individual.

# THYMUS

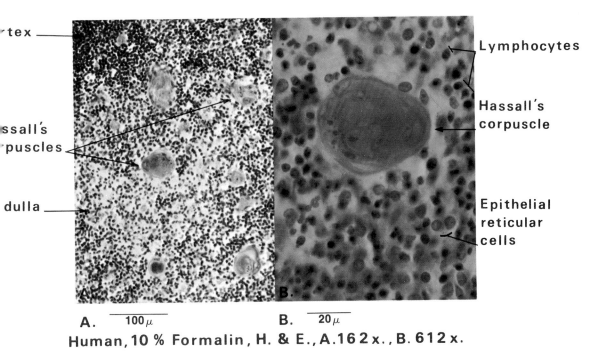

tex

ssall's
puscles

dulla

Lymphocytes

Hassall's
corpuscle

Epithelial
reticular
cells

A. ‾‾100μ‾‾        B. ‾‾20μ‾‾

Human, 10 % Formalin, H. & E., A. 162 x., B. 612 x.

In *A*, note the cortex of the thymic lobule, composed of densely packed lymphatic tissue, and the medulla, composed of looser lymphatic tissue containing Hassall's corpuscles. The latter are diagnostic for the thymus. They vary in size and are formed of concentrically arranged polygonal or flattened cells with a hyalinized degenerated core.

In *B*, a Hassall's corpuscle is seen at higher magnification. Note also the abundance of lymphocytes and the epithelial reticular cells. The latter are characterized by a large pale nucleus and are derived from embryonic entoderm rather than from mesenchyme.

## SPLEEN
Capsule

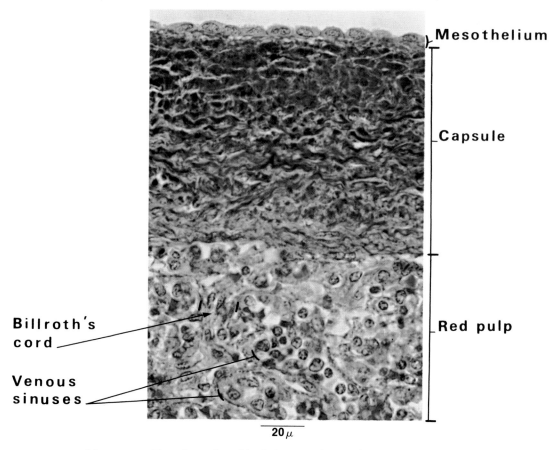

Mesothelium

Capsule

Red pulp

Billroth's cord

Venous sinuses

20 μ

**Human, Zenker's fluid, Mallory's stain, 612 x.**

**Mesothelium:** A single layer of mesothelial cells which covers the free surface of the spleen except at the hilum.

**Capsule:** Dense fibroelastic tissue containing some smooth muscle fibers.

**Red pulp:** Loosely textured lymphatic tissue. Formed of anastomosing cords of tissue (Billroth's or splenic cords) rich in cells which separate the venous sinuses.

See also Plate 154.

The spleen is concerned with the production of lymphocytes and monocytes, storage of red blood corpuscles, destruction of aged and damaged red blood corpuscles by lining cells of the sinuses and the macrophages of the splenic cords, preservation of the iron freed from the breakdown of hemoglobin stored in the reticular cells and used subsequently in the formation of new hemoglobin, clearance of particulate materials from the blood, production of antibodies to antigens carried in the blood, and storage of blood lipids in the reticular cells.

## SPLEEN

White
pulp

Central
artery

Red pulp

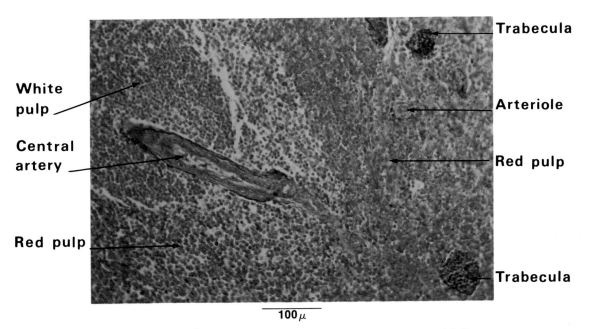

Trabecula

Arteriole

Red pulp

Trabecula

100 μ

## Human, Helly's fluid, Mallory-Azan stain, 162 x.

**White pulp:**   A mass of compact lymphatic tissue filled with lymphocytes surrounding the central artery.

**Central artery:**   A misnomer, as it is invariably eccentrically placed in the white pulp. A branch of the splenic artery, it gives off numerous capillaries before leaving the white pulp to enter the red pulp.

**Red pulp:**   So called because of its color during life. Red color is imparted by the abundant erythrocytes. Lymphatic tissue of the red pulp is not as compact as that of the white pulp with which it blends. Apparent compactness in fixed preparations is attributed to the collapse of sinusoids after death.

**Trabecula:**   Collagenous connective tissue projections from the capsule. Branches repeatedly, and imperfectly divides the spleen into anastomosing chambers.

**Arteriole:**   Terminal branches of the central artery in the red pulp. Has no investment of compact lymphatic tissue.

## SPLEEN
## White pulp
## splenic nodule

Lymphocytes

Central
arteriole

White pulp

Red pulp

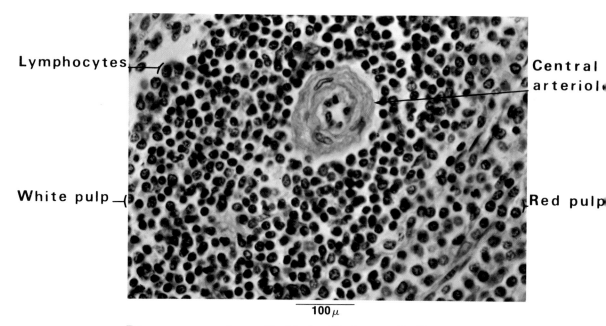

100 μ

Rhesus monkey, Helly's fluid, H. & E., 162 x.

**White pulp:** Compact lymphatic tissue sheath surrounding the central arteriole. This sheath forms ovoid enlargements at intervals. The enlargements, known as lymphatic nodules, splenic nodules or Malpighian corpuscles, may have germinal centers. Blends into the adjacent red pulp. Lymphocytes are the predominant cellular element, but plasma cells, macrophages and other free cells are found.

**Red pulp:** Less compact lymphatic tissue. Traversed by venous channels (sinusoids), imparting to it a reddish color in the fresh or unfixed state. Looks somewhat compact in fixed preparation because of the collapse of sinusoids.

**Lymphocytes:** Large, medium and small lymphocytes constitute the principal cell types found in the white pulp. They are compactly arranged in the white pulp and more loosely arranged in the red pulp.

**Central arteriole:** Courses in the white pulp. Adventitia is replaced by reticular tissue which is infiltrated by lymphocytes in the white pulp. Supplies capillaries to the white pulp.

## SPLEEN
### Red pulp

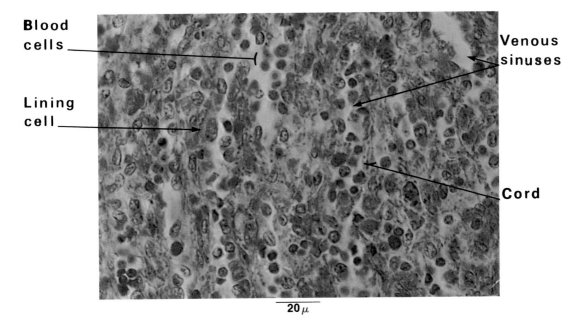

Blood cells

Lining cell

Venous sinuses

Cord

20 μ

## Human, Zenker's fluid, Mallory's stain, 612 x.

**Venous sinuses:**  Form an anastomosing plexus through the red pulp between the pulp cords. Highly distensible in the living state.

**Cords:**  Loose lymphatic tissue arranged in anastomosing cords and plates characterizes the red pulp of the spleen. Also termed Billroth or splenic cords. The cords contain varying numbers of red blood corpuscles, lymphocytes, plasma cells and monocytes. Between cords are the venous sinusoids.

**Blood cells:**  Fill the venous sinusoids and impart the red color to the pulp in the fresh unfixed state.

**Lining cells:**  Sinusoids are lined by phagocytic reticular cells belonging to the widespread macrophage (reticuloendothelial) system. Shape changes with state of distension of the sinus.

# Section 10    The Digestive System

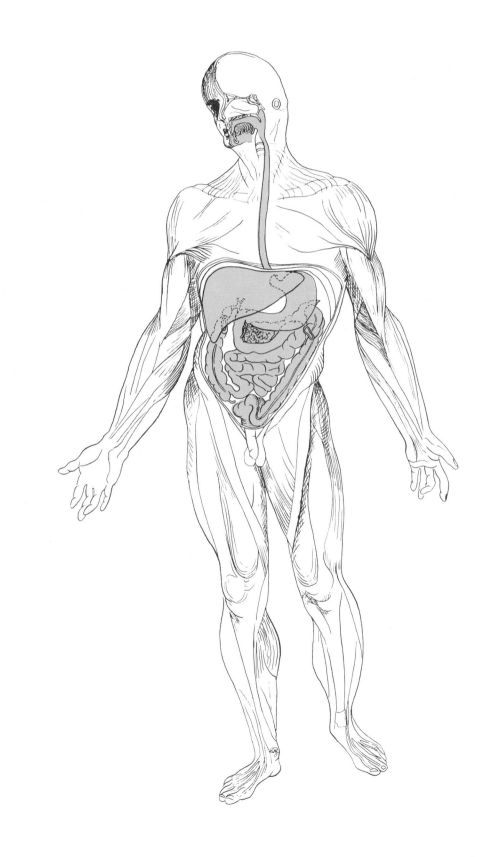

# The Digestive System

The digestive system includes the mouth, pharynx and the digestive tube. Various regions of the digestive system display structural specializations related to their specific function. In addition, several glands deliver their secretory products into the digestive tract, where regionally specific functions are performed.

The digestive process begins in the mouth as the food is chewed and ground to reduce the size of the pieces of ingested food. As the food is chewed the salivary glands secrete saliva which moistens it and initiates the digestion of starch and glycogen contained within the disrupted plant and animal cells, respectively (Plates 180, 181, 182 and 183). The tongue moves the food within the mouth to the teeth and is essential in the chewing process. In addition, the sense of taste is received by, and transmitted to, the central nervous system by taste buds located on the tongue (Plates 157 and 247). The tongue directs the bolus of chewed food to the pharynx as an initial step in the swallowing mechanism. The pharynx is a conical chamber through which both air and food pass. The role of the pharynx in swallowing is involuntary.

The bolus of food passes into the esophagus which conducts it to the stomach. This process is accomplished by muscular contraction and gravity. The muscularis of the esophagus contains both striated and smooth muscle fibers. See Plate 163. The epithelium which lines the digestive system to this point is nonkeratinized stratified squamous epithelium. An abrupt change in the epithelium takes place in the stomach, where it now appears as columnar mucous secretory cells which form the cardiac glands (Plate 162). These are followed by the gastric glands, composed of four epithelial cell types: (1) mucous neck cells; (2) chief cells; (3) parietal cells; and (4) argentaffin cells (Plates 165, 166 and 172). At the distal end of the stomach, mucus-secreting pyloric glands are found and these are structurally similar to the cardiac glands.

The glands of the mucosa rest upon a basement membrane and a scanty lamina propria surrounding the gastric glands. Underlying this connective tissue layer is the thin muscularis mucosa, composed of two layers of smooth muscle fibers, an inner circular and an outer longitudinal layer. Beneath the mucosa there is a loose connective tissue layer called the submucosa. It contains large blood vessels, lymphatics and nerves. Surrounding the submucosa are three irregularly arranged layers of smooth muscle constituting the muscularis: an inner oblique, a middle circular and an outer longitudinal layer. At the distal opening of the stomach is the valve designated the pyloric sphincter, which is a special thickening of the circular layer of smooth muscle. The outermost covering of the stomach is termed the serosa and is composed of a loose fatty connective tissue surfaced by mesothelium; this is the visceral peritoneum.

The intestine is a hollow tube which extends in a coiled course between the pylorus and anus. The intestine, like the stomach, is composed of four distinct layers (in sequence from the inside): the mucosa, submucosa, muscularis and serosa if the intestine is contained within a peritoneal fold of mesentery, or adventitia if it is incompletely covered and lies behind the peritoneum attached to the dorsal abdominal wall.

The mucosa of the small intestine is covered by a simple epithelium which lines the distinctive villi and intestinal glands. Four types of lining cells are found throughout the intestinal mucosa (lining epithelium and glands): (1) simple columnar cells; (2) goblet cells; (3) Paneth cells; and (4) argentaffin cells. The structure and function of these cell types are included in the legends of Plates 170, 171 and 172. The intestinal mucosal glands are the pitlike crypts of Lieberkühn. Surrounding the intestinal glands and forming the core of each intestinal villus is the lamina propria, which characteristically contains lymphatic aggregates, loose lymphocytes, plasma cells, eosinophils and mast cells, and scattered smooth muscle fibers derived from the underlying muscularis mucosa. See Plates 28, 169 and 173. The lamina propria has a rich capillary network and a lymphatic capillary in the core of each villus called the central lacteal. Located in the outermost layer of the lamina propria is a band of smooth muscle, the muscularis mucosa, composed of inner circular and outer longitudinal layers.

A diagnostic feature of the duodenum is the location in the submucosa of the mucous glands of Brunner, whose ducts open into the lumina of intestinal glands (see Plate 167). The muscularis is composed of an inner circular and an outer longitudinal coat. Between these two layers is the myenteric nerve plexus of Auerbach (Plate 174). The intestine is contained primarily within a fold of the peritoneum (mesentery) and is covered superficially by a mesothelial cell layer.

The intestine is divided anatomically into two major subdivisions, the small and large intestine. The small intestine, about 23 feet long in man, is further subdivided into three regions: the proximal (structurally distinctive) duodenum, middle jejunum and distal ileum. The large intestine, about 5 feet in length, is approximately twice the diameter of the small intestine, and includes four anatomically defined regions: the caecum, appendix, colon and rectum. The inner lining of the large intestine lacks the villi which characterize the small intestine (Plates 164 and 178). The intestinal glands are tightly packed and appear more conspicuous due to the lack of villi, but are composed of the same cell types as the small intestine. Only quantitative differences exist in epithelial cell populations.

The large intestine begins at the ileocaecal valve, which is formed by two folds of the mucosa and submucosa and circular smooth muscle. The caecum is a pouch from which the fingerlike vermiform appendix extends. The surface epithelium is primarily a simple columnar epithelium with some goblet cells. Lymphoid tissue in the form of solitary lymphatic nodules forms a conspicuous part of the lamina propria of the mucosa. A distinctive feature of the caecum and colon, but not of the appendix, is the arrangement of the smooth muscle of the muscularis. The inner muscular layer is circular but the outer longitudinal layer is aggregated into three equally spaced thick bands named the taeniae coli. Between the taeniae the longitudinal layer is a very thin but complete layer. The rectum is similar in structure to the colon but lacks the taeniae or ribbonlike bands of longitudinal smooth muscle. At the rectal-anal junction the surface epithelium changes, to become a nonkeratinized stratified squamous epithelium, which then changes at the anal orifice to its keratinized form (epidermis). At this most distal end of the digestive tube cutaneous glands (large apocrine glands) and hair appear. The submucosa has an extremely rich vascular supply (hemorrhoidal vessels) and the circular smooth muscle of the muscularis forms the internal anal sphincter. Striated muscle in close association with the smooth muscle layer forms the external anal sphincter.

Associated with the digestive tube are eight major glands: the three paired salivary glands, the pancreas and the liver.

The major salivary glands are the parotid, the submandibular and the sublingual. These large glands are structurally compound tubuloalveolar, whose ducts open into the oral cavity. The parotid gland is composed of serous cells (exclusively in man) and the submandibular and sublingual glands are mixed serous and mucous glands (Plates 180,181,182 and 183). The secretory alveoli of these glands are linked to the oral cavity by a system of ducts which are divided into three segments (leading from the secretory cells): intercalated ducts, composed proximally of squamous cells and distally of cuboidal cells; secretory ducts, composed of columnar cells with basal striations; and excretory ducts, which begin as columnar cells and terminate as tubes lined by stratified squamous epithelium continuous with the same epithelium lining the oral cavity. The duct system is most conspicuous in the parotid gland and least conspicuous in the sublingual gland in which some modifications appear. The intercalated ducts of the sublingual gland are composed primarily of mucous cells in the form of tubules and are linked to very short secretory ducts. The final excretory segment is similar in all three glands.

The pancreas has both an exocrine and an endocrine function. The exocrine or digestive enzyme-producing part of the gland will be considered here, and the endocrine portion will be considered in the section on endocrine glands. The pancreas is a compound tubuloalveolar gland with purely serous alveoli. It is covered by a sheath of areolar connective tissue from which thin fibrous septa extend into the gland to subdivide it into many distinct lobules. The parenchyma is a glandular epithelium consisting of pyramidal cells which secrete zymogen granules into a system of ducts (Plates 25 and 184). An unusual feature of the pancreas is the existence of the centroalveolar or centroacinar cells which are interposed between the secretory cells and the lumen of the alveolus (Plate 184). The centroalveolar cells are in continuity with the intercalated or intralobar ducts composed of cuboidal epithelium. The intercalated ducts join the excretory or interlobar ducts lined with simple columnar epithelium. These ducts join the main excretory duct, which empties into the lumen of the duodenum. The stroma is composed of delicate connective tissue supporting the parenchymal cells, nerve fibers, blood and lymphatic vessels.

The liver is the largest gland of the body. It is composed of four incompletely separated lobes covered by a connective tissue capsule (Glisson's capsule) and incompletely invested by a reflection of peritoneum. The parenchyma of this organ is composed of lobules and an anastomosing series of hepatic cords. In histologic sections, the hepatic cords radiate outward from the central vein much like the spokes of a wheel. The cells are actually arranged in sheets one cell thick. Located between the cellular sheets are sinusoids approximately 9 to 12 $\mu$ in width which receive blood at the periphery of the lobule from the portal vein and hepatic artery and, after traversing the lobule, discharge the blood into the central vein at the center of the lobule (Plates 185 and 186). The sinusoids are lined with endothelial cells and contain the stellate cells of von Kupffer. Kupffer cells are phagocytes belonging to the widely distributed system of fixed macrophages. At the interface between adjacent hepatic cells minute bile capillaries (canaliculi) are formed which drain toward the periphery of the hepatic lobule into a bile duct in the portal canal (Plates 185, 188 and 189). This fundamental structural unit of the liver, the hepatic lobule, is repeated throughout the liver. The smaller bile ducts converge within the liver to form the hepatic duct outside the liver. The gall bladder and its cystic duct join with the hepatic duct to form the common bile duct, which drains into the lumen of the duodenum. The bladder stores up to 90 ml of bile between meals. Bile is secreted continuously by the liver, with a total daily output of about 500 cc.

# TONGUE

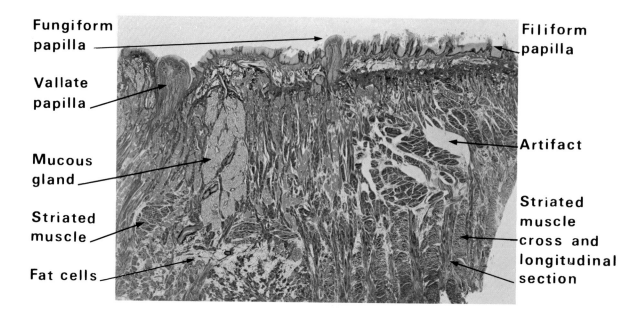

Fungiform papilla

Filiform papilla

Vallate papilla

Mucous gland

Artifact

Striated muscle

Striated muscle cross and longitudinal section

Fat cells

**Human, Zenker's fluid, Phosphotungstic acid hematoxylin stain, 5.6 x.**

The epithelium of the dorsal surface of the tongue has three types of papillae: fungiform, filiform and circumvallate (vallate).

**Fungiform papillae:** Few in number, scattered among the filiform papillae. Larger than the filiform papillae. Wider at the top than at the base, resembling a mushroom, hence their name. Epithelial covering may possess taste buds.

**Filiform papillae:** Threadlike papillae much more numerous and smaller than fungiform papillae. Each papilla is made up of a thin core of vascularized connective tissue covered by a cornified stratified squamous epithelium. They do not have taste buds.

**Vallate papillae:** Large, surrounded by moats. Stratified squamous noncornified epithelium covers a connective tissue core and contains taste buds. The serous or gustatory glands of von Ebner are closely associated with vallate papillae and empty into the circumvallate groove.

**Mucous gland:** Pure mucous glands occur in the root and in the posterior part of the tongue. Their ducts open onto the dorsum of the tongue.

**Striated muscle:** The core of the tongue contains interlacing bundles of striated fibers that run in three planes, longitudinal, transverse and vertical.

**Fat cells:** Part of the areolar fatty tissue in which muscles of the tongue are embedded.

**Artifact:** Spaces between muscle bundles are artifacts of fixation and/or embedding of the tissue prior to sectioning.

The tongue is innervated by four cranial nerves, the fifth or trigeminal, the seventh or facial, the ninth or glossopharyngeal, and the twelfth or hypoglossal. The trigeminal nerve supplies the anterior two-thirds of the tongue and is concerned with general sensibility. The facial nerve serves the same region but is concerned with taste or gustatory sensibility. The posterior one-third of the tongue is innervated by the glossopharyngeal nerve serving both general and gustatory sensibility. The hypoglossal nerve is the motor nerve supplying the striated (somatic) skeletal musculature of the tongue. General sensibility refers to touch, pressure, pain, temperature, sense of position and movement. Taste or gustatory sense, smell, sight, hearing, head position and movements are termed the special senses.

# TONGUE
## Fungiform and filiform papillae

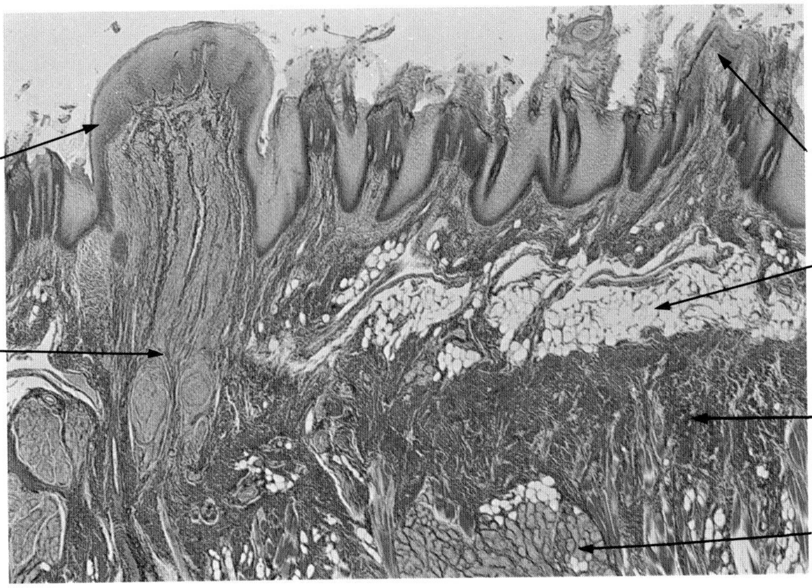

Fungiform papilla

Nerve fibers

Filiform papilla

Fat cells

Collagenous connective tissue

Serous gland acini

**Human, Zenker's fluid, phosphotungstic acid hematoxylin, 26x.**

**Fungiform papillae:** Mushroom-like. Larger but much less frequent than filiform papillae. Has a stratified squamous noncornified epithelial covering and a highly vascularized connective tissue core giving it a red hue in the living state. Although not seen here the epithelium may contain taste buds. Small secondary papillae are formed beneath the superficial epithelial cover of the primary connective tissue papillae.

**Filiform papillae:** Threadlike. Smaller and much more numerous than the fungiform variety. Epithelial lining is keratinized stratified squamous and is devoid of taste buds. Thin connective tissue core.

**Nerve fibers:** Thinly myelinated sensory fibers that arborize under the epithelium.

**Fat cells:** Part of the fatty (adipose) tissue underlying the lamina propria.

**Collagenous connective tissue:** A fibrofatty connective tissue which forms a bed for glands and skeletal muscle fibers and serves to anchor them.

**Serous gland acini:** Mixed serous and mucous glands are scattered among the connective tissue and muscle fascicles in the anterior two-thirds of the tongue close to its ventral surface. Their ducts open onto the ventral surface of the tongue.

## TONGUE
### Vallate papilla

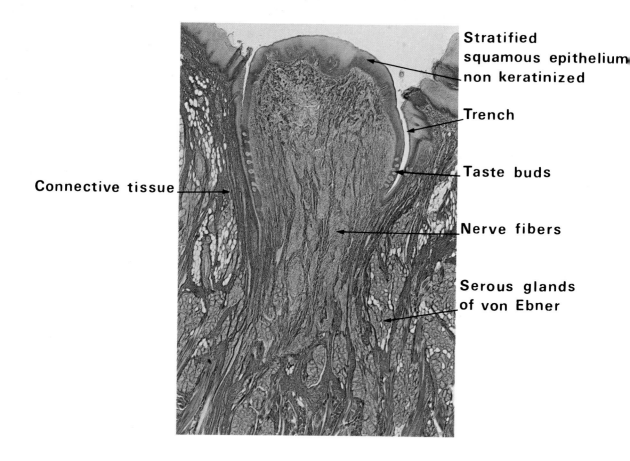

Stratified
squamous epithelium
non keratinized

Trench

Taste buds

Connective tissue

Nerve fibers

Serous glands
of von Ebner

### Human, Zenker's fluid, Phosphotungstic acid hematoxylin stain, 26x.

Vallate papillae line the V-shaped boundary between the anterior two-thirds and posterior one-third of the tongue. They are shaped like an inverted cone.

**Stratified squamous epithelium:** Covers the tong surface and dips into the trenches between papillae.

**Trench:** A moat or groove that surrounds each vallate papilla.

**Taste buds:** The organs of taste. Oval structures located in the lateral wall of vallate papillae and less frequently in the outer wall of the trench.

**Nerve fibers:** Myelinated nerve fibers, 1 to 6 $\mu$ in diameter, branch profusely within the papillae, lose their myelin, penetrate the basement membrane and form a plexus around the receptor cells of taste buds.

**Serous glands of von Ebner:** Limited to the posterior part of the tongue in the neighborhood of the vallate papillae. Ducts open into the circumvallate groove surrounding the vallate papillae.

**Connective tissue:** Forms the core of the papillae and supports the underlying glands. This connective tissue is rich in collagenous and elastic fibers.

## TONGUE
### Mucous and Serous glands

Fat cells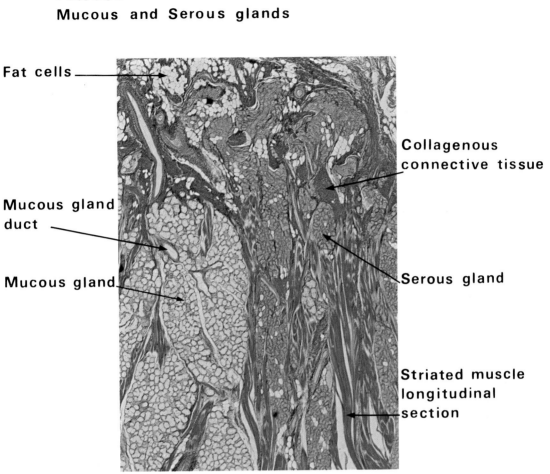

Collagenous
connective tissue

Mucous gland
duct

Mucous gland

Serous gland

Striated muscle
longitudinal
section

**Human, Zenker's fluid, Phosphotungstic acid
hematoxylin stain, 26×.**

Mixed serous and mucous glands (glands of Nuhn) are found in the anterior two-thirds of the inferior surface of the tongue. They are shown here intermixed with striated muscle fibers, collagenous connective tissue and fat.

**Fat cells:** Appear empty because their lipid c͡    ͟ʳ has been lost in tissue preparation.

**Collagenous connective tissue:** Surrounds and supports the glands and encompasses muscle fibers to form fascicles.

**Mucous glands:** Embedded between muscle fascicles. Appear lightly stained.

**Mucous gland ducts:** Several are seen in this figure. They open primarily on the surface of the tongue.

**Serous glands:** Scattered among muscle fascicles. The cytoplasm stains more deeply here than in mucous glands.

**Striated muscle longitudinal section:** Interlacing muscle fibers of the tongue run in three directions: longitudinal, transverse and vertical. The muscle fibers located between glands are inserted in the dense connective tissue beneath the surface epithelium.

## LINGUAL GLANDS
### A. Mucous gland
### B. Serous gland

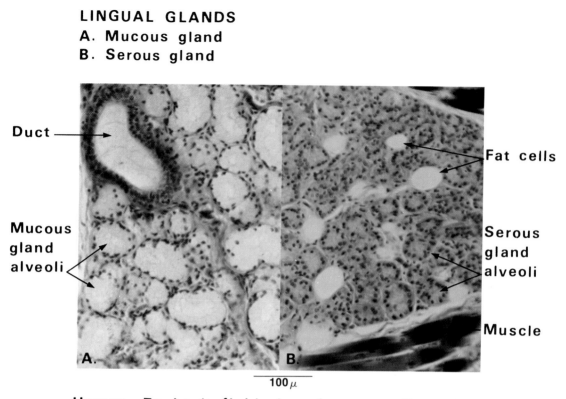

Duct

Fat cells

Mucous gland alveoli

Serous gland alveoli

Muscle

A.

B.

100 μ

Human, Zenker's fluid, Iron hematoxylin and aldehyde fuchsin stains, 162 x.

The tongue has three groups of glands, serous, mucous, and mixed serous and mucous.

Mucous glands are interspersed between muscle bundles and serous glands. Their ducts terminate on the surface of the tongue. The mucous glands are most numerous in the root of the tongue. Their ducts open into the crypts of the lingual tonsil.

The serous glands (of von Ebner) are located in the region of the vallate papillae. They extend into the muscle layer as shown in this figure. Ducts open into trenches of vallate papillae. Fat cells are scattered among the alveoli. The secretion of these glands moistens the epithelium and taste buds and flushes the trenches around the vallate papillae. These are important functions for taste discrimination.

Note that the serous cells forming the alveoli are wedge-shaped and well stained, and the lumina are narrow. In contrast, the mucous cells are pale and the lumina are much wider. Note that serous cell nuclei, although basally located, are not flattened like mucous cell nuclei.

## DEVELOPING TOOTH

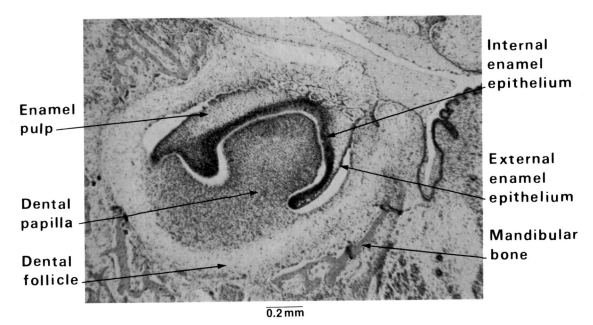

Internal enamel epithelium

External enamel epithelium

Mandibular bone

Enamel pulp

Dental papilla

Dental follicle

0.2 mm

Cat, 10 % Formalin, H. & E., 50 x.

**Internal enamel epithelium:** A single layer of columnar cells which become the enamel-producing ameloblasts.

**External enamel epithelium:** A single layer of cuboidal epithelium.

**Enamel pulp:** A collection of loosely arranged branching cells. Also called stellate reticulum.

**Dental papilla:** Proliferation and condensation of mesenchyme which constitutes the primordium of the enamel pulp.

**Dental follicle:** It is also called the dental sac and is composed of mesenchyme surrounding the dental papilla and enamel organ. The part adjacent to the dental papilla forms the future periodontal membrane. Its peripheral part becomes the periosteum of the wall of the future alveolus.

**Mandibular bone:** In which the tooth is embedded.

## DEVELOPING TOOTH

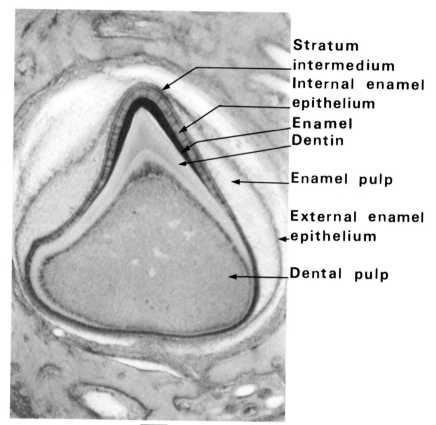

Stratum
intermedium
Internal enamel
epithelium
Enamel
Dentin

Enamel pulp

External enamel
epithelium

Dental pulp

0.2 mm

Kitten, 10% Formalin, H. & E., 40 x.

**Internal enamel epithelium:** A single layer of columnar cells. Cells here become the enamel-producing ameloblasts. A basement membrane separates the internal enamel epithelium from the dental pulp.

**External enamel epithelium:** A single layer of cuboidal epithelium.

**Stratum intermedium:** Two or more layers of cuboidal or squamous cells that separate the inner enamel epithelium from the stellate cells of the enamel pulp.

**Enamel pulp:** Or stellate reticulum, a collection of loosely arranged branching cells.

**Enamel:** Hardest substance in the body, composed of calcium salts in the form of apatite crystals and only 3 per cent organic material.

**Dentin:** Deposited by odontoblasts derived from dental pulp.

**Dental pulp:** Origin from dental papilla. Popularly but incorrectly called the nerve of the tooth.

# ESOPHAGUS—STOMACH JUNCTION
## Longitudinal section

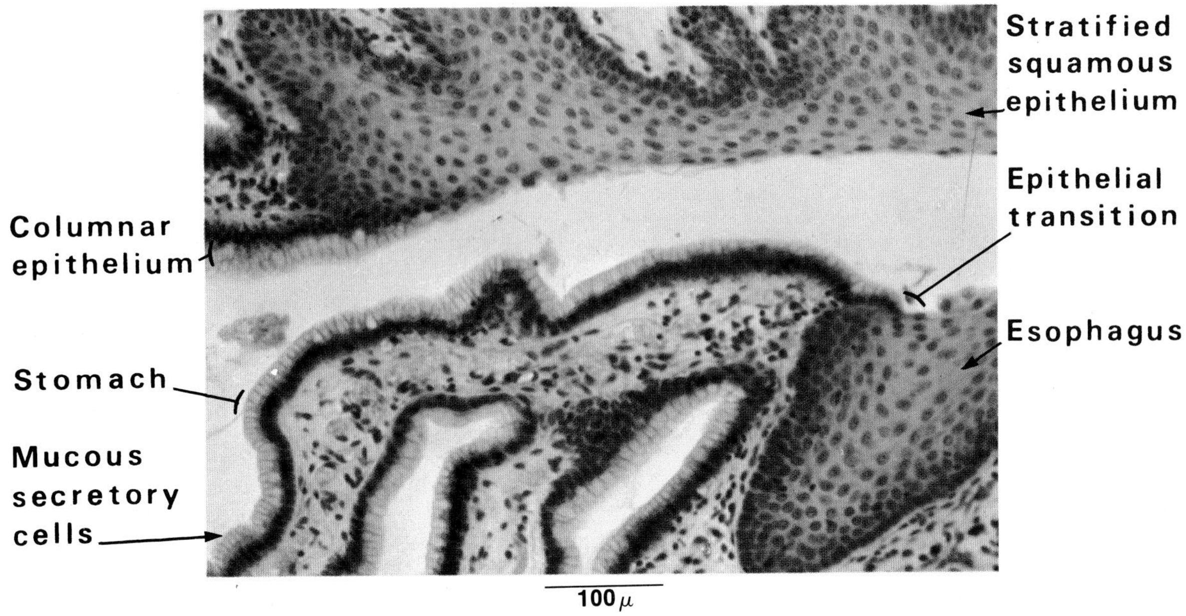

Stratified squamous epithelium

Epithelial transition

Esophagus

Columnar epithelium

Stomach

Mucous secretory cells

100 μ

Dog, Helly's fluid, H. & E., 162 x.

**Stratified squamous epithelium:** Lines the esophagus. Indented by connective tissue papillae.

**Epithelial transition:** From the stratified squamous epithelium of the esophagus to the columnar epithelium of the stomach. Note that the transition is abrupt and that only the basal cells of the esophagus continue into the stomach.

**Columnar epithelium:** Tall simple columnar with basal nuclei. Continuous with the basal layers of esophagus epithelium. These cells secrete protective mucus constantly.

## ESOPHAGUS
### Muscularis externa

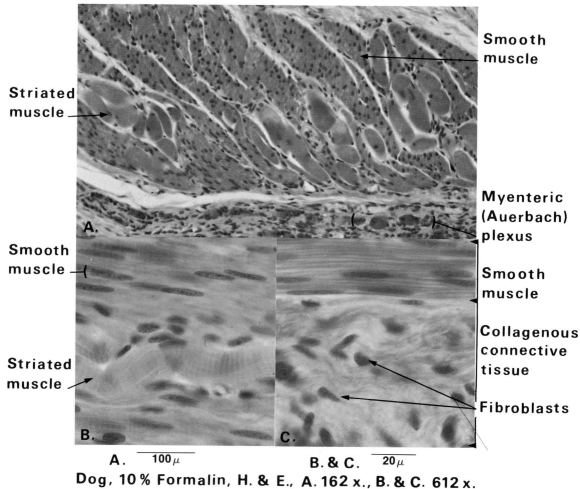

Striated muscle

Smooth muscle

Myenteric (Auerbach) plexus

Smooth muscle

Smooth muscle

Collagenous connective tissue

Striated muscle

Fibroblasts

A.    $\overline{100\,\mu}$      B. & C.    $\overline{20\,\mu}$

**Dog, 10% Formalin, H. & E., A. 162 x., B. & C. 612 x.**

The external muscular coat of the esophagus is made up entirely of skeletal muscles in the upper third; of skeletal and smooth muscles in the middle third (*A* and *B*); and of purely smooth muscle in the lower third (*C*). Outside the muscle layer is a layer of collagenous connective tissue with fibroblasts, the adventitia (*C*). The orientation of muscle fibers also varies. Typically, an inner circular and outer longitudinal layer exist but many bundles are arranged obliquely or in a spiral fashion. Between the two layers of muscle is a nerve plexus associated with numerous small ganglia, the myenteric plexus of Auerbach (*A*). This is mainly a parasympathetic plexus with some postganglionic sympathetic nerves. It is named after Leopold Auerbach, a German anatomist, who described it in 1862.

## MUCOSA
### Surface view

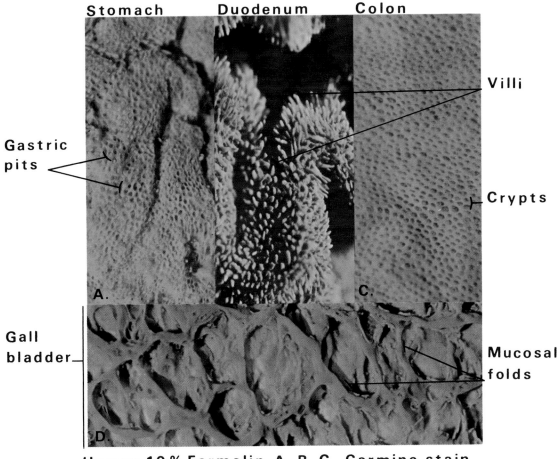

Stomach     Duodenum     Colon

Villi

Gastric pits

Crypts

Gall bladder

Mucosal folds

Human,10 % Formalin, A.,B.,C., Carmine stain, D. Unstained,10x.

    Striking differences in the surface of the mucosa of the stomach, duodenum, colon and gall bladder are illustrated in this plate.

    The mucosal surface of the stomach contains numerous cylindrical openings, the gastric pits. The cells lining the gastric pits secrete their products into the lumina of the gastric pits and the secretions flow onto the surface of the mucosa. In contrast, the surface of the intestinal mucosa is thrown into folds (the plicae circularis), with fingerlike projections, the intestinal villi, which characterize the small intestine. The villi and mucosal folds markedly increase the surface area of the absorptive and secreting surfaces of the small intestine. The surface of the colon (large intestine) lacks villi and is pitted like the stomach. Tubular glands (crypts of Lieberkühn) extend from the surface through the thickness of the mucosa. The mucosal surface of the gall bladder is also thrown into numerous folds, giving it a honeycomb appearance. Cross sections of these same organs are seen in Plates 165, 167, 178 and 191.

PLATE 165

# STOMACH
## Fundus

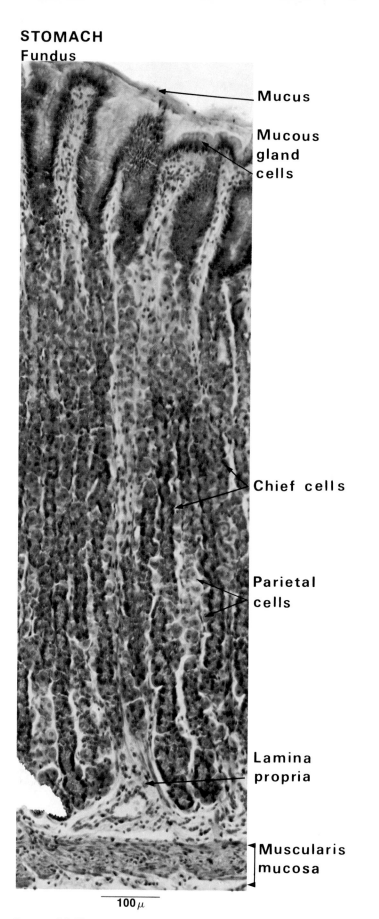

Mucus

Mucous
gland
cells

Chief cells

Parietal
cells

Lamina
propria

Muscularis
mucosa

100μ

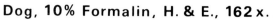

**Dog, 10% Formalin, H. & E., 162 x.**

Although this figure is labeled fundus, it shows the characteristic glands found in most of the wall of the stomach. The term "fundic" as applied to this type of gland is a misnomer since it is not limited to the fundus of the stomach but is found throughout most of the stomach wall except the cardiac and pyloric ends. Another term applied to these glands is "gastric." The fundic or gastric glands are simple (sometimes slightly branched), long tubular glands that extend throughout the mucosa down to the muscularis mucosa. Note the secreted mucus covering the surface of the epithelium and the mucous cells with their characteristic basal nuclei and clear cytoplasm. Fundic or gastric glands contain chief and parietal cells. The former are the more abundant, and have basally located nuclei and basophilic cytoplasm. They secrete pepsinogen and possibly a mucoprotein which enhances the absorption of Vitamin $B_{12}$. The parietal cells are larger and less abundant than the chief cells among which they are scattered. Their cytoplasm is eosinophilic and nuclei are centrally placed. They secrete HCl. See Plates 5 and 166.

The lamina propria is scanty and fills in the narrow spaces between glands.

The muscularis mucosa is thin and arranged in layers. Delicate muscular strands extend between glands.

## STOMACH
### Chief and parietal cells

Parietal cells

Chief cells

Mitochondria

Zymogen
granules
(pepsinogen)

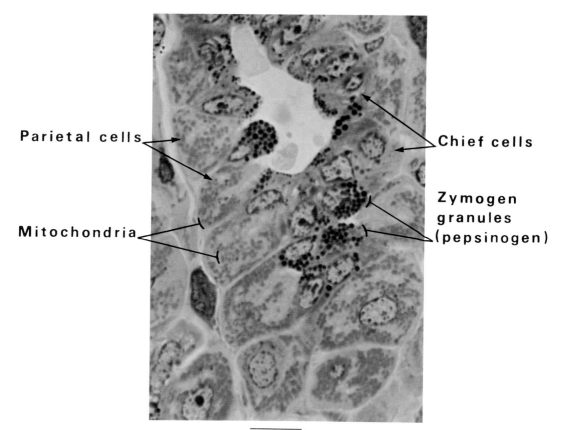

10μ

### Rhesus monkey, Glutaraldehyde – osmium
### fixation, Toluidine blue stain, 1416 x.

**Chief cells:**   Most numerous of gastric gland cells. Cuboidal or pyramidal in shape. Nucleus in basal half of the cell. Rich in cytoplasmic ribonucleic acid. Synthesizes zymogen granules containing pepsinogen.

**Parietal cells:**   Larger than chief cells, oval or polygonal in shape. Nuclei are spherical and centrally located. Cytoplasm is finely granular due to an abundance of mitochondria. Parietal cells secrete the hydrochloric acid of the gastric juice.

Note the cytological detail seen in this one-micron thin section and compare with Plate 5.

# DUODENUM AND JEJUNUM
## Cross section

Mucosa

Submucosa
Brunner's glands

Muscularis

Mucosa

Lamina propria

Lymph nodule

Submucosa

Muscularis

A.

B.

0.2 mm

## Human, 10% Formalin, H. & E., 50 x.

The basic pattern and arrangement of layers in the intestinal wall are seen in both the duodenum and jejunum. In each there is a mucosa, submucosa, muscularis and serosa.

The mucosa has fingerlike projections, the villi, lined by simple columnar epithelium. Villi of the duodenum tend to be flattened while those of the jejunum are more rounded. The core of the villus is composed of loose connective tissue, blood vessels, a lymphatic vessel, smooth muscle fibers and other cells of the connective tissue (see Plates 28, 170 and 173). This portion of the mucosa is named the lamina propria. The lamina propria terminates at the muscularis mucosa, which is composed of a band of smooth muscle fibers a few layers thick. Located within the mucosa are simple tubular intestinal glands, the crypts of Lieberkühn, and lymphatic nodules. Lymphatic nodules are found more frequently in the jejunum than in the duodenum.

The submucosa is composed of loose connective tissue and contains, in the duodenum but not the jejunum, the compound tubular mucous glands of Brunner. They are a continuation of the pyloric glands found in the stomach.

The muscularis contains an inner circular and an outer longitudinal layer of smooth muscle fibers. The two layers are separated by reticular and collagenous connective tissue containing nerve fibers and parasympathetic ganglion cells (Auerbach's plexus).

Surrounding the muscularis is the serosa, which consists primarily of loose connective tissue containing nerves, blood and lymphatic vessels. Wherever the intestine is not bound to the posterior abdominal wall the serosa continues into the suspending mesentery and is covered with mesothelium.

See also Plate 174

# DUODENUM AND JEJUNUM
## Submucosa

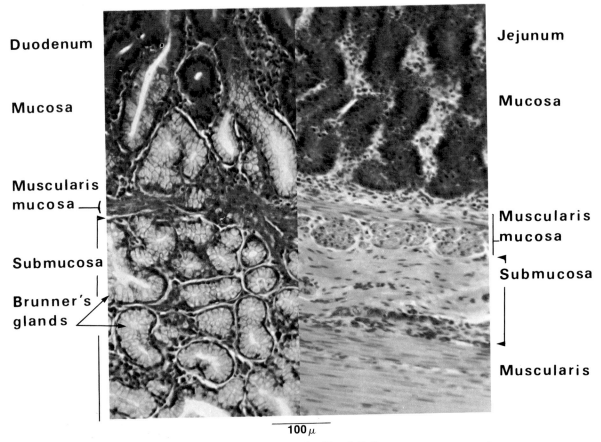

Duodenum

Jejunum

Mucosa

Mucosa

Muscularis
mucosa

Submucosa

Muscularis
mucosa

Submucosa

Brunner's
glands

Muscularis

100 μ

## Human, 10 % Formalin, H. & E., 162 x.

In this plate the structure of the duodenum and the jejunum can be compared. Both segments contain simple tubular glands composed of columnar epithelium separated by the connective tissue of the lamina propria. In the duodenum, note the presence of Brunner's glands in the submucosa which are diagnostic for this segment of the small intestine. Brunner's glands are compound tubular and are composed of low columnar cells which secrete mucus. The secretory cells closely resemble the cells of the pyloric glands, which also secrete mucus.

Although these glands were first described in 1679 by J. J. Wepfer, Brunner's father-in-law, credit is given to Johann Brunner, the Swiss anatomist, who drew attention to them in his dissertation in 1687.

See also Plate 167.

## DUODENUM
### Villi

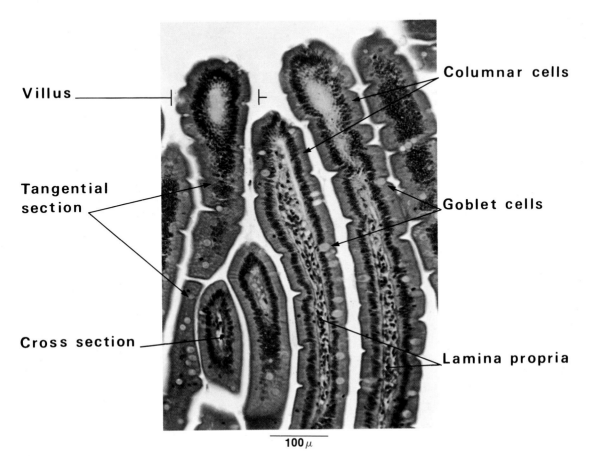

Villus

Tangential
section

Cross section

Columnar cells

Goblet cells

Lamina propria

100 μ

### Cat, Helly's fluid, Mallory's stain, 162x.

Fingerlike projections of the mucosa into the intestinal lumen characterize the small intestine. Note the simple columnar absorptive epithelial covering with basally located nuclei and the delicate basement membrane. Interspersed among the columnar absorptive cells are goblet cells which are unicellular mucous glands. The core of each villus is composed of loose, delicate connective tissue (lamina propria). See also Plate 170.

## DUODENUM
### Villus

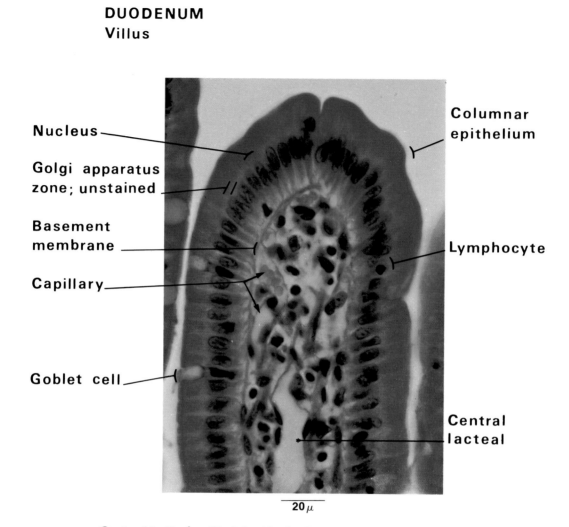

Nucleus

Golgi apparatus
zone; unstained

Basement
membrane

Capillary

Goblet cell

Columnar
epithelium

Lymphocyte

Central
lacteal

20 μ

### Cat, Helly's fluid, H. & E., 612 x.

The word villus is of Latin origin, meaning shaggy hair or a tuft of hair. The intestinal villi project from the intestinal wall like hairs or the nap on cloth. The term villus was first coined for the intestinal projections by Berengarius in 1524.

**Columnar epithelium:** Covers the surface of the villus. Surface of the epithelium has a striated border (microvilli by electron microscopy) to increase its absorptive surface. Products obtained from the extracellular digestive process, salts, vitamins and other substances are carried through the cytoplasm of these cells and delivered to the connective tissue to enter the blood vessels or lymphatics. The surface epithelial cells are being continuously shed from the apex of the villus (extrusion zone) and replaced by migrating cells from the bottom of the crypts (Plates 28 and 173).

**Nucleus:** Ovoid, located in the lower half of the columnar cell.

**Golgi apparatus zone:** Relatively pale area in this preparation. Specific stains are needed to demonstrate the Golgi apparatus which lies between the nuclei and free surface.

**Lymphocytes:** One of the cell types commonly found in the lamina propria. Seen migrating into the epithelial layer to be extruded into the lumen. See Plates 28 and 173.

**Goblet cell:** Dispersed among the columnar absorptive epithelial cells. They appear empty because some mucin is lost during the preparation of the specimen. The residual mucin stains poorly with the H. & E. stain. Nucleus is basally located. Compare the small number of goblet cells in this preparation with their abundant number in another region of the intestine (Plate 178).

**Basement membrane:** A delicate membrane which supports the epithelium. Composed primarily of reticular fibers embedded in an amorphous protein polysaccharide ground substance.

**Central lacteal:** A lymph vessel situated near the center of the villus. Note its endothelial lining. The lacteals become distended during absorption of fat.

**Capillary:** Capillaries of the villus form a network which lies underneath the basement membrane of the lining epithelium.

## DUODENUM

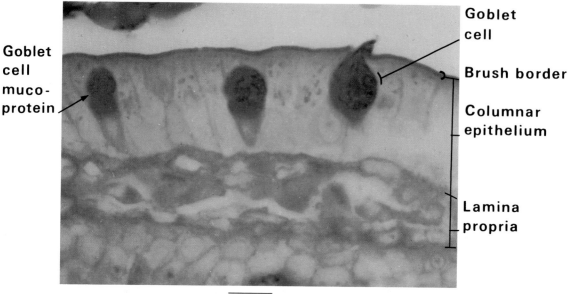

Goblet
cell
muco-
protein

Goblet
cell

Brush border

Columnar
epithelium

Lamina
propria

20 μ

Rhesus monkey, Helly's fluid, Periodic acid -
Schiff stain, 612 x.

The method used in this preparation stains protein polysaccharides (mucin) which are synthesized and excreted by goblet cells. The striated border and goblet cells are very well outlined, while the absorptive columnar epithelium and the lamina propria are not as intensely stained. The relatively unstained basal portion of the goblet cell represents the nuclear region and its surrounding narrow stem of cytoplasm.

# DUODENUM
## Intestinal gland
## Lamina propria

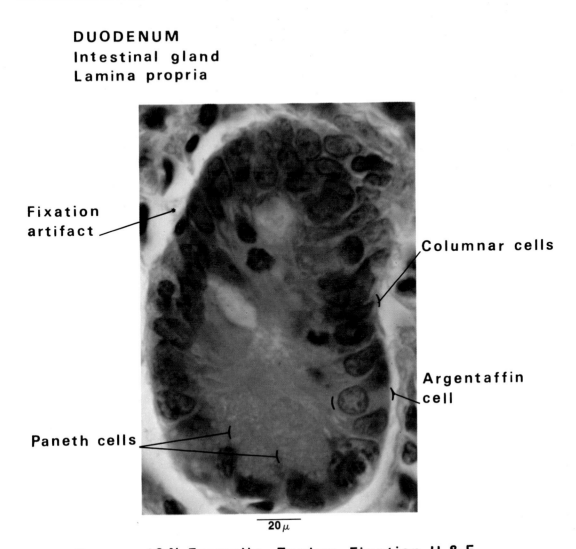

Fixation artifact

Columnar cells

Argentaffin cell

Paneth cells

20μ

Human, 10% Formalin—Zenker Fixation, H. & E., 612x.

Intestinal glands are simple tubular glands located in the mucous membrane. These glands are surrounded by a cell-rich connective tissue, the lamina propria. Intestinal glands of Lieberkühn secrete the so-called intestinal juice (succus entericus).

**Columnar cells:** Shorter than the columnar absorbing cells of the villi. Poorly developed striated border. Source of the surface epithelial cells at the apex of the villus.

**Argentaffin cells:** Also known as enterochromaffin cells. Fairly common in duodenum. Located among epithelial cells lining the crypts of Lieberkühn (intestinal glands). Contain fine granules stainable by silver salts (argentophilic) and by dichromate, and located in the abluminal portion of the cell between the nucleus and the basement membrane. Argentaffin cells are identified with the production of serotonin (5-hydroxytryptamine), which is secreted into the lamina propria rather than the intestinal lumen. Serotonin is a powerful stimulant of smooth muscle, resulting in contraction, and may play a role in stimulating peristaltic activity of the intestine.

**Paneth cells:** Coarsely granular cells in the depth of the intestinal gland. Acidophilic granules apically placed. The base of the cell is dark staining and basophilic. Acidophilic granules accumulate during fasting and disappear during digestion. The exact function of this cell is not established but it has been suggested that they may secrete digestive enzymes (lipoenzyme or a peptidase, or both).

231

## LAMINA PROPRIA
### Duodenum

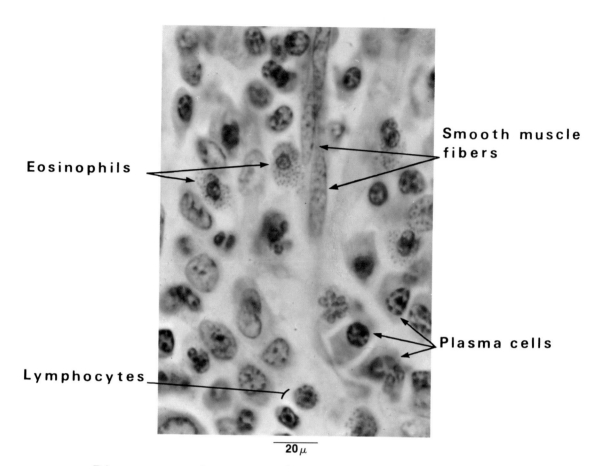

Eosinophils

Smooth muscle fibers

Plasma cells

Lymphocytes

20 μ

Rhesus monkey, Helly's fluid, H. & E., 612 x.

Lamina propria forms the connective tissue core of the villus and fills the spaces between glands. Primarily a reticular tissue framework with numerous lymphocytes, eosinophils and plasma cells. Single smooth muscle fibers derived from the muscularis mucosa are oriented longitudinally. Eosinophilic leucocytes and lymphocytes migrate from blood vessels. The lymphocytes seen here are of the small variety which are immunologically competent. The abundant plasma cells manufacture most of the antibody proteins.

## JEJUNUM
### Cross section

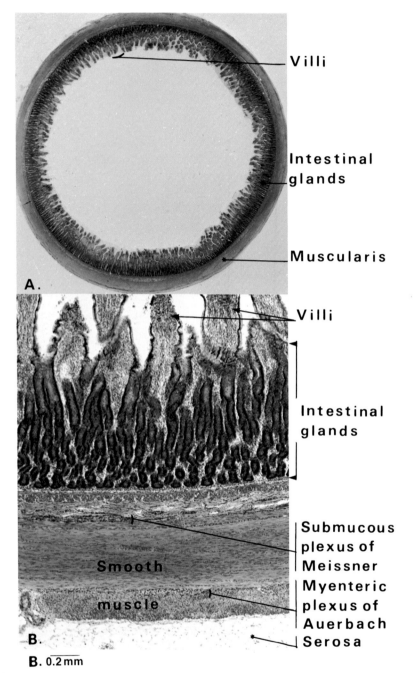

Villi

Intestinal glands

Muscularis

A.

Villi

Intestinal glands

Submucous plexus of Meissner

Smooth

Myenteric plexus of Auerbach

muscle

Serosa

B.

B. 0.2 mm

Cat, 10 % Formalin, H. & E., A. 3.8 x., B. 40 x.

*See text on following page.*

*A,* Low magnification plate of a cross section of the jejunum. Note the prominent fingerlike villi projecting into the lumen, and the darker intestinal glands beneath them. The prominent muscularis is seen outside the intestinal glands.

*B,* Higher magnification, showing some details of the structure of the jejunal wall. Each villus is covered by simple columnar epithelium and the connective tissue composing its core also fills spaces between intestinal glands. Note that the epithelium covering the villi continues into the intestinal glands. New cells are formed in the depth of these glands and migrate upward to the surface of the villi.

Note the plexus of Meissner in the submucosa and the myenteric plexus of Auerbach between the two layers of the muscularis. These plexuses contain autonomic ganglia that receive preganglionic parasympathetic fibers from the vagus nerve and sacral outflow. Postganglionic fibers pass to the muscles and vessels of the gut wall and stimulate muscular contraction and intestinal secretion. The two layers of the muscularis (inner circular and outer longitudinal) are well defined. The serosa is a connective tissue sheath on the outside of the intestinal wall, covered by mesothelial cells and continuous with the mesentery.

## JEJUNUM
## Muscularis mucosa
## submucosal plexus of Meissner

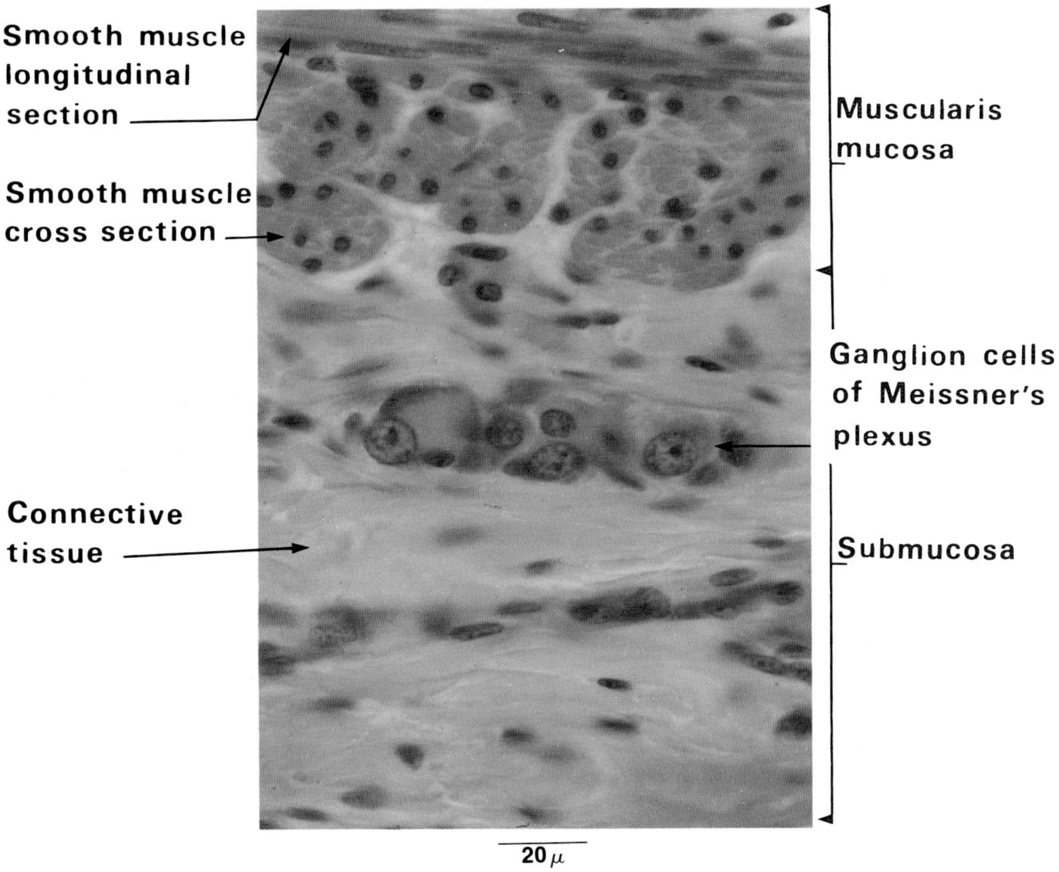

Smooth muscle
longitudinal
section ——————

Smooth muscle
cross section ——→

Connective
tissue ——————→

Muscularis
mucosa

Ganglion cells
of Meissner's
plexus

Submucosa

20 μ

## Cat, 10 % Formalin, H. & E., 612 x.

This is a section of part of the wall of the jejunum showing the muscularis mucosa and submucosa. In the muscularis mucosa note the two layers of smooth muscle, inner circular and outer longitudinal. The submucosa is composed of loose connective tissue and contains the ganglion cells of Meissner's plexus. These cells receive preganglionic parasympathetic vagal fibers. Postganglionic fibers pass to the muscles of the gut wall and its vessels. They excite muscular (peristaltic) activity and intestinal secretion.

## JEJUNUM

Lamina propria —

Paneth cells —

Muscularis mucosa

Submucosa

Crypt of Lieberkühn

Paneth cells

Smooth muscle

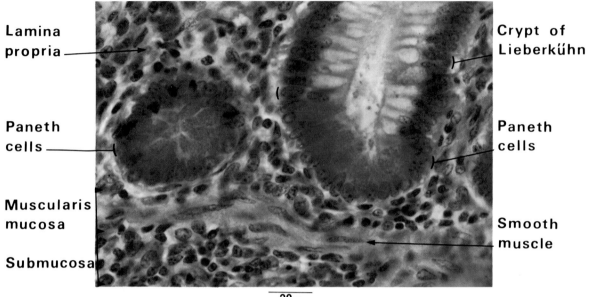

$\overline{20\,\mu}$

## Human, 10 % Formalin, H. & E., 612 x.

**Crypt of Lieberkühn:** Simple tubular intestinal glands in the mucosa which extend through the lamina propria to the level of the muscularis mucosa. The simple columnar epithelium of these glands is continuous with the surface epithelium lining the villi. Undifferentiated epithelial cells of the crypts give rise to the surface epithelial cells covering the villi. In addition to goblet cells, Paneth cells are found in the crypts. The latter contain coarse acidophilic granules that probably represent zymogen. See Plate 172. These cells are located in the depth of the crypt.

**Smooth muscle:** Circularly arranged in the muscularis mucosa.

**Lamina propria:** Connective tissue stroma filling the spaces between the crypts. Also see Plates 28 and 168.

**Submucosa:** Connective tissue coat, containing an abundance of lymphocytes.

## APPENDIX

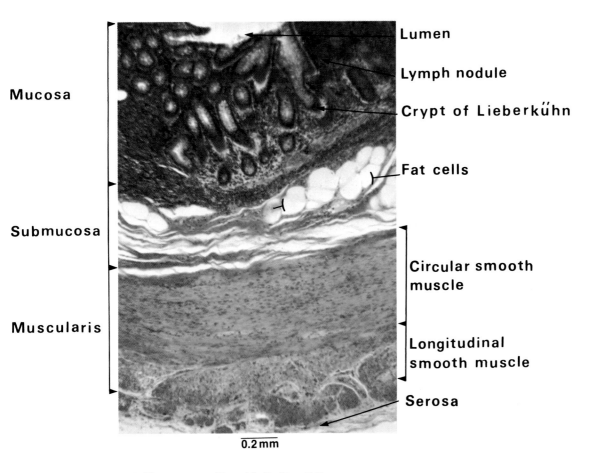

Mucosa

Submucosa

Muscularis

Lumen

Lymph nodule

Crypt of Lieberkühn

Fat cells

Circular smooth muscle

Longitudinal smooth muscle

Serosa

0.2 mm

Human, 10 % Formalin, H. & E., 50 x.

The histologic structure of the appendix resembles that of the colon. The lumen is, however, much smaller than that of the colon and often is obliterated by debris.

**Mucosa:** Consists of the lining columnar epithelium (which lacks villi), simple tubular intestinal glands (crypts of Lieberkühn), muscularis mucosa, and conspicuous lymph nodules.

**Submucosa:** Thick and rich in fat cells.

**Muscularis:** Relatively thin and composed of two layers of smooth muscle, inner circular and outer longitudinal.

**Serosa:** Loose areolar connective tissue coat continuous with a mesentery that surrounds the appendix.

## COLON

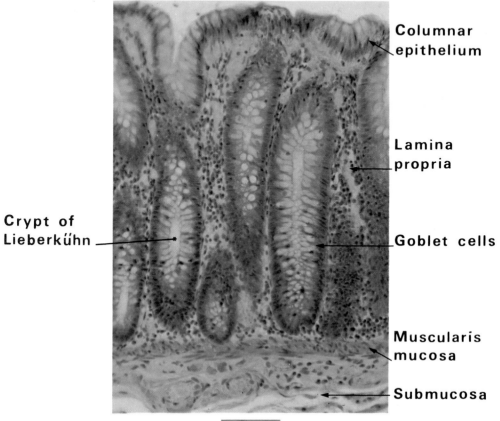

Columnar epithelium

Lamina propria

Crypt of Lieberkühn

Goblet cells

Muscularis mucosa

Submucosa

100 μ

## Human, 10 % Formalin, H. & E., 162 x.

**Columnar epithelium:** Tall columnar epithelium lines the absorbing surface of the colon. Goblet cells are interspersed among the columnar absorbing cells. These columnar cells are primarily concerned with the absorption of water and possibly other substances (*e.g.*, vitamins) from the colon.

**Goblet cells:** Interspersed among the superficial columnar cells. They are very numerous in the depth of the crypts. Produce the copious mucus needed in the colon to facilitate passage of dehydrated undigested materials through the digestive tract.

**Lamina propria:** Connective tissue (rich in plasma cells, lymphocytes, eosinophils and other cells) located between glands.

**Muscularis mucosa:** Note the two layers of smooth muscle (inner circular and outer longitudinal).

**Submucosa:** Loose connective tissue stroma containing vessels and nerves.

**Crypts of Lieberkühn:** The name of the simple tubular glands opening into the intestine. They were described by Johann Lieberkühn in a memoir on the small intestine published at Leyden in 1745. Although named after him, they were first noted by Malpighi in 1688.

## RECTUM AND ANAL CANAL

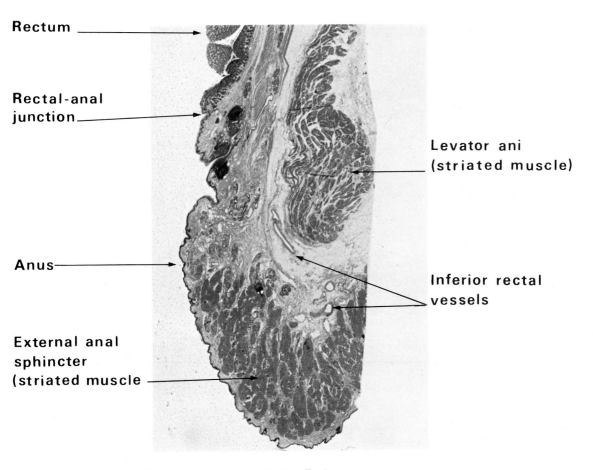

Rectum

Rectal-anal junction

Levator ani (striated muscle)

Anus

Inferior rectal vessels

External anal sphincter (striated muscle

Cat, 10% Formalin, H. & E., 5.4 x.

This plate shows the changes that take place at the recto-anal junction. Note the transition in the type of epithelium from the simple columnar of the rectum to a stratified epithelium in the anal canal. The nonkeratinized stratified squamous epithelium of the anal canal changes into epidermis at the anal orifice. The external anal sphincter surrounds the whole length of the anal canal and keeps the anal canal and anus closed. During defecation, the sphincter is relaxed. Note the levator ani muscle at the recto-anal junction. This striated muscle fuses with the longitudinal smooth muscle coat of the rectum. Inferior rectal vessels supply the muscles and skin of the anal region.

## PAROTID GLAND

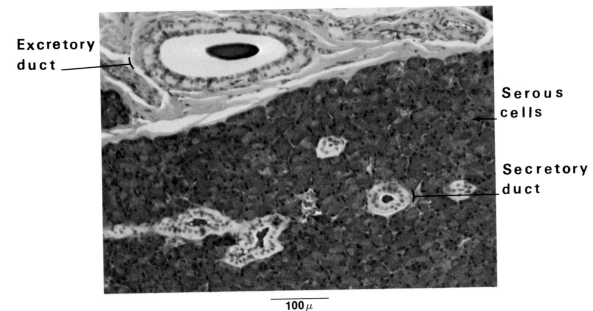

Excretory duct

Serous cells

Secretory duct

$\overline{100\,\mu}$

Rhesus monkey, Zenker's fluid, H.& E., 162 x.

**Excretory duct:** In the connective tissue septa. Simple columnar epithelial lining. Gradation to stratified epithelium occurs as the duct approaches the main outlet.

**Secretory duct:** Cuboidal to low columnar epithelial lining depending on location and size. Found in connective tissue septa between and within lobules of the gland.

**Serous cells:** Form a circular cluster of pyramidal cells with a central lumen (acinus). Acini of the human parotid gland are pure serous. The serous secretion is watery and contains salts, proteins and amylase. Amylase is an enzyme which splits starch and glycogen into smaller carbohydrates, dextrins and maltose. Acinar cells have basal nuclei and secretory granules which are found between the free or luminal surface and the nucleus.

Salivary secretion is essential to the swallowing process and for taste. In addition, the salivary secretion continuously rinses the oral cavity and is antimicrobial. Digestion begins in the mouth, where the food is mixed with saliva, and continues in the stomach, within the bolus of chewed and moistened food, until the acid gastric juices penetrate the bolus. The parotid gland produces about one-fourth of the daily output of 1 liter of saliva. In man and dog the watery secretion of parotid gland acini is modified by the striated ducts through the absorption of sodium and chloride, producing a saliva hypotonic with respect to blood. With increased flow of saliva, the reabsorption of these salts fails to keep pace and the sodium concentration increases. The epithelium of the parotid ducts also excretes iodide into the saliva.

The secretion of salivary glands is dependent upon their innervation, and each major gland is supplied by both sympathetic and parasympathetic nerves. Although the specific role of the sympathetic innervation is still uncertain it would appear that under normal circumstances the sympathetic fibers are inhibitory and parasympathetic stimulation is secretory.

## PAROTID GLAND

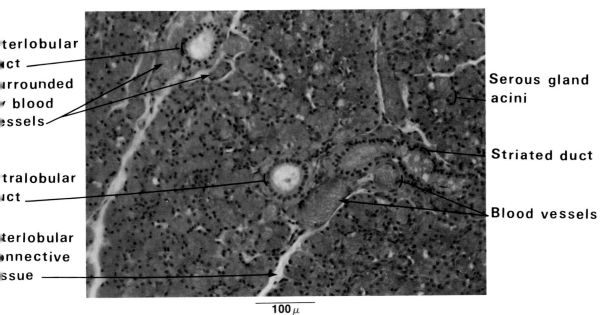

terlobular
uct
urrounded
blood
essels

tralobular
uct

terlobular
onnective
ssue

Serous gland
acini

Striated duct

Blood vessels

100μ

Human, 10% Formalin, H. & E., 162 x.

**Interlobular duct surrounded by blood vessels:** Located in the septa separating lobules. Lining epithelium cuboidal to low columnar.

**Intralobular duct:** Located within the lobules. Lined by cuboidal epithelium.

**Interlobular connective tissue:** Septa that extend from the capsule separate lobes and lobules of the parotid gland. Carry ducts, nerves, blood and lymph vessels.

**Serous gland acini:** The parotid gland of man is purely serous. Individual acini are lined by pyramidal cells with basal nuclei and a small, hardly visible lumen.

**Striated duct:** So named because some segments of the intralobular duct show basal striations. These ducts are believed to be secretory in nature and contribute water and calcium salts to the gland secretions.

# SUBMANDIBULAR GLAND
## Striated ducts

Mucous cells

Serous cells

Mixed alveolus

Striated ducts

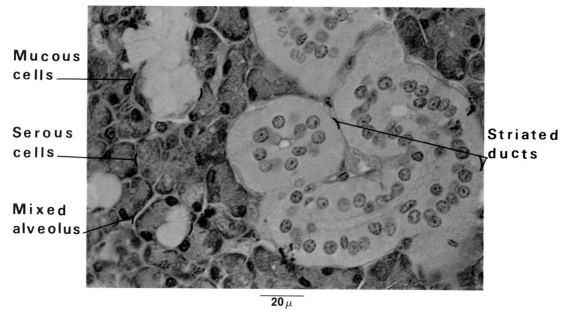

20 μ

## Human, Zenker's fluid, H. & E., 612 x

**Mucous cells:** Nuclei flattened and pushed to the basal part of the cell by secretory droplets. Purely mucous alveoli are not frequent in human submandibular gland.

**Serous cells:** Pyramidal in shape, darkly staining, with indistinct cell boundaries. Nuclei are more rounded and are pushed to the base of the cell by secretory droplets (zymogen granules) in some cells.

**Mixed alveolus:** Made up of serous and mucous cells. In mixed alveoli, serous cells cap mucous alveoli (so-called demilune) or line terminal portions of mucous alveoli.

**Striated ducts:** So called because of prominent basal striations. These ducts are long and very conspicuous in sections of the submandibular gland. Lined by columnar cells with apically placed nuclei. Electron microscopy reveals the striations to be invaginations of the basal plasma membrane, with rows of elongated mitochondria in the pockets thus formed. The striated ducts play a role in secretion and absorption of salts and thereby modify the composition of the saliva produced by the secretory cells. The secretory product enters the oral cavity near the frenulum of the tongue. The submandibular gland produces about two-thirds of the daily output of 1 liter of saliva. The saliva from this gland is a viscid solution containing mucin, salts and the enzyme amylase.

## SUBLINGUAL GLAND

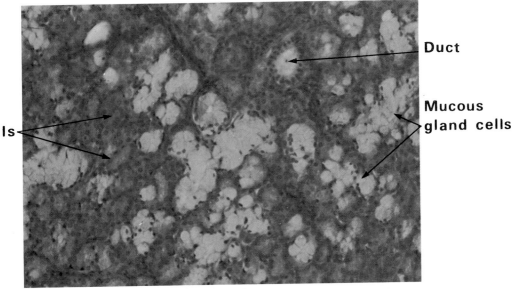

Serous gland cells

Duct

Mucous gland cells

100 μ

## Human, 10% Formalin, H. & E., 162 x.

The sublingual gland of man is a mixed gland with a preponderance of mucous gland cells. Most of the secretory units are either pure mucous or mixed mucous and serous. Pure serous units are not common. Ducts of the sublingual gland are short and are not commonly seen in sections.

## PANCREAS
### Acinar and centroacinar cells

Cytoplasmic
basophilia
of acinar
cells

Acinar
cells

Centro-
acinar cell

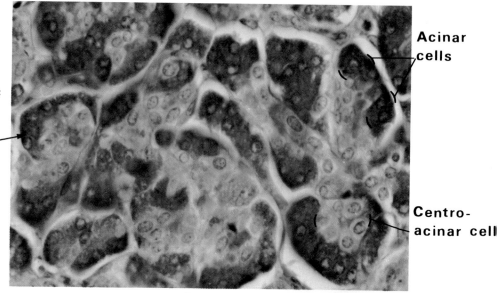

20 μ

### Human, 10 % Formalin, Toluidine blue and eosin stains, 612 x.

**Acinar cells:**   Cells forming the alveoli or acini of the pancreas. Pyramid-shaped cells arranged around a central lumen. Alveoli are packed close together with intervening delicate connective tissue. Cytoplasm of individual acinar cells is densely basophilic and the nucleus is spherical and basally located. The cytoplasmic basophilia (RNA) is a reflection of the specialization of these cells for protein synthesis and secretion of zymogen.

**Centroacinar cells:**   Belong to the duct system. Smaller than the surrounding acinar cells. Centroacinar cells stain lighter than acinar cells and are squamous to cuboidal. Centroacinar cells occur only in the pancreas.

**LIVER**
Portal canal

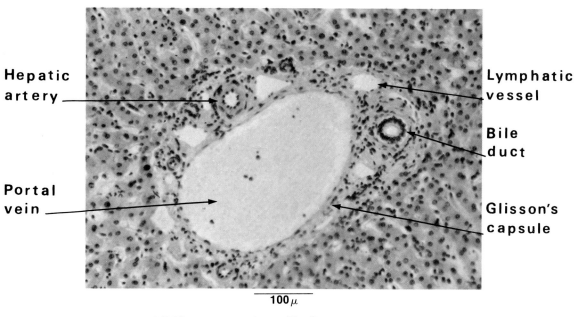

Hepatic artery

Lymphatic vessel

Bile duct

Portal vein

Glisson's capsule

100 μ

**Human, 10% Formalin, H. & E., 162 x**

The portal canals are located at the periphery of the hepatic lobule and contain the triad composed of branches of the hepatic artery, a thin-walled portal vein and a bile duct. A small lymphatic vessel is usually found in addition. The portal canal is surrounded by Glisson's capsule, composed of dense collagenous fibers. The bile duct is lined with cuboidal or low columnar epithelium.

# LIVER

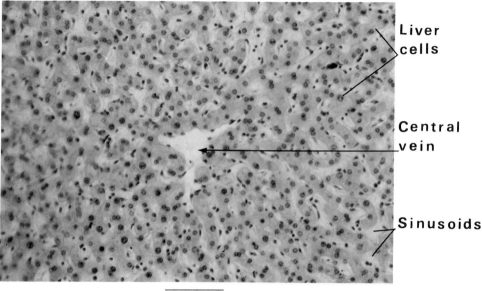

Liver
cells

Central
vein

Sinusoids

100 μ

## Human, 10% Formalin, H. & E., 162x.

**Liver cells:**  Polyhedral cells with a round central nucleus. Arranged in cords and plates radiating in a spoke-like manner from the central vein.

**Central vein:**  Forms the axis of the hepatic lobule. Receives blood from the hepatic sinusoids and drains into intercalated (sublobular) veins.

**Sinusoids:**  Form an extensive fenestrated system of vascular channels which radiate from the central vein. Lined with endothelial cells and Kupffer phagocytic cells. Receive blood from the interlobular branches of the portal vein and hepatic artery at the periphery of the lobule. Blood flows toward the center of the lobule and is drained by the central vein. Also see Plates 8, 36, 187 and 190.

The liver is essential to life and, although it is the largest gland in the body, only a fraction of its total mass is required. The liver can be considered both an exocrine gland, secreting bile via a system of bile ducts into the duodenum, and an endocrine gland, synthesizing and releasing a variety of organic compounds into the blood stream. The importance of the liver can be appreciated by considering the blood supply to the organ. The liver receives blood directly from the digestive tract, which is rich in absorbed carbohydrates, amino acids, salts and vitamins; from the pancreas, containing the hormones insulin and glucagon; and from the spleen, breakdown products of red blood cell destruction. The liver metabolizes digestion products, synthesizes other substances for use or storage elsewhere, stores glycogen and fat, maintains blood glucose levels, synthesizes blood proteins, degrades or detoxifies harmful substances and eliminates them in the bile, and secretes bile, which plays an important role in the digestive process.

## LIVER

**Hepatic cords** 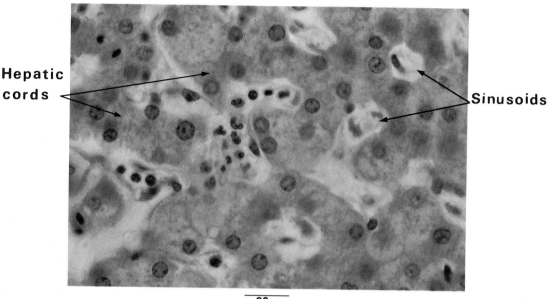 **Sinusoids**

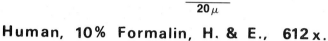

$\overline{20\,\mu}$

## Human, 10% Formalin, H. & E., 612x.

**Hepatic cords:**  Sheets or plates of hepatic cells, one cell thick. Note the large polyhedral liver cells with round nuclei and prominent nucleoli.

**Sinusoids:**  Tortuous channels connecting vessels at the periphery of the lobule with the central vein. Course between hepatic cords.

See legend of Plate 186 for discussion of liver functions.

## BILE CANALICULI
### Liver cells

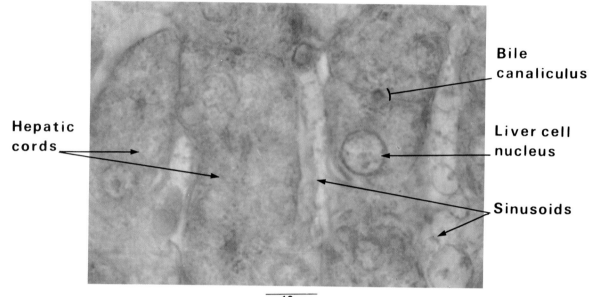

Bile canaliculus

Hepatic cords

Liver cell nucleus

Sinusoids

10 μ

**Human, Zenker's fluid, Mallory's stain, 1416 x.**

**Hepatic cords:**  See Plate 187.

**Liver cell nucleus:**  Large and centrally placed.

**Sinusoids:**  See Plate 187.

**Bile canaliculi:**  Seen in cross section, these are channels between rows of cells within hepatic cords. Bile flows toward the periphery of the lobule to enter the system of bile ducts and gall bladder. Also see Plate 189.

## LIVER
### Bile canaliculi

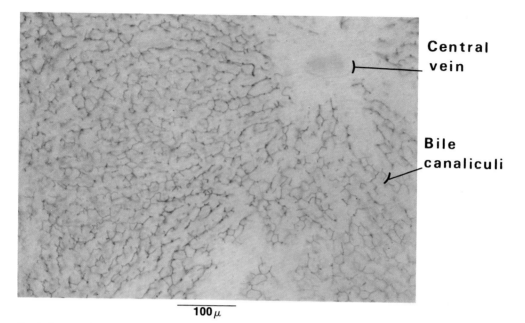

Central vein

Bile canaliculi

100 μ

**Rabbit, Golgi method, rapid process, 162 x.**

**Central vein:** In the center of the hepatic lobule. Receives the blood from all the sinusoids of the lobule. Also see Plates 186 and 190.

**Bile canaliculi:** Minute anastomosing channels formed by adjacent hepatic cells into which bile is secreted. Also see Plate 188.

Bile is secreted by the hepatic cells and is composed of water, bile salts, bile pigments, cholesterol, lecithin, fat and inorganic salts. Bile secreted into the duodenum produces an acceleration in the action of pancreatic and intestinal lipases and facilitates the absorption of fats from the intestine. Bile salts are absorbed during digestion and returned to the liver for reutilization. It is believed that the bile salts are secreted twice during the digestion of a single meal (enterohepatic circulation).

## LIVER
### Phagocytic Kupffer cells

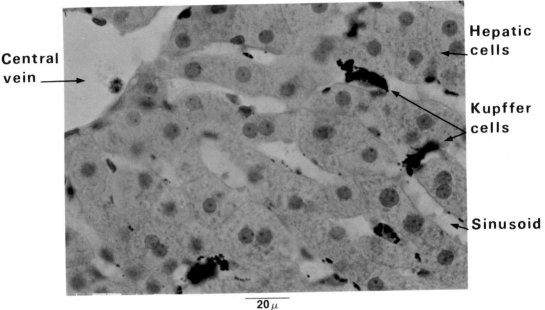

Central vein →

Hepatic cells

Kupffer cells

Sinusoid

20 μ

**Rabbit, 10% Formalin, H. & E., 612 x.**

**Hepatic cells:** Arranged in cords. Note the binucleate hepatic cells.

**Sinusoids:** Vascular channels between hepatic cords. Blood flows in them toward the central vein.

**Central vein:** In the center of the lobule. Receives blood from the sinusoids.

**Kupffer cells:** Reticuloendothelial cells in the walls of the sinusoids of the liver were described by Kupffer, a German anatomist, in 1876. His observations led to a better understanding of the so-called reticuloendothelial (macrophage) system. The Kupffer cells belong to the group of mixed macrophages. They act to clear the blood of foreign particles, aging and damaged red blood cells and other cellular debris. They are also said to play a role in fat metabolism and in the formation of bile pigment.

# GALL BLADDER

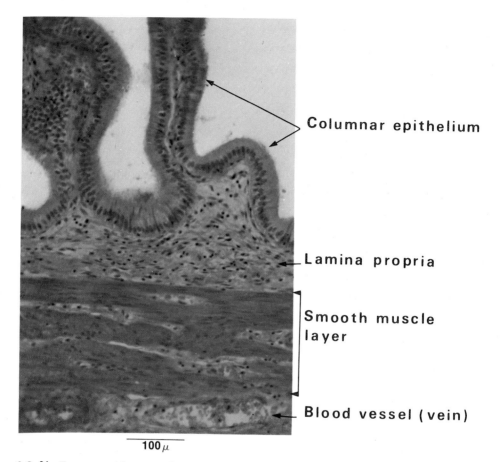

Columnar epithelium

Lamina propria

Smooth muscle layer

Blood vessel (vein)

$\overline{100\,\mu}$

**Human, 10% Formalin, H. & E., 162 x.**

The wall of the gall bladder consists of a mucosa composed of surface epithelium and lamina propria, a layer of smooth muscle and a perimuscular connective tissue and serosa.

The mucosal lining of the bladder is markedly folded. The lining epithelium of the folds is composed of tall columnar pale-staining cells with ovoid, basally located nuclei. The folds have a core composed of a delicate, richly vascular connective tissue. The gall bladder wall does not have a submucosa. Note the muscular layer next to the lamina propria. This is formed of interlacing bundles of smooth muscle fibers, most of which are circularly disposed and separated by fibroelastic tissue. The blood vessels outside the muscular layer are located in the perimuscular connective tissue.

# Section 11    The Respiratory System

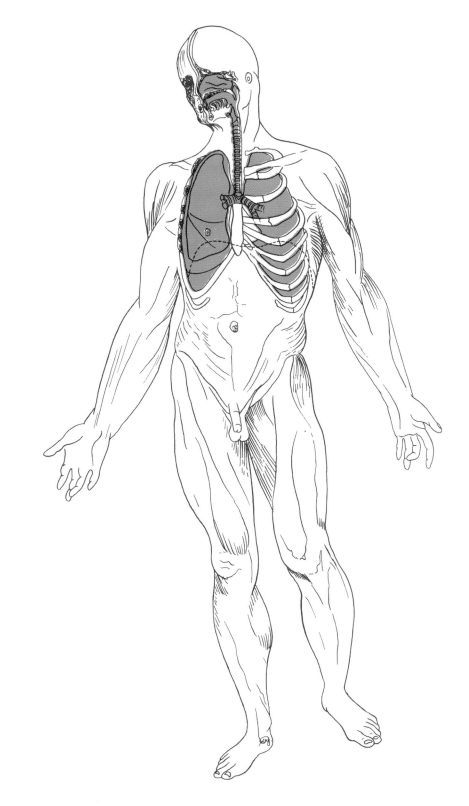

# The Respiratory System

The respiratory system is composed of conducting and respiratory passages which serve several functions. The primary function of this system is the exchange of oxygen and carbon dioxide; secondary functions are phonation and olfaction.

The conducting portion of the respiratory system includes the nasal cavity, paranasal sinuses, nasopharynx, larynx, trachea and bronchi. The conducting portion, from the nostrils to the lungs, warms, humidifies and filters the air. The mucus secreted by goblet cells (approximately 1 liter per day) entraps particulate matter, and the cilia of the pseudostratified columnar epithelial lining help to remove the mucus from the respiratory system.

The trachea is a relatively rigid tube about 11 cm in length and 2.5 cm in diameter. At the inferior border of the superior mediastinum of the thorax the trachea bifurcates into two primary bronchi which are structurally similar to the trachea. The mucosa of these tubes is supported by incomplete cartilaginous rings. Three layers of the wall are recognizable. (1) The mucosa is composed of a ciliated pseudostratified columnar epithelium and numerous goblet cells, both of which rest on a prominent, thick basement membrane. A thin lamina propria is composed of collagenous, elastic and reticular fibers and may contain accumulations of lymphocytes. There is no muscularis mucosa. (2) The submucosa contains seromucous glands, located primarily at the interspaces between the cartilaginous rings, and some fat cells. (3) The adventitia contains the cartilaginous rings interconnected by connective tissue. Each ring is composed of hyaline cartilage, appears in the form of the letter C or Y, and is open posteriorly. The open ends are connected by fibroelastic tissue and a band of smooth muscle (the trachealis muscle). This soft tissue band on the posterior surface of the trachea, which faces the esophagus, is capable of yielding to esophageal dilation resulting from the passage of food or liquid. The cartilaginous rings mechanically hold the airway open but also give it flexibility. By preventing the collapse of the conducting pathway respiration is not impeded (Plates 192 and 194).

The lungs are contained within the paired pleural cavities in the thorax. The lungs lie free within the pleural sac but are firmly attached at the hilus to the mediastinum, where a primary bronchus and the pulmonary vessels are located.

Beginning with the bronchus, the designated subdivisions of the respiratory tree within the lung include: bronchiole, respiratory bronchiole, alveolar duct, alveolar sacs and alveoli.

The epithelium of the bronchus is pseudostratified columnar ciliated, with numerous goblet cells. The subsequent branching and reduction in size of the bronchi result in a change in the epithelium to simple columnar ciliated, with abundant goblet cells. The lamina propria is encircled by a smooth muscle layer, which when contracted gives the tube a folded appearance. The connective tissue outside the muscle contains seromucous glands. Solitary lymph nodules may be present in the mucosa and in the connective tissue around the cartilage. The adventitia contains hyaline cartilage in the form of plates rather than rings.

The bronchiole is a smaller subdivision of the conducting tube and varies in size from about 0.5 to 1 mm in diameter. The ciliated epithelium is columnar, and diminishes to a cuboidal form as the branching to successively smaller bronchioles continues. The muscle layer becomes the dominant structure, and is composed of smooth muscle fibers and elastic tissue. Within the adventitia there is a reduction and then elimination of the cartilaginous plates, glands and lymph nodules. The mucosa of the smaller bronchioles may be highly folded due to the loss of firm supporting structures. (See Plates 29, 194 and 195.)

The respiratory segments include the respiratory bronchioles, alveolar ducts, alveolar sacs and alveoli. These crucially important segments of the lung mark the transition from the conducting to the respiratory passages, where oxygen and carbon dioxide are exchanged.

The epithelium of the respiratory bronchiole is primarily cuboidal and may be ciliated. Goblet cells are absent. The epithelium is supported by a thin collagenous layer, in which smooth muscle and some elastic fibers are found. Alveoli appear as small pockets which interrupt the main wall. Alveoli become more numerous distally. The respiratory bronchiole branches to form alveolar ducts. These thin walled, fibroelastic tubes are lined with a squamous epithelium and possess alveoli which appear as outpockets of the main wall. The main wall between alveoli contains smooth muscle. The terminal portion of the respiratory duct (atrium) gives rise to the alveolar sacs, composed of a variable number of alveoli which appear as small compartments opening into the alveolar sac. The alveoli are the smallest and most numerous subdivisions of the respiratory system. The alveolar wall is lined by a thin squamous epithelium covered with a thin film of fluid rich in hydrophilic lipid. The epithelium rests upon a basement membrane which, in turn, is intimately associated with capillaries of the pulmonary vascular system. The extremely thin wall and rich capillary bed favor the transfer of oxygen to the red blood corpuscles and the release and transfer of carbon dioxide to the alveolar airway. (See Plates 198 and 199.)

Several important structural arrangements are essential to respiratory function. The lungs are enclosed in the pleural cavities, which enlarge as the thorax expands during inspiration. This results in a negative pressure within the respiratory tree and air enters the system. During the filling of the lungs, the rich elastic network throughout the system becomes stretched, expanding and elongating the alveolar ducts and drawing oxygen-rich air into, and mixing it with, the carbon dioxide-rich air already contained within the alveoli. During expiration, air is expelled from the system by elastic recoil as the thoracic cavity decreases in size. During muscular exercise skeletal muscles assist in this process.

If the pleural cavities are exposed to air from the outside through an artificial opening in the thoracic wall, the lungs will collapse and will not fill during inspiration owing to the equalization of the air pressure inside and outside the lungs.

## TRACHEA

Ciliated
pseudostratified
columnar
epithelium

Lamina
propria

Perichondrium

Hyaline
cartilage

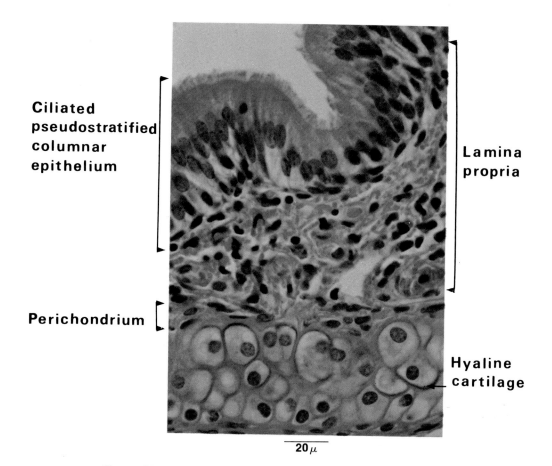

20 μ

### Rat, Helly's fluid, H. & E., 612 x.

This is a section of the wall of the trachea showing the ciliated pseudostratified columnar epithelial lining, the fibrous lamina propria and a small segment of hyaline cartilage with its perichondrium. The cartilage forms an irregular C- or Y-shaped ring around the trachea. The free ends are joined by a band of smooth muscle and face dorsally adjacent to the esophagus.

# CILIATED PSEUDOSTRATIFIED COLUMNAR EPITHELIUM
## Trachea

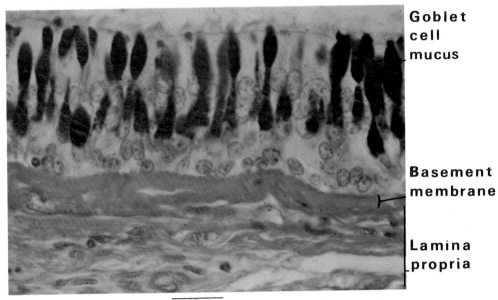

Goblet
cell
mucus

Basement
membrane

Lamina
propria

10 μ

**Human, Helly's fluid, Periodic acid – Schiff and hematoxylin stain, 1416 x.**

**Goblet cell:** Mucin-secreting, nonciliated columnar cell. The secretion of these cells collects inhaled particulate materials.

**Ciliated cells:** Tall columnar; central nucleus; form the ciliated pseudostratified epithelium of the trachea. Cilia extend into the lumen of the trachea and sweep particulate material away from the respiratory alveoli and out of the respiratory tree.

**Basement membrane:** Unusually thick and prominent. Composed of reticular fibers and protein polysaccharides. The apparent thickness of the basement membrane in this location is attributed to closely applied elastic fibers.

**Lamina propria:** Thin, fibrous layer with abundant elastic fibers.

See also Plates 19 and 192.

## BRONCHUS and BRONCHIOLE

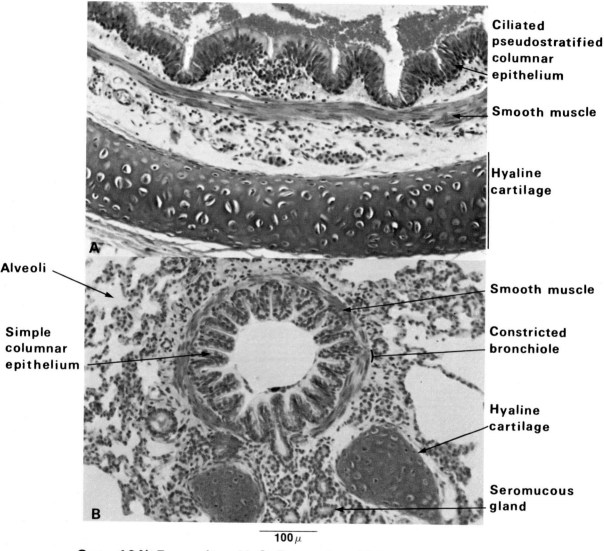

Ciliated pseudostratified columnar epithelium

Smooth muscle

Hyaline cartilage

Alveoli

Simple columnar epithelium

Smooth muscle

Constricted bronchiole

Hyaline cartilage

Seromucous gland

A

B

100 μ

Cat, 10% Formalin, H. & E. stain, 162 x.

In *A*, part of a bronchus can be seen. Bronchi are lined by pseudostratified columnar epithelium with goblet cells. The thickness and layering of the epithelium decreases gradually with the decrease in size of bronchi. A smooth muscle layer encircles a thin connective tissue lamina propria. In contrast to the trachea, the smooth muscle of the bronchus is arranged in interlacing spirals around the bronchus. Between the smooth muscle layer and the cartilage is the submucosa, which may contain seromucous glands, not seen in this preparation. The hyaline cartilage is arranged in discontinuous plates around the bronchus.

In *B*, a bronchiole is seen in the midst of respiratory tissue. The epithelium is simple columnar ciliated. The lamina propria is replaced by the muscle layer which encircles the bronchiole. In man, cartilage and glands are characteristically present until bronchioles decrease in size to approximately 0.5 mm in diameter.

## BRONCHIOLE

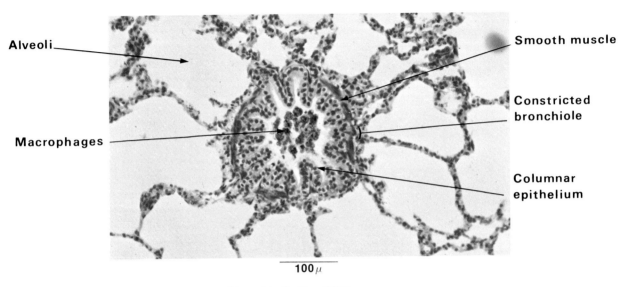

Alveoli

Smooth muscle

Macrophages

Constricted
bronchiole

Columnar
epithelium

100 μ

**Cat, 10% Formalin, H. & E., 162 x.**

This is a cross section of a bronchiole surrounded by respiratory tissue. Note the low columnar epithelial lining, the prominence of smooth muscle fibers in the lamina propria and the absence of cartilaginous plates and glands. Macrophages filled with black carbon particles are seen in the lumen of the bronchiole. The elastic spongework of respiratory tissue surrounding the bronchioles prevents their collapse during inspiration. Every inspiratory movement exerts a pull on the wall of the bronchiole protecting it from collapse, hence there is no need for cartilage rings or plates.

## LUNG
### Respiratory bronchioles

**Pulmonary blood vessels**

**Respiratory bronchiole**

**Visceral pleura**

**Alveolar ducts**

**Alveolar sacs**

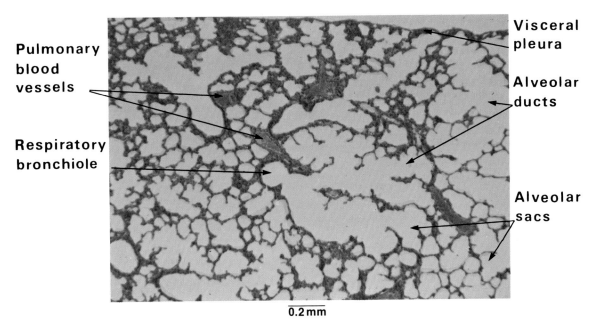

0.2mm

### Cat, 10% Formalin, H. & E., 50x.

**Respiratory bronchioles:** A branch of the terminal bronchiole. Alveoli arise as outpouchings of the bronchiole. Pulmonary arteries and veins are found adjacent to the bronchiole, but only capillaries extend beyond the respiratory bronchiole.

**Alveolar ducts:** Arise by branching of respiratory bronchioles; walls made up of alveolar sacs and alveoli.

**Alveolar sacs:** Cluster of alveoli which open into the lumen of the alveolar ducts. Composed of squamous epithelial cells, basement membrane and capillaries. Site of respiratory exchange.

**Visceral pleura:** A serous membrane that intimately covers the surface of the lung.

## RESPIRATORY BRONCHIOLE, DUCT AND ALVEOLI

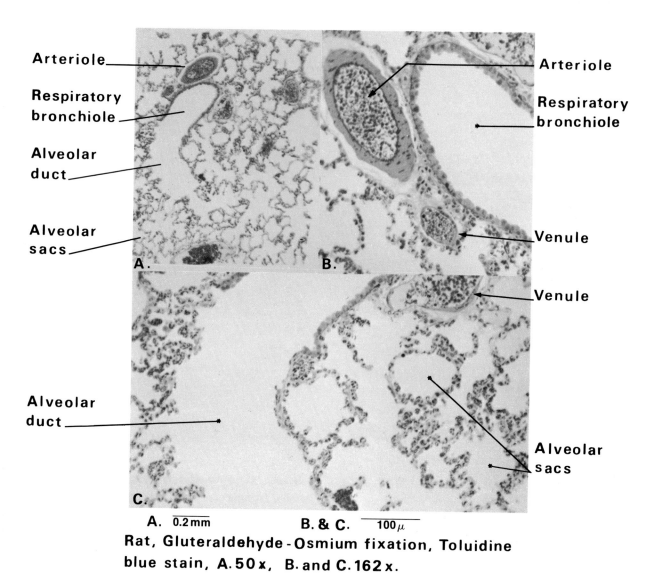

A. ‾0.2mm‾     B. & C. ‾100μ‾

Rat, Gluteraldehyde-Osmium fixation, Toluidine blue stain, A.50x, B. and C.162x.

**Respiratory bronchiole:** A branch of the terminal bronchiole. Epithelium low columnar to low cuboidal. Cilia present in the larger tubes only. Thin supporting wall of collagenous and elastic fibers and smooth muscle. Differs from the terminal bronchiole in having alveoli as outpouchings of its wall. Accompanying arterioles and venules are seen in the wall of the bronchiole. Note that large arterioles and venules are not seen at a level below the respiratory bronchiole.

**Alveolar duct:** Arises by branching of respiratory bronchioles; wall made up of alveolar sacs and alveoli. Lining epithelium is reduced to flattened cells with occasional cuboidal cells.

**Alveolar sacs:** Cluster of alveoli which open into the lumen of the alveolar duct. Individual alveoli are lined by thin squamous cells (Pneumocyte I) and cuboidal cells which bulge into the alveolus (Pneumocyte II). The latter cell is responsible for the production of surfactant, which maintains the configuration and stability of the alveolus and plays a role in fluid transport across the alveolocapillary membrane. Site of respiratory exchange.

# ALVEOLAR DUCT AND ALVEOLAR SACS

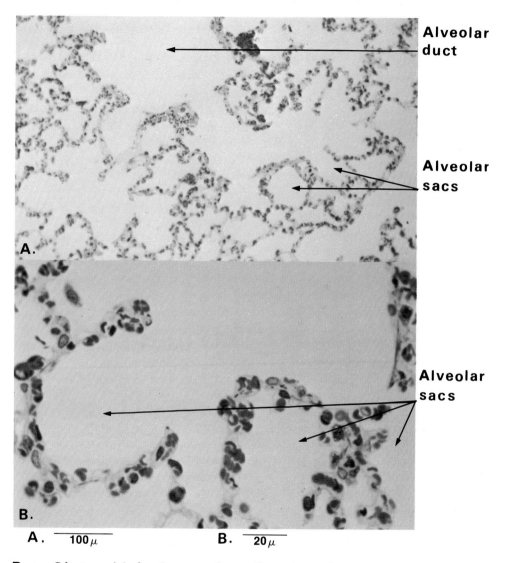

Alveolar
duct

Alveolar
sacs

Alveolar
sacs

A. $\overline{100\,\mu}$     B. $\overline{20\,\mu}$

**Rat, Gluteraldehyde-osmium fixation, Toluidine blue stain, A. 162 x, B. 612 x.**

**Alveolar duct:** A branch of the respiratory bronchiole. The duct is composed of alveolar sacs and alveoli. See Plates 196 and 197.

**Alveolar sacs:** Cluster of alveoli opening into the main lumen of the sac. Individual alveoli are lined by a thin squamous and cuboidal epithelium. A closely applied capillary network is separated from the epithelium by a thin basement membrane. It is across this trilaminar wall that oxygen, carbon dioxide and other inspired gases are exchanged in respiration.

## ALVEOLUS

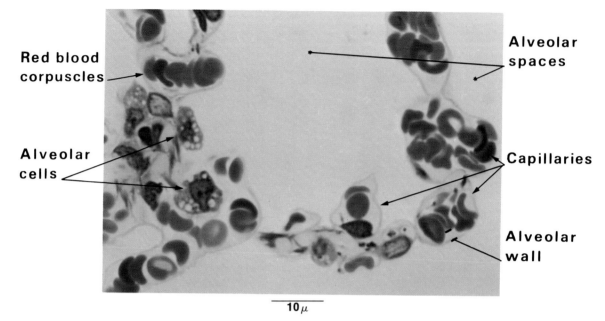

Red blood corpuscles

Alveolar cells

Alveolar spaces

Capillaries

Alveolar wall

10 μ

**Rat, Glutaraldehyde – osmium fixation, Toluidine blue stain, 1416 x.**

The partition between adjacent alveoli is shown in this plate. Note that capillaries form a major part of the partition, the very thin alveolar wall and the alveolar cells. The alveolar wall has been shown by electron microscopy to be composed of an epithelial cell, basement membrane and an endothelial cell. The alveolar cells (also known as septal cells) are cuboidal in shape and appear to have empty vacuoles in their cytoplasm. The vacuoles, as shown by electron microscopy, frequently contain osmiophilic bodies with concentric lamellae (cytosomes). Cytosomes are believed to contribute to the pulmonary surfactant that coats the alveolar epithelium in order to reduce the surface tension and keep the alveoli from collapsing. Through the alveolar wall gaseous exchange takes place between blood and air.

# The Urinary System

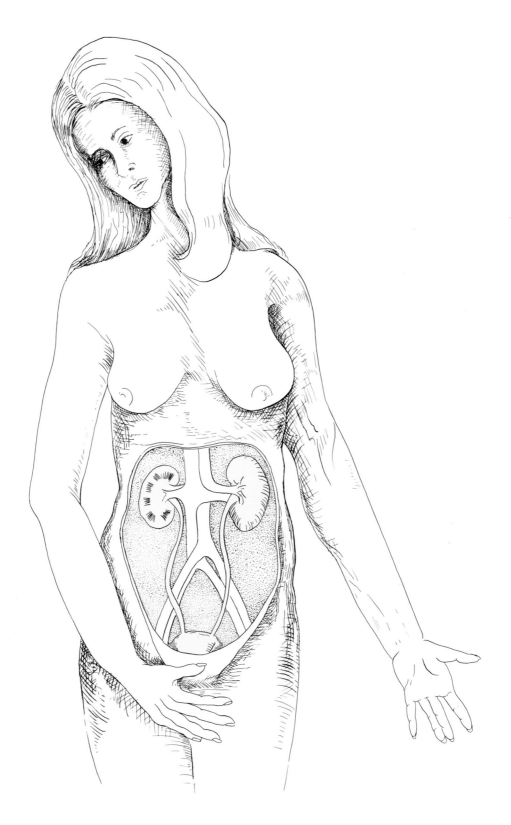

# The Urinary System

The urinary system consists of the kidneys, ureters, urinary bladder and urethra.

The volume and composition of body fluids are maintained remarkably constant regardless of fluid and solute intake. The regulation of the body fluid and the constancy of the internal environment is the primary role of the kidneys. Every minute approximately one-fourth of the cardiac output of blood enters the kidneys. As the blood flows through the glomerular capillaries about one-fifth of the plasma water leaves the capillaries and enters Bowman's space and the proximal tubules. The blood remaining in the capillaries flows into the efferent arterioles which break up into capillary peritubular networks closely applied to the renal tubules.

The plasma water is termed the glomerular filtrate and normally contains all the major ions, amino acids, glucose, urea and other substances in approximately the same concentration that exists in the blood plasma. This ultrafiltrate does not normally contain red blood corpuscles or significant amounts of protein.

Within the renal tubules both water and solutes are reabsorbed through the tubule cells to the fluid-filled interstitial space and into the peritubular capillaries to re-enter the blood stream. This is called tubular reabsorption. Other substances leave the peritubular capillaries, enter the interstitial fluid and are transported through the tubule cells, where they enter the tubule to be added to the glomerular filtrate. This is called tubular secretion.

The proximal tubule reabsorbs the filtered glucose and amino acids, and some of the sodium, chloride and bicarbonate ions. This active process results in an osmotic gradient which causes the passive reabsorption of water. The content of the proximal tubule is isotonic with respect to blood plasma. The distal end of the proximal tubule is in continuity with the thin loop of Henle, which extends into the kidney medulla and returns to the cortex. The content of the descending limb becomes increasingly hypertonic as sodium ions are actively transported from the ascending limb into the interstitial space to the descending loop. Unlike the descending limb, the ascending limb of the loop of Henle is impermeable to water and the content of the ascending limb of the tubule becomes increasingly hypotonic as sodium ions are actively transported from it. Sodium ions are actively reabsorbed and water is passively reabsorbed in the distal tubule.

The ascending limb of the thin loop is in continuity with the distal tubule. The distal tubule and the collecting duct are engaged primarily in the regulation of acid-base and potassium ion balance. Sodium ions are conserved and exchanged for hydrogen or potassium ions, or both.

The final concentration of urine, by passive reabsorption of water to form a hypertonic urine, occurs in the collecting ducts as they pass through the region of increasing osmolality in the medulla produced by the thin loop of Henle. The urine leaves the kidney via papillary ducts, enters the ureter and is stored in the urinary bladder. Contraction of the urinary bladder forces the urine into the urethra to be eliminated from the body.

## KIDNEY AND ADRENAL GLAND
Fetal

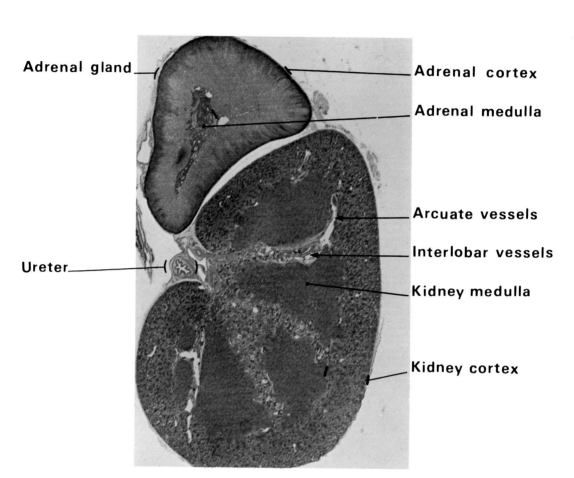

Adrenal gland — | Adrenal cortex

Adrenal medulla

Arcuate vessels

Interlobar vessels

Ureter — | Kidney medulla

Kidney cortex

**Rhesus monkey, 10% Formalin, H. & E., 6 x.**

In this plate the gross histologic features of the adrenal gland and the kidney are seen. Note the location of the adrenal gland, riding the superior pole of the kidney. Within the kidney note the hilum where the ureter is seen in cross section and where vessels are seen entering and leaving the kidney. The divisions of the kidney into cortex and medulla are clearly seen. Note the peripheral location of the cortex and the cortical columns that dip between the medullary pyramids. The latter are pyramid-shaped medullary structures, with the base of the pyramid resting against the peripheral cortex and the apex toward the hilum. Between the pyramids note the interlobar vessels. The interlobar artery is a branch of the renal artery. The interlobar veins form the renal vein. In the marginal zone, between the cortex and base of the pyramids, course the arcuate arteries and veins, which are tributaries of the interlobar vessels.

In the adrenal gland note the subdivisions into cortex and medulla.

## KIDNEY
### Cortex

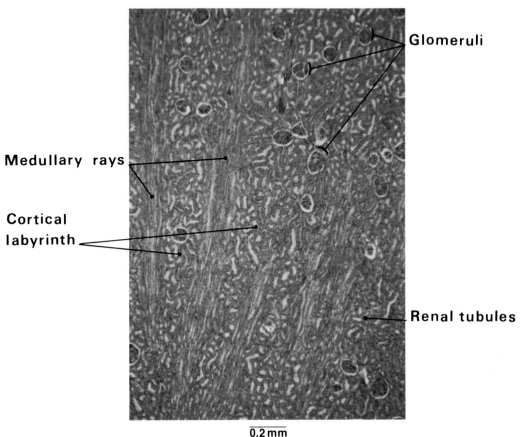

Glomeruli

Medullary rays

Cortical
labyrinth

Renal tubules

0.2 mm

**Rhesus monkey, 10% Formalin, H. & E., 50 x.**

In this plate the various constituents of kidney cortex are shown. The cortex is composed of radiating columns of straight renal tubules (medullary rays) alternating with regions containing glomeruli and convoluted renal tubules (cortical labyrinth). Other names for these two divisions are pars radiata or the processes of Ferrein for the medullary rays, and the pars convoluta for the cortical labyrinth. The cortical labyrinths contain glomeruli, proximal and distal convoluted tubules and the arched collecting tubules. The medullary rays contain the straight portions of proximal tubules (medullary segments), the thick segments of ascending arms of Henle's loops and the straight collecting tubules.

# KIDNEY
## Vascular system
## cortex

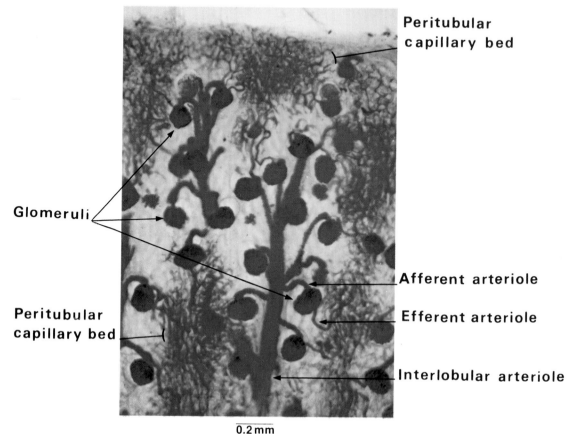

Peritubular
capillary bed

Glomeruli

Peritubular
capillary bed

Afferent arteriole

Efferent arteriole

Interlobular arteriole

0.2 mm

**Cat, Vascular injection (gelatin), Carmine, 50 x.**

This is an injected specimen to demonstrate some aspects of vascular supply of the kidney. The interlobular arteries are branches of the arcuate arteries. The latter are located in the zone separating the cortex from the base of the medullary pyramids. The interlobular arteries ascend perpendicularly to the surface of the kidney and provide numerous short lateral branches (afferent arterioles) that enter one or more renal corpuscles (glomeruli). The interlobular arteries terminate at the periphery of the cortex as afferent arterioles and each supplies a glomerulus. From every glomerulus an efferent arteriole leaves and divides into a system of capillaries called the peritubular plexus around the tubules of the cortex. The injected carmine gelatin illustrates the larger size of the lumen of the efferent arterioles. This relative size difference presumably increases the glomerular filtration pressure.

# KIDNEY
## Cortex

Arteriole

Distal tubule

Capillary

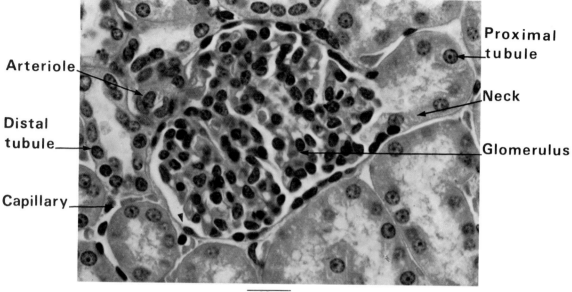

Proximal tubule

Neck

Glomerulus

20 μ

**Rhesus monkey, Zenker's fluid, H. & E., 612 x.**

**Proximal tubule:** Lumen continuous with that of glomerular capsule (Bowman's space). Large cuboidal cells, abundant eosinophilic cytoplasm and large spheroidal nuclei. Brush border.

**Neck:** The first part of the proximal tubule leading away from the glomerulus. Narrow and straight.

**Distal tubule:** Wider lumen, shorter cells, without brush border.

**Glomerulus:** A tuft of winding capillaries surrounded by epithelial cells and few connective tissue cells.

**Arteriole:** Afferent arteriole breaks up into many capillary loops inside the glomerulus. From these capillaries the efferent arteriole is formed.

**Capillary:** Surrounds the renal tubules. These capillaries are branches of the efferent arteriole.

# KIDNEY

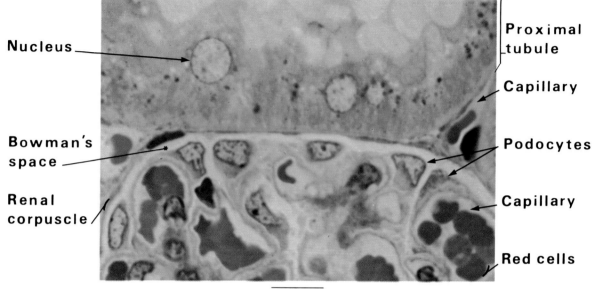

Nucleus

Bowman's space

Renal corpuscle

Proximal tubule

Capillary

Podocytes

Capillary

Red cells

10 μ

Cat, Glutaraldehyde – osmium fixation, Toluidine blue stain, **1416** x.

**Proximal tubule:**   Single layer of cuboidal cells with irregular surface. Rounded nucleus. Granular cytoplasm (see also Plate 15).

**Capillary:**   Within the renal corpuscle. Filled with red blood cells.

**Podocytes:**   The name given to cells of the visceral epithelium of Bowman's capsule. They have many foot-like processes (podia) resting upon the basement membrane covering the capillaries.

**Bowman's space:**   Space between the parietal and visceral layer of Bowman's capsule in continuity with the lumen of the proximal tubules. See also Plate 203.

**Renal corpuscle:**   Includes Bowman's capsule plus the glomerulus formed of capillaries. Also known as Malpighian body.

# KIDNEY
## Cortex

Distal
tubule

Bowman's
capsule

Afferent
arteriole

Juxta-
glomerular
cells

Proximal
tubule

Vascular
pole

Efferent
arteriole

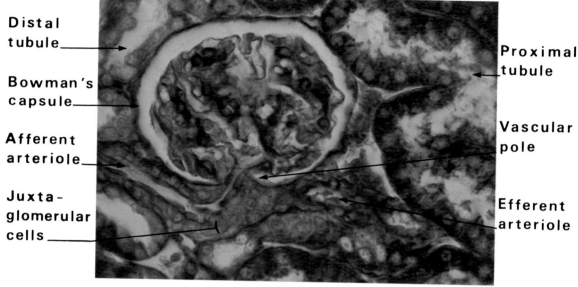

20 μ

Rhesus monkey, Zenker's fluid, Mallory's stain, 612x.

**Bowman's capsule:** Squamous epithelium forming a double-walled cup surrounding the glomerular capillaries. The portion of the wall applied to the capillaries is termed the visceral epithelium and can be seen in Plate 204. The visceral epithelium is separated from the outer wall by Bowman's space (Plate 203). The outer wall is continuous with the proximal tubule, and Bowman's space is continuous with the lumen of the proximal tubule at the urinary pole of the capsule.

**Vascular pole:** The point of entry of the afferent arteriole into Bowman's capsule which immediately forms the tuft of glomerular capillaries and the point of origin of the efferent arteriole from glomerular capillaries which leaves Bowman's capsule.

**Afferent arteriole:** Carries blood to the glomerular capillaries.

**Efferent arteriole:** The arterial vessel which carries blood away from the glomerular capillaries. Uniquely, in the kidney, a capillary bed is interposed between arterial vessels. The efferent arteriole leads to the cortical inter-tubular capillary network (see Plate 202).

**Juxtaglomerular cells:** Myoepithelioid cells replace typical smooth fibers in the wall of the afferent arteriole as it approaches the glomerulus. These cells secrete a hypertensive factor, renin. See also Plates 206 and 207.

**Proximal tubule:** Single layer of cuboidal cells with an irregular brush border.

**Distal tubule:** Cuboidal cells without a brush border which stain less intensely than the proximal tubule cells.

# KIDNEY
## Cortex

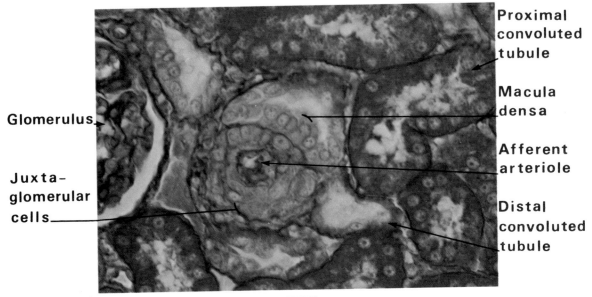

Glomerulus

Juxta-
glomerular
cells

Proximal
convoluted
tubule

Macula
densa

Afferent
arteriole

Distal
convoluted
tubule

20 μ

## Rhesus monkey, Zenker's fluid, Mallory's stain, 612 x.

**Afferent arteriole:**  Seen here in cross section. Its proximity to the glomerulus (not seen here) which it serves is indicated by the presence of cells containing conspicuous granules which replace smooth muscle fibers normally found in the wall of arterioles.

**Juxtaglomerular cells:**  Rich in cytoplasmic granules containing renin. Renin secreted into the blood is known to play a role in the formation of a hypertensive substance known as angiotensin II.

**Glomerulus:**  Tuft of capillaries having their origin from the afferent arteriole and surrounded by Bowman's capsule. The glomerulus, together with Bowman's capsule, comprises the renal corpuscle.

**Proximal convoluted tubule:**  Outlet of Bowman's capsule approximately 14 mm long with many small loops near the renal corpuscle. It ultimately straightens and runs toward the medulla in the medullary rays.

**Distal convoluted tubule:**  This portion of the renal tubule has many short loops in close association with the proximal convoluted tubule and the glomerulus. It is about one-third the length of the proximal tubule. The distal tubule is continuous with the collecting tubules.

**Macula densa:**  Specialized region of the distal convoluted tubule with tightly packed tubule cells in contact with the afferent arteriole. The bases of the cells of the macula densa are consistently found in intimate association with the juxtaglomerular cells in the wall of the afferent arteriole. Because this structural relationship suggests a functional relationship (supported experimentally), the macula densa and the juxtaglomerular cells together are referred to as the juxtaglomerular apparatus.

# KIDNEY
## Juxtaglomerular cells

Lumen of
Bowman's
capsule

Afferent
arteriole

Juxta-
glomerular
cells

Proximal
convoluted
tubule

Macula
densa

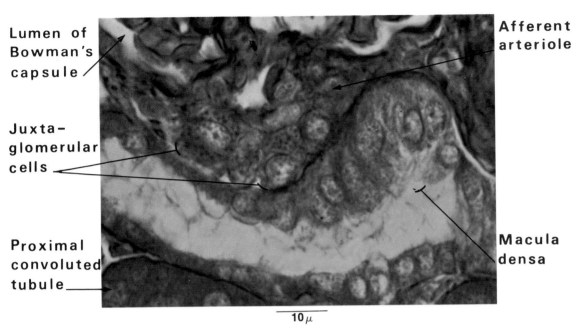

10 μ

Rhesus monkey, Zenker's fluid, Mallory's stain, 1416 x.

**Afferent arteriole:**  Terminal branch of the interlobular artery entering the glomerulus. The renal afferent arterioles are volume receptors and are sensitive to changes in perfusion (blood) pressure.

**Juxtaglomerular cells:**  Granular variety of myoepithelioid cells in the wall of the afferent arteriole. Replace the typical smooth muscle cells of the tunica media of the artery. A decrease in afferent arterial volume secondary to low perfusion pressure results in the release of renin. Renin is an enzyme which is released into the blood and acts upon blood proteins to produce a potent vasoconstrictor, angiotensin, which can under abnormal conditions elevate blood pressure to dangerous levels. Hypertension of renal origin in humans can be cured by removal of the diseased or ischemic kidney. Renin also affects blood volume and osmolarity by initiating a chain of events leading to the release of the hormone aldosterone by the cells of the zona glomerulosa of the adrenal cortex. Aldosterone acts upon the renal tubules to enhance sodium reabsorption. A second system unrelated to the kidney involves the hypothalamus of the brain and the posterior lobe of the pituitary (neurohypophysis) also regulates the volume and osmolarity of the extracellular fluid of the body. See Plates 104 and 206.

**Macula densa:**  A group of specialized cells of the straight portion of the distal tubule, in contact with the afferent arteriole and in relation to the juxtaglomerular cells. The cells are taller, thinner and tightly packed compared to other distal tubule cells. These cells are functionally related to the juxtaglomerular cells, although their exact role is undefined. The macula densa marks the origin of the convoluted portion of the distal tubule.

**Lumen of Bowman's capsule:**  Located between the parietal and visceral epithelial layers. Receives the ultrafiltrate of blood plasma circulating through the glomerular capillaries. The glomerular filtrate traverses the glomerular endothelium, the basal lamina (basement membrane) and the visceral epithelium to reach Bowman's space. Bowman's space is continuous with the lumen of the proximal convoluted tubule.

**Proximal convoluted tubule:**  Deeply staining cuboidal cells surrounded by a thin basal lamina (basement membrane).

# KIDNEY
## Medulla

Collecting
tubule

Capillary

Ascending
limbs of
Henle's
loop

Thin
segments
of Henle's
loop

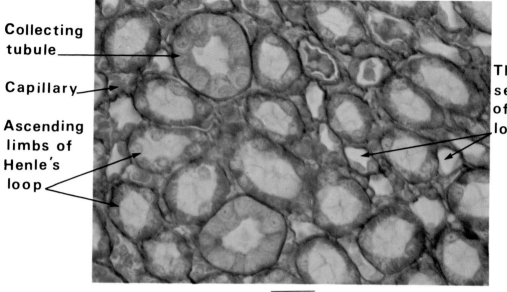

20 μ

## Rhesus monkey, Zenker's fluid, Mallory's stain, 612 x.

**Collecting tubule:** Cuboidal or columnar lining. Nuclei round and dark. Cytoplasm clear with distinct cell outlines.

**Capillary:** Filled with red cells.

**Ascending limb of Henle's loop:** Lined by cuboidal cells.

**Thin segments of Henle's loop:** Cells flattened, single layer, nuclei bulge into lumen.

See also Plate 14.

## KIDNEY
### Papilla, Area cribrosa, Minor calyx

Medulla

Papillary ducts

Minor calyx

Area cribrosa

Transitional epithelium

Connective tissue

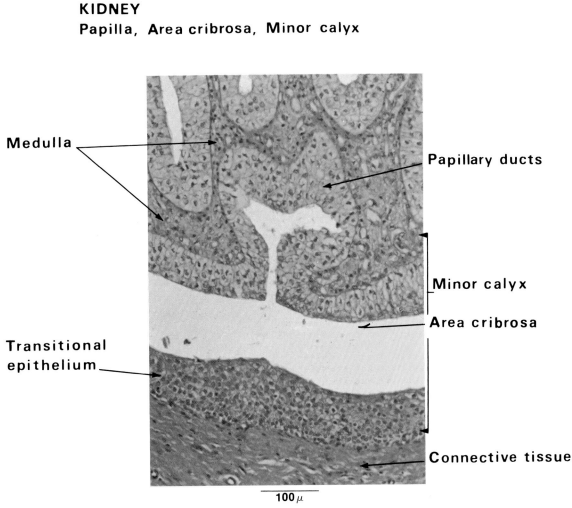

$100\,\mu$

### Rhesus monkey, Helly's fluid, H. & E., 162 x.

**Papillary ducts (of Bellini):** Named after Lorenz Bellini, the Italian anatomist, who described them in 1662. Arise by convergence of collecting tubules in the medulla near the pelvis. These ducts have large lumina and open at the area cribrosa at the apex of the papilla. Note the tall columnar epithelium lining the ducts. Cytoplasm of epithelial cells is clear; nuclei are dark and basally located. The tops of cells tend to bulge into the lumen.

**Minor calyx:** Subdivision of a major calyx in the pelvis of the kidney. The minor calyx is an infolded tube forming a double-walled cup. The inner wall of the calyx fits over the papilla of a pyramid. The transitional epithelium of the minor calyx is continuous with the columnar epithelium of the papillary ducts. The lamina propria is made up mostly of collagenous connective tissue and lacks papillae.

**Area cribrosa:** The sievelike appearance of the papilla is produced by the large number of collecting tubules passing through it.

# URETER
## Cross section
## contracted

Lumen

Transitional epithelium

Lamina propria

Muscular layer

Adventitia

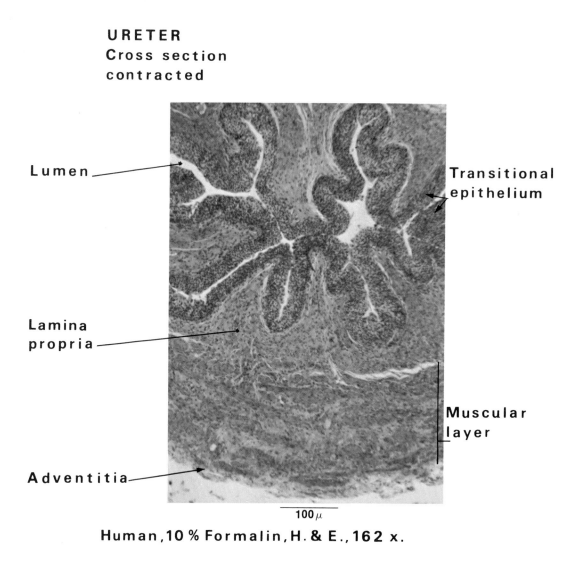

100 μ

## Human, 10 % Formalin, H. & E., 162 x.

The ureter extends from the renal pelvis to the urinary bladder and constitutes the main excretory duct of the kidney. The ureteral wall is composed of a mucosa which includes the epithelium and the lamina propria, a poorly defined submucosa of loose connective tissue containing some elastic fibers, a muscularis and an adventitia.

**Transitional epithelium:**  Characteristic epithelium found only lining the renal pelvis, ureter and urinary bladder. The thickness of this epithelium varies with the degree of distention of the ureter. See also Plate 23.

**Lamina propria:**  Located beneath the epithelium and composed primarily of collagenous and some elastic fibers. The junction between the epithelium and the lamina propria is smooth and devoid of connective tissue papillae. Diffuse lymphatic tissue is frequently found in the cell-rich connective tissue layer.

**Muscular layer:**  The muscular tunic or coat consists of an inner longitudinal and an outer circular layer of smooth muscle. Near the urinary bladder the ureter gains an additional outermost layer of longitudinally arranged smooth muscle.

**Adventitia:**  The ureter lies behind the peritoneum and, as a result, it is neither enclosed in a mesentery nor covered by a mesothelial cell outer lining. This layer is called, therefore, the adventitia. It appears in sections as an irregular, ragged fibrous coat because it is removed from surrounding connective tissue with which it is loosely joined. The adventitia contains blood vessels which supply the wall of the organ. In addition, motor nerves pass through this fibrous layer to supply the muscular layer.

## URINARY BLADDER

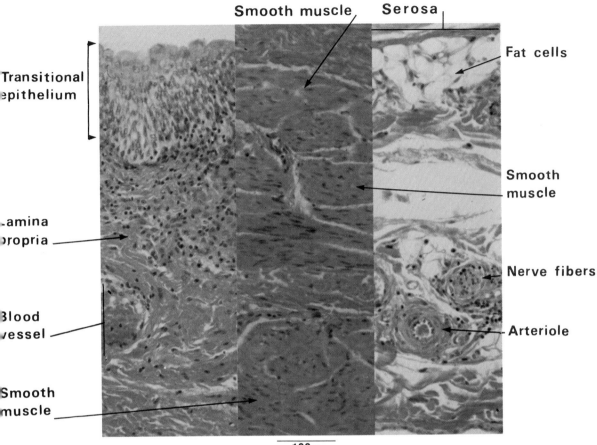

Smooth muscle — Serosa

Fat cells

Transitional epithelium

Smooth muscle

Lamina propria —

Nerve fibers

Blood vessel —

Arteriole

Smooth muscle

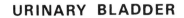

100 μ

Human, 10% Formalin, H. & E., 162 x.

This plate, in three sections, illustrates the component parts of the wall of the urinary bladder. Note the transitional epithelial mucosal lining. The number of layers and the shape of cells vary with the state of fullness of the bladder. The lamina propria is composed of loosely arranged connective tissue containing blood vessels and many lymphocytes. Beneath the mucosa is the muscle coat, made of interlacing bundles of smooth muscle fibers. Three layers can generally be recognized, inner longitudinal, middle circular and outer longitudinal. The serosa is composed of a loosely arranged fibrofatty connective tissue containing many large blood vessels and nerves.

# URETHRA
Female

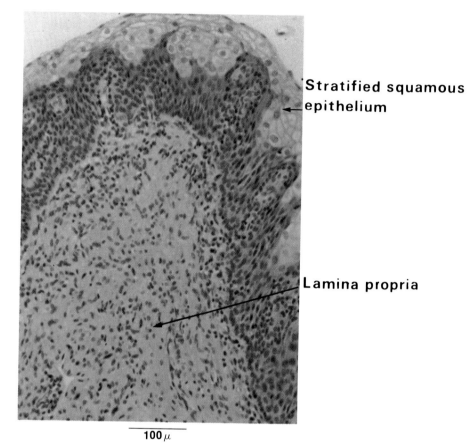

Stratified squamous ←epithelium

Lamina propria

100 μ

Human, 10% Formalin, H. & E., 162 x.

This is a section of female urethra showing the mucosa. The lining epithelium here is stratified squamous. The type of epithelium lining the urethra is variable at different sites. It is transitional near the urinary bladder and stratified squamous throughout most of its extent except for interrupted segments of stratified columnar or pseudostratified epithelium. The lamina propria of loose connective tissue lacks papillae.

## URETHRA
## Cavernous portion
## penis

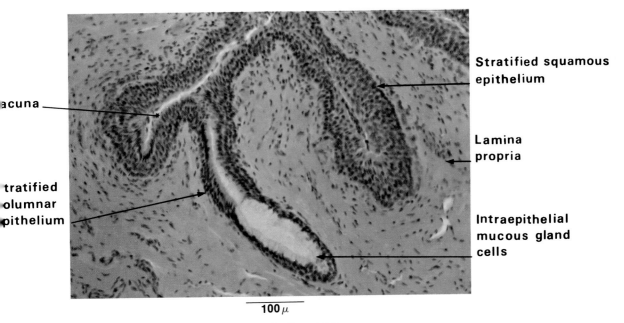

Stratified squamous epithelium

Lamina propria

Intraepithelial mucous gland cells

acuna

tratified olumnar pithelium

100 μ

Human, 10% Formalin, H.& E., 162 x.

This plate shows the histology of the cavernous portion of the male urethra. This portion of the urethra extends throughout the penis to open at the end of the glans. Note the stratified columnar epithelium mucosal lining intermixed with stratified squamous epithelium. The latter type of epithelium is found in interrupted areas throughout the extent of the urethra and is the only epithelial type found at the external opening of the urethra.

Note the deep recesses of the mucosal surface known as lacunae of Morgagni. Isolated intraepithelial mucous gland cells are seen interspersed between the stratified columnar cells lining the lacunae.

The lamina propria is made up of loose connective tissue rich in elastic fibers.

# The Female
# Reproductive System

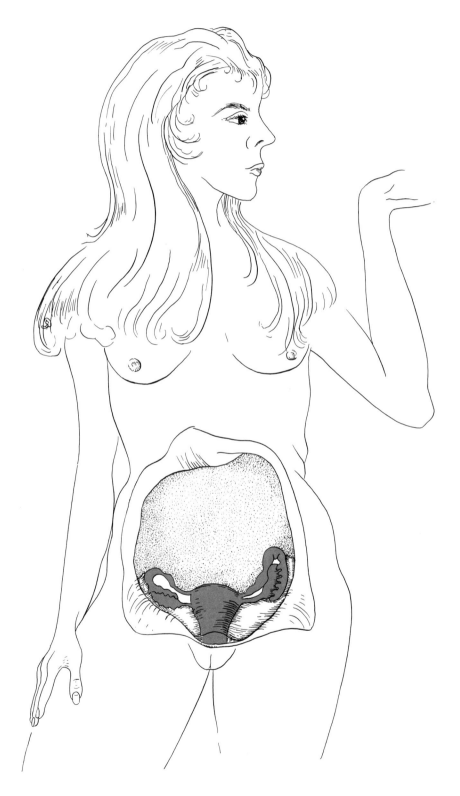

# The Female Reproductive System

The female reproductive system consists of the ovaries, the uterine tubes, uterus, vagina and external genitalia. The ovaries perform both an exocrine function by producing ova and an endocrine function by producing estrogen and progesterone.

The ovaries are ovoid structures lying on each side of the uterus within the pelvis. The ovary consists of a cortical zone composed of a dense stroma which contains follicles with ova. In the mature functional ovary many follicles are quiescent while others show progressive or regressive changes and specialized end products of follicular development. The medulla consists primarily of connective tissue and an extremely rich vascular supply.

The immature ova or oogonia are spherical cells, about 30 $\mu$ in diameter, which, when fully mature, increase in size to about 120 $\mu$ and are designated primary oocytes. The nucleus of an oocyte is large, about 25 $\mu$ in diameter, vesicular, and contains a prominent nucleolus. The cytoplasm is rich in nutritive material called the yolk.

The primordial or primary follicles number over 200,000 in each human fetal ovary and these decline in number until very few or none are left at about the 50th year. The primordial follicle is an ovum enclosed in a single layer of cells, follicle cells, and measures about 40 $\mu$ in diameter. The transition from an inactive primordial follicle to a growing and maturing primary follicle involves changes in the oocyte, the follicular cells and the adjacent connective tissue. As the oocyte enlarges the single layer of follicular cells increases in number through mitotic division and gives rise to granular (granulosa) cells that form a stratified epithelium. A distinctive feature of the multilaminar follicle is the interposition of a highly refractile zona pellucida interposed between the oocyte and granulosa cells. Along with the development of the granulosa cells a sheath of stroma cells (theca folliculi) develops around the follicle and subsequently forms two layers. The inner layer is a highly vascular capillary plexus composed of secretory cells, the theca interna, and an outer layer of connective tissue, the theca externa. The cells of the theca interna are believed to secrete the female sex hormones, the estrogens. Secondary follicles can be identified when about 0.2 mm in diameter and can be recognized by the presence of irregular spaces among the granulosa cells filled with a clear liquid (liquor folliculi) which increases with increased growth of the follicle. Eventually the ovum is seen eccentrically placed in the follicle on a mound of granulosa cells, the cumulus oophorus, and through the confluence of the smaller spaces a large, single, crescent-shaped, fluid-filled space (antrum) appears around the cumulus oophorus.

Although the ovum has stopped growing the follicle may enlarge until it reaches approximately 10 mm in diameter. A follicle in which an appreciable amount of follicular fluid has accumulated is termed a vesicular follicle or a Graafian follicle. The growth of a primordial follicle to full maturity takes about

10 to 14 days. The enlarged follicle now occupies the full thickness of the cortex of the ovary and bulges out from the free surface of the ovary prior to ovulation. The thecae folliculi, particularly the theca interna, reach their highest development in relation to the mature follicle.

Following ovulation and discharge of the liquor folliculi, the walls of the follicle collapse and the granular cell lining becomes folded. Rupture of blood vessels in the theca interna is associated with bleeding into the partially collapsed follicle, and a clot is formed. The cells of the granulosa layer and the theca interna undergo a cellular transformation and are renamed granulosa lutein and theca cells, respectively. These changes in the follicle following ovulation result in a new but transitory organ, the corpus luteum, which secretes the hormone progesterone. If the secreted ovum fails to be fertilized the corpus luteum remains functional for about 14 days and then is reduced to a scar, the corpus albicans. In the event of fertilization the corpus luteum enlarges and persists as a functional endocrine gland throughout most of pregnancy but begins to involute after the sixth month. Its ultimate fate after the termination of pregnancy is to become a scarred mass, the corpus albicans.

Vast numbers of follicles never develop into mature follicles since that number is limited to about 400 (or 1 out of every thousand follicles) during the period of human sexual maturity. The process by which follicles degenerate and disappear is termed follicular atresia. This process can begin at any stage of follicular development. The smallest follicles leave no trace of their dissolution, but larger follicles may leave the zona pellucida as a persistent marker. In larger vesicular follicles the earliest signs of atresia include the loosening and shedding of the granulosa cells, the invasion of the granulosa layers by vascular tissue and wandering cells, and the collapse or partial collapse of the follicle.

The oviduct (the uterine or Fallopian tube) receives the ovum; here it may be fertilized and conveyed to the uterus for subsequent development. The uterine tube shows four regional divisions: (1) the infundibulum, which flares and bears fringed folds called the fimbria; (2) the ampulla, a dilated midportion of the tube, where fertilization takes place; (3) the isthmus, which is a slender tube connecting the duct with the uterus; and (4) the interstitial portion of the duct which passes through the uterine wall. The epithelium of the mucosa is mostly simple columnar and some cells are ciliated. The muscularis of the uterine tube, composed of two layers, becomes progressively thicker as the tube approaches the uterus.

The uterus lies between the bladder and the rectum and is a hollow, pear-shaped organ that opens into the vagina. The uterus is composed of a mucosa given the special name of endometrium, a muscularis termed the myometrium and the serosa or perimetrium. The uterine mucosa undergoes cyclic changes which are in correlation with ovarian secretory activity. The surface epithelium is simple columnar with patches of ciliated columnar cells. Uterine glands, lined with a similar columnar epithelium, open to the surface and secrete mucus. The endometrial stroma has a framework consisting of reticular fibers and stromal cells. Lymphocytes and granular leucocytes are also found in the stroma. The endometrium is composed of two parts, the superficial functionalis, which changes during the menstrual cycle and is shed during menstruation, and the basalis, which does not undergo cyclic changes and remains intact during menstruation.

The myometrium is a thick coat containing smooth muscle and abundant connective tissues. The smooth muscles of the uterus, in response to female sex hormones, undergo cyclic variation in length and diameter, and in functional activity. Three layers of smooth muscle are recognized: an inner longitudinal layer, a middle circular and oblique layer and an outer longitudinal layer.

The following cyclic changes occur in the uterine endometrium during the menstrual cycle. (1) The proliferative or estrogenic phase extends from about the fourth to the fifteenth day of the cycle. This period involves re-epithelization of the raw endometrial surface and the growth in thickness of the endometrium and glands. The glands are initially straight but begin to coil toward the end of this phase. Estrogen is the dominant hormonal influence during this phase. (2) The secretory, progestational or luteal phase constitutes days 16 to 28 of the cycle. During this period the uterine glands become highly coiled and irregularly sacculated in the middle of the endometrium. The glandular epithelium secretes a mucoid fluid rich in glycogen. The endometrium becomes edematous and may reach a thickness of 6 mm. Progesterone is the primary hormonal influence during this phase. On the twenty-seventh or twenty-eighth day the uterus enters the ischemic phase during which the arterial supply constricts intermittently. At this point glandular secretion is interrupted. (3) The menstrual phase involves the extravasation of blood and the detachment of patches of blood-soaked endometrium until the entire functionalis is sloughed. The basal layer remains intact during this phase and is the source of the regenerating functional layer during the proliferative phase. The menstrual phase lasts from days 1 to 4 or 5.

The outlet of the uterus is the vagina, a fibromuscular sheath lined with thick stratified squamous epithelium. The underlying lamina propria is also thick and contains numerous lymphocytes and other wandering cells which invade the epithelium. The muscularis is irregularly arranged in two layers: an inner circular or spiral layer and an outer longitudinal layer. The vagina does not possess a muscularis mucosa or glands in the lamina propria. The adventitia is a dense collagenous tissue which merges with the adventitia of the bladder and rectum and is highly vascular.

In the event of pregnancy an important but temporary organ, the placenta, is formed in the uterus. The placenta is of both maternal (uterus) and fetal origins. The maternal component is the endometrium; the fetal contribution consists of the chorionic plate and its branching villi which are of two types: the anchoring villi, which extend from the chorionic plate to the decidua basalis, and the free villi formed by branches from the anchoring villi. A villus has a fibromuscular core with fetal blood vessels and is covered by an epithelium named the trophoblast. The trophoblast is arranged in two layers: an outer layer without cell boundaries, the syncytial trophoblast, and an inner cuboidal cell layer, the cytotrophoblast. In the late stages of pregnancy the cellular layer disappears.

The fetal and maternal blood do not mix. The fetal blood is contained entirely within small vessels and capillaries while the maternal blood leaves arterial vessels, enters the placenta, and flows around the fetal villi (anchoring and free villi). Here, oxygen, carbon dioxide, nutrients and waste products are exchanged across the trophoblastic epithelium. Maternal blood is drained by veins from the intervillous spaces of the placenta.

## OVARY
### Uterine ducts

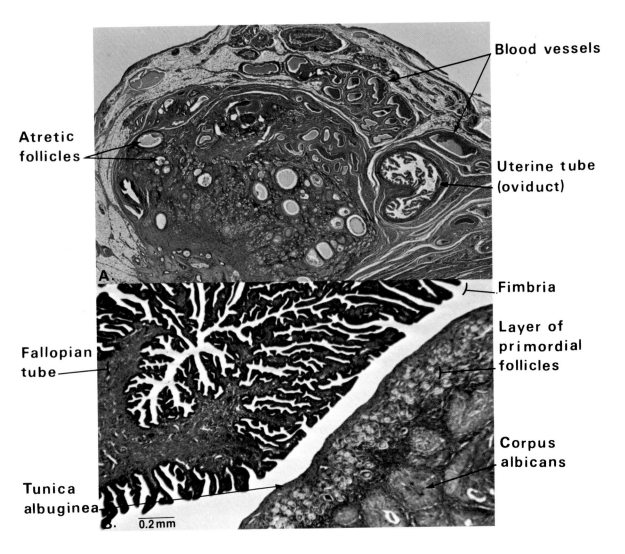

Rhesus monkey, Helly's fluid, H. & E., A. 9x.,
B. 50x.

The upper part of the plate (*A*) shows a section of the ovary and uterine (Fallopian) tubes. Note the blood vessels in the medulla of the ovary. These vessels are branches of ovarian and uterine vessels. Many atretic follicles are seen in the ovary. Additional features of the uterine tube are seen in *B*, which shows a section of the infundibular region of the uterine tube characterized by the presence of fimbria. The lining epithelium of the tube is simple columnar. In the ovary adjacent to the uterine tube in *B*, note the outer layer of primordial follicles and the scarred whitish corpus albicans. Note also the tunica albuginea of the ovary. This is a dense fibrous layer of the ovarian stroma underneath the germinal epithelium. It is composed of relatively few cells and packed fibers.

## OVARY
### Cortical region

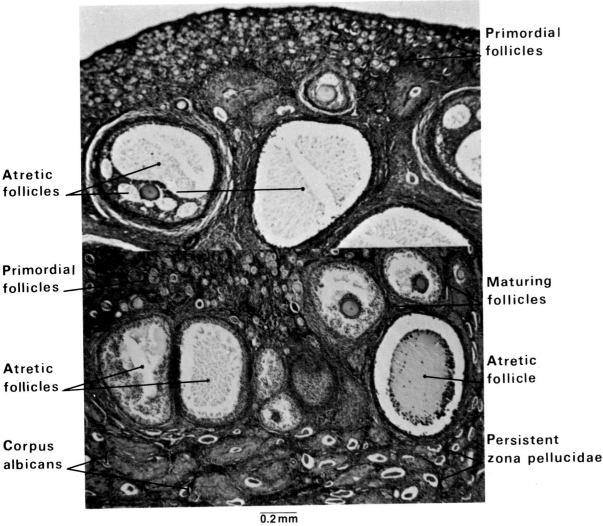

Rhesus monkey, Helly's fluid, H. & E., 50 x.

0.2 mm

**Primordial follicles:** Consist of an ovum surrounded incompletely by a single layer of low cuboidal or flattened epithelium (follicular or granulosa cells). Note the distribution in peripheral layers of the cortex.

**Maturing follicle:** Note the multilayered follicular cells, the increased size, the eccentric position of the ovum, and the prominent connective tissue capsule. Maturing follicles occupy deeper zones of the cortex. Note the vesicular nucleus and the deeply staining small nucleolus. The ovum is pushed to the side of the follicle by the accumulation of follicular fluid.

**Atretic follicle:** Follicles that do not reach maturity degenerate and are called atretic follicles. Nucleus becomes pyknotic and later fragments. Follicular cells also degenerate. Atretic follicles are later resorbed and are replaced by a connective tissue stroma. The zona pellucida of atretic follicles stains deeply and may persist by itself in the stroma.

**Corpus albicans:** A hyaline scar resulting from the degeneration of corpus luteum of ovulation.

289

## OVARY

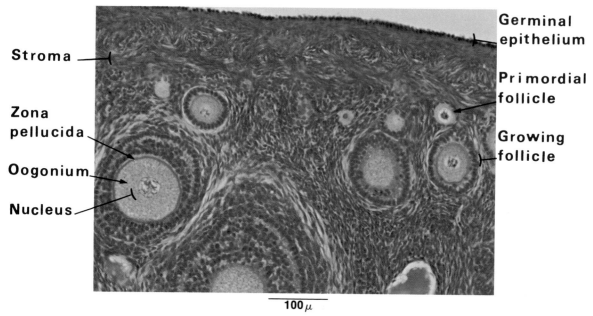

Stroma

Zona pellucida

Oogonium

Nucleus

Germinal epithelium

Primordial follicle

Growing follicle

100 μ

Rabbit, 10 % Formalin, H. & E., 162 x.

**Germinal epithelium:** Forms the surface layer of the ovary and consists of a specialized peritoneal mesothelium. Misnomer since there is no convincing evidence that it is the source of germ cells.

**Stroma:** Connective tissue stroma, richly cellular and compact. Stroma cells are spindle-shaped with elongated nuclei. The ovarian follicles are scattered within the stroma.

**Primordial follicle:** Consists of an ovum surrounded by a single layer of low cuboidal epithelium.

**Growing follicle:** At the initiation of follicular growth the follicle cells assume a cuboidal shape, divide and become multilayered.

**Zona pellucida:** Thick membrane surrounds the growing ovum. Rich in polysaccharides.

**Oogonium:** Primordial ovum containing the somatic number (diploid) of chromosomes. Divides mitotically to produce primary oocytes.

**Nucleus:** The nucleus of a primordial ovum is large and contains a prominent nucleolus.

## OVARY
## Theca interna
## growing follicle

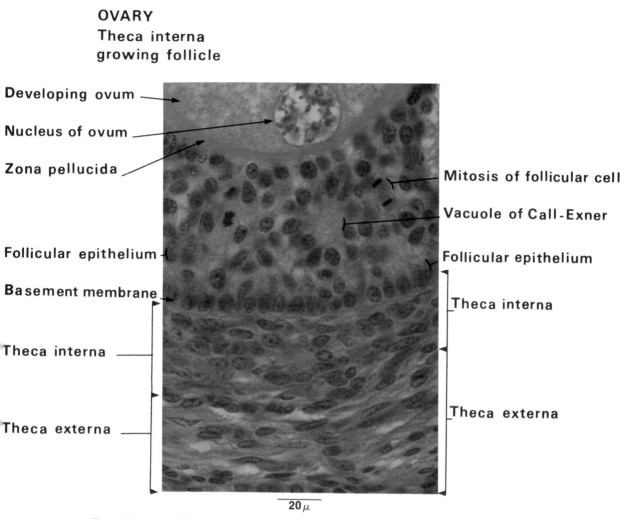

Developing ovum

Nucleus of ovum

Zona pellucida

Mitosis of follicular cell

Vacuole of Call-Exner

Follicular epithelium

Follicular epithelium

Basement membrane

Theca interna

Theca interna

Theca externa

Theca externa

20 μ

**Rabbit, 10% Formalin, H. & E., 612 x.**

This plate shows a rather advanced stage in the maturation of the ovarian follicle. Note the increase in size of the ovum and the follicular cells in comparison to that seen in the primary follicle (Plate 216). The nucleus of the ovum is large and has a sparse reticulated chromatin network. The cytoplasm of the ovum is granular. A thick membrane, the zona pellucida, incompletely separates the ovum from the follicular cells. This tough membrane is rich in polysaccharides and is believed to be elaborated by the ovum and/or the follicular cells. It persists even after the degeneration of the ovum during atresia of the follicle (Plate 215). The follicular cells have formed a stratified epithelial layer at this stage of growth. Mitotic figures are frequent, indicating continued active proliferation. Accumulations of densely staining material are seen among follicular cells. These are vacuoles of Call-Exner. They are believed to represent droplets within the cytoplasm of follicular cells. They stain positively with PAS and may be the precursors of follicular fluid. The stroma around the follicular epithelium is composed of an inner theca interna and an outer theca externa. A basement membrane separates the follicular cells from the theca interna while a distinct boundary is not evident between the theca interna and externa. The cells of the theca interna have epithelioid characteristics and are believed to elaborate estrogen. Note the ovoid or round nuclei of the theca interna. The theca externa is composed of spindle-shaped cells and is more fibrous. Both thecae are connective tissue derivatives.

## CORPUS LUTEUM

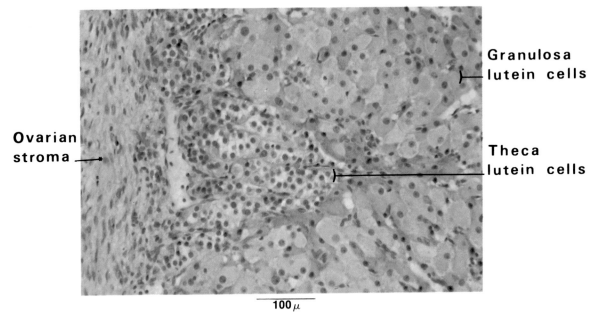

Granulosa lutein cells

Theca lutein cells

Ovarian stroma

100 μ

## Human, 10% Formalin, H. & E., 162 x.

The corpus luteum (yellow body) is a stage in the transformation of an ovarian follicle following ovulation.

**Granulosa lutein cells:** Larger in size, more centrally located; nuclei less densely stained and cytoplasm more abundant. They are transformed cells of the stratum granulosum of the ovarian follicle.

**Theca lutein cells:** Smaller, have less cytoplasm, are more peripherally located and nuclei stain more densely. They are transformed cells of the theca interna of the ovarian follicle.

Both types of cells are epithelioid and produce progesterone. Progesterone induces changes in the uterine endometrium (secretory phase), in preparation for the implantation of a fertilized ovum, and inhibits spontaneous contractions of the smooth muscle of the uterus so that gestation can be maintained. The vacuoles seen in some cells are due to the lipid droplets dissolved during processing of tissue.

**Ovarian stroma:** Connective tissue stroma, remnant of theca externa of the ovarian follicle. Sends fine septa into the parenchyma.

## OVARY

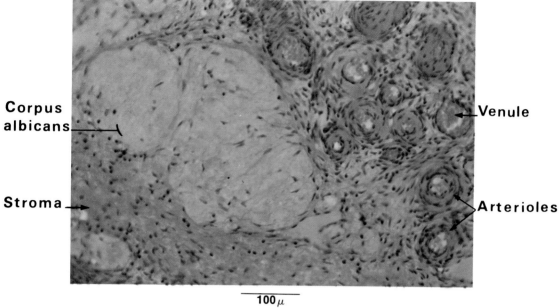

**Corpus albicans** —

**Stroma** →

**Venule**

**Arterioles**

100 μ

Rabbit, 10 % Formalin, H. & E., 162 x.

**Corpus albicans:** A hyaline scar resulting from the degeneration of the corpus luteum.

**Arterioles:** Arteries enter the medulla of the ovary at the hilum and spiral their way through to the cortex.

**Venules:** Rich plexus of veins accompanies the arteries and leaves the ovary at the hilum.

**Stroma:** Compact connective tissue. Spindle-shaped cells with elongated nuclei and fine reticular connective tissue fibers.

## UTERUS
### Endometrium
### A. early post menstrual, B. proliferative phase, C. secretory phase

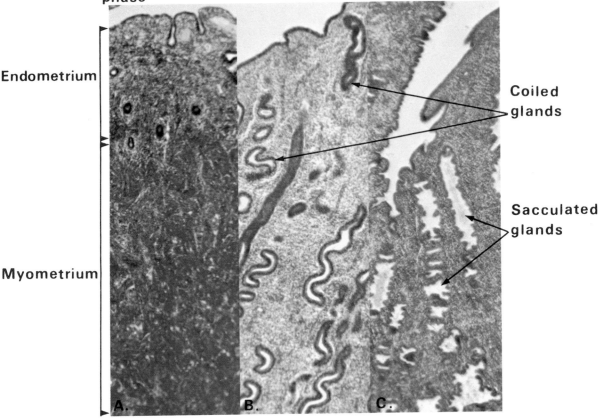

Endometrium

Coiled glands

Myometrium

Sacculated glands

A. B. C.

0.2 mm

**Human, 10% Formalin, H. & E., 50x.**

The uterine wall undergoes four phases during the menstrual cycle. These are the (1) resurfacing, (2) proliferative, (3) secretory and (4) ischemic phases.

The first three phases are shown in this plate. In *A*, the resurfacing phase, corresponding to days 5 and 6 of the cycle, is shown. During this stage remnants of the glands in the basal zone of the mucosa proliferate and migrate to cover the raw surface of the endometrium denuded from its mucosa by menstrual flow. The thick myometrium is shown. This is a massive coat of smooth muscle fibers arranged in three concentric layers.

In *B*, the proliferative or follicular phase of the menstrual cycle, which lasts from the seventh to the fourteenth day of the cycle, is shown. During this stage, the mucosal glands become longer and assume a curved or coiled configuration. The stroma between glands also increases by proliferation of connective tissue cells. The proliferative phase is induced by estrogen (see also Plate 217).

In *C*, the third or secretory phase, corresponding to days 15 to 27 of the menstrual cycle, is shown. This is also known as the progravid or luteal phase. During this stage, glands stop proliferating and begin to distend and secrete abundantly. In the middle region of the mucosa, saccular outpouchings of the glands are seen. The changes observed in this stage are induced by progesterone following estrogen priming.

## VAGINA

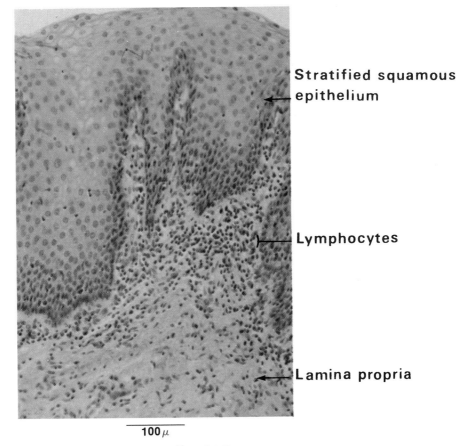

Stratified squamous epithelium

Lymphocytes

Lamina propria

100 μ

Human, 10% Formalin, H. & E., 162 x.

This is a section of part of the wall of the vagina showing the mucosa. Note the stratified squamous nonkeratinized epithelium. The lamina propria consists of loose connective tissue and is rich in lymphocytes. Occasional lymph nodules (not seen here) are found. The vaginal epithelium undergoes cyclic changes during the menstrual cycle.

## MAMMARY GLAND
### A. Inactive,  B. Proliferation,  C. Lactation

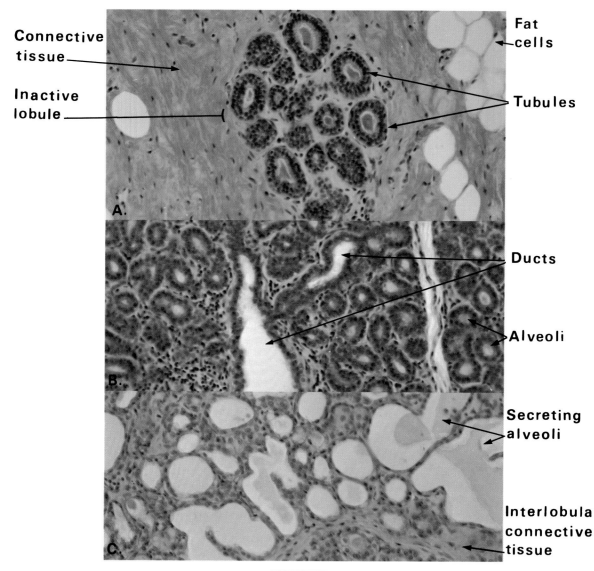

Connective tissue

Inactive lobule

Fat cells

Tubules

A.

Ducts

Alveoli

B.

Secreting alveoli

Interlobula connective tissue

C.

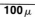
100 μ

## Human,  10% Formalin,  H. & E.,  126 x.

This figure shows the structure of the mammary gland in the inactive condition, in the proliferative phase and during lactation.

In *A*, the inactive gland is shown. The lobules are small and made up primarily of a group of epithelial ducts lined by cuboidal or columnar cells. The intralobular connective tissue between ducts is loose and devoid of fat cells. In contrast, the interlobular connective tissue around the lobules is abundant, dense and rich in fat cells.

The active proliferative gland seen in *B* is characterized by abundant alveoli lined by simple cuboidal epithelium. These alveoli arise by budding off from the ends of existing ducts. With the formation of alveoli, the intra- and interlobular connective tissue becomes markedly reduced. The active or proliferative gland is associated with pregnancy.

In the active lactating stage, seen in *C*, the alveoli become saccular, and distend with secretion products (milk). Secretory alveoli in different stages of secretion are seen in this figure. Some secretory alveoli are seen to be fully distended with flattened epithelium while others are less distended and have a thicker wall and smaller lumen. The interlobular connective tissue is reduced to thin septa between lobules.

PLATE 223

## PLACENTA

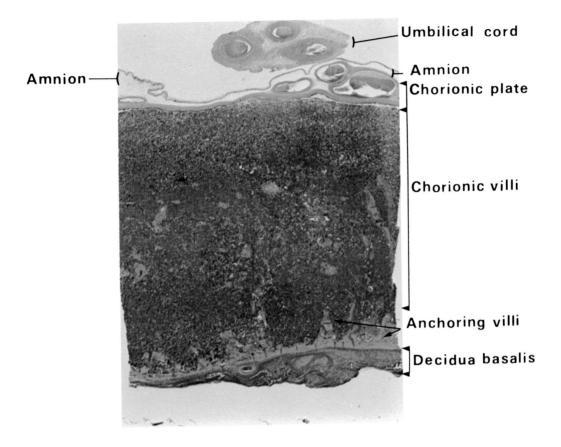

Umbilical cord

Amnion

Amnion

Chorionic plate

Chorionic villi

Anchoring villi

Decidua basalis

**Rhesus monkey, 10% Formalin, H. & E., 3.5 x.**

The components of the placenta are seen at low magnification in this plate. The maternal contribution is the decidua basalis. This is the part of the endometrial mucosa lying beneath the embryo between the embryo and the myometrium. The fetal contribution is the chorionic plate and its villi. The chorionic plate is a portion of the chorionic sac about the embryo. Chorionic villi arise from the chorionic plate and lie in the spaces through which maternal blood circulates. Many villi are free floating, others attach to the decidua basalis as anchoring elements. Villi receive their blood from the umbilical arteries and drain into the umbilical vein. Outside the chorionic plate note the amnion which lines the amniotic cavity containing the umbilical cord. The embryo is not seen.

# Section 14    The Male Reproductive System

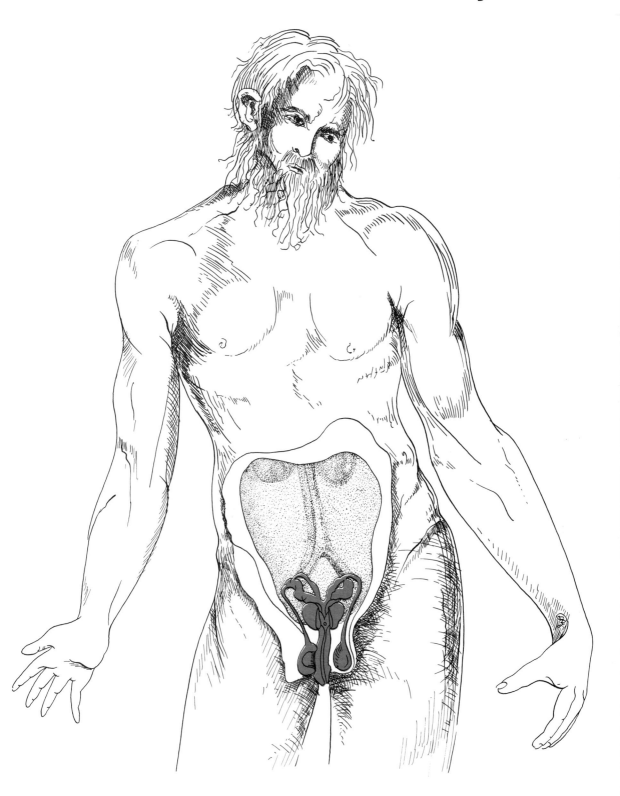

# The Male Reproductive System

The male reproductive organs include the primary sex glands, the testes, the various excretory ducts, the accessory glands and the penis.

The testes, contained within twin cavities and covered by a specialized skin (the scrotum), are compound tubular glands with both exocrine and endocrine functions. The exocrine function is the formation of the mature male germ cell (spermatozoa) and the endocrine function is the production of the male sex hormone testosterone. The testes are ovoid glands approximately 4.5 cm in length and are covered by a thick capsule (tunica albuginea) composed primarily of collagenous connective tissue with some elastic fibers. The tunica albuginea thickens posteriorly to form the mediastinum testis, which is the area where the ducts, blood vessels and nerves leave or enter. From the mediastinum, thin, incomplete and branching fibrous septa and associated blood vessels radiate into the testis and divide it into about 250 lobules. These incomplete pyramidal spaces contain the seminiferous tubules embedded in a fibrous stroma rich in vascular and cellular elements. Of particular interest are the interstitial cells (of Leydig), located in the stroma, which secrete testosterone, the male sex hormone, into the surrounding capillary bed.

The epithelium of the seminiferous tubules is stratified and is called the germinal epithelium. It consists of two types of cells, the maturing germ cells and the sustentacular or Sertoli cells.

The cells which comprise the germinal epithelium, and, through cell division and maturation, give rise to mature spermatozoa, are given special names. The spermatogonia lie on the basement membrane and contain, in humans, 23 pairs (a total of 46) of chromosomes. These cells divide mitotically, and each resulting daughter cell possesses 23 pairs of chromosomes. Primary spermatocytes are the largest of the maturing germ cells, and division of both the primary and secondary spermatocytes (the daughter cells of primary spermatocytes) is by meiosis and results in only a single set of 23 chromosomes, one of which being an X or a Y chromosome in each daughter cell. Spermatids are the daughter cells of secondary spermatocytes and are about half their size. These cells do not divide, but through a cellular transformation become mature spermatozoa. The nucleus forms most of the head which is pear-shaped and flattened. The Golgi apparatus contributes to the acrosome located at the apex of the sperm head. Other organelles and components of the spermatid, such as the mitochondria, centrioles and some of the cytoplasm, contribute to the structure of the mature spermatozoön. Human spermatozoa are about 60 $\mu$ in length. The head and middle piece are each 5 $\mu$ and the tail is about 50 $\mu$ in length.

The Sertoli or sustentacular cells, crowded between the sex cells, are pillarlike, with an irregular shape. They possess distinctive nuclei by which they can be identified.. These nuclei are ovoid, are finely granular and possess prominent nucleoli. Sertoli cells are considered to act as supporting cells and spermatids and maturing spermatozoa attach themselves to the apices of these cells in great numbers.

Leading from the seminiferous tubules are the tubuli recti or straight tubules lined only with Sertoli cells. The straight tubules open into the rete testis, a network of irregular anastomosing channels lined with a simple cuboidal or columnar epithelium, which may possess a single flagellum. The efferent ductules (10 to 15 in man) emerge from the rete testis and join to form the epididymis. Each appears as a coiled mass lined with ciliated columnar cells alternating with ciliated cuboidal cells. The ductus epididymis in man is a highly coiled tube about 5 m in length. It is lined with a pseudostratified epithelium with tall columnar cells and round basal cells. The columnar cells possess long nonmotile stereocilia. The ductus deferens is continuous with the ductus epididymis and extends to the prostatic urethra. The lumen of the ductus deferens increases in size and the wall thickens as it extends distally. Near the prostate gland the ductus is enlarged to form the ampulla and immediately thereafter is joined by the seminal vesicles. After this union the ductus deferens, now called the ejaculatory duct, continues to the urethra. It is lined with a pseudostratified or simple columnar epithelium.

Three glands are associated with the male reproductive system: the seminal vesicles, the prostate gland and the bulbourethral glands. The seminal vesicles develop as outgrowths of the ductus deferens. Each is a glandular sac honeycombed by thin branching folds of the mucosa lined with a pseudostratified columnar or cuboidal epithelium. The prostate gland encircles the urethra adjacent to the neck of the bladder and is formed of 30 to 50 tubuloalveolar glands grouped into lobes. The glandular epithelium consists of simple cuboidal or columnar cells. Prostatic concretions (corpora amylacea) are prominent constituents of the alveoli. The bulbourethral glands are compound tubuloalveolar glands which secrete a clear, viscous mucoid product. The secretory epithelium is cuboidal to columnar. The ducts of the gland enter the cavernous urethra.

The penis serves as an outlet for urine and semen and as a copulatory organ. The penis is made up of three cylinders of erectile tissue composed of a labyrinth of blood sinuses. The cavernous urethra is contained within the corpus spongiosum, which enlarges distally into the glans penis. Parallel with, and dorsal to, the corpus spongiosum are the paired corpora cavernosa, which extend distally to the glans. The corpora cavernosa are united distally by a median partition, the pectiniform septum. All three structures are surrounded by a thick fibrous tunica albuginea and a subcutaneous connective tissue layer covered by a thin skin.

## TESTIS

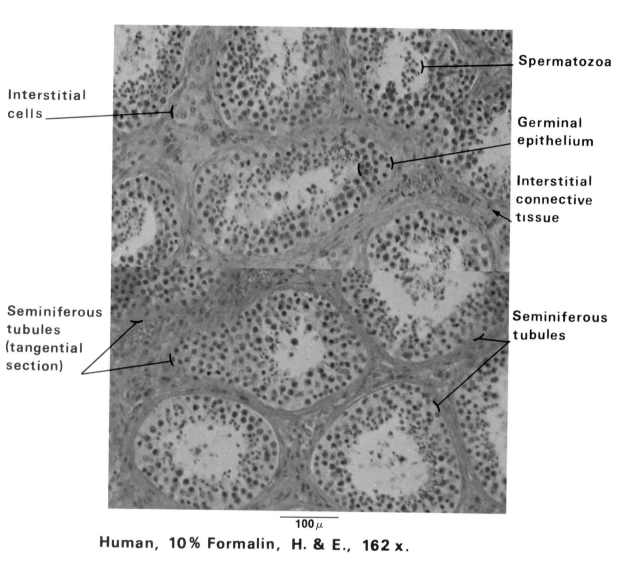

Spermatozoa

Interstitial cells

Germinal epithelium

Interstitial connective tissue

Seminiferous tubules (tangential section)

Seminiferous tubules

100 μ

**Human, 10% Formalin, H. & E., 162 x.**

This is a section of the testis showing the seminiferous tubules separated by interstitial connective tissue. The seminiferous tubules are lined by a stratified epithelium, the germinal epithelium, composed primarily of sex cells with some supporting cells. The epithelium rests on a basement membrane that varies in thickness with age. The lumina of the seminiferous tubules contain mature sex cells (spermatozoa). Seminiferous tubules are separated by an interstitial stroma made up of loose connective tissue and contain the interstitial cells of Leydig. These large ovoid cells that occur in groups are believed to secrete testosterone, the male sex hormone.

## SEMINIFEROUS TUBULE

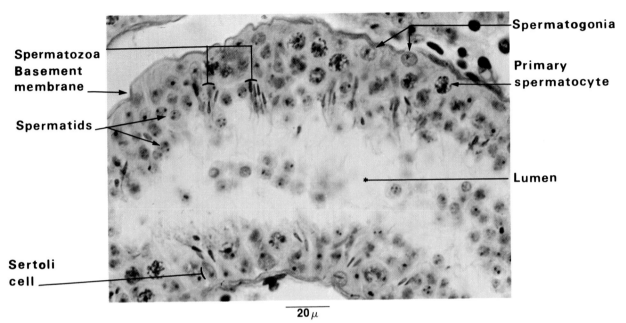

Spermatozoa
Basement
membrane

Spermatids

Sertoli
cell

Spermatogonia

Primary
spermatocyte

Lumen

20 μ

### Rhesus monkey, Helly's fluid, Iron hematoxylin and Orange G. stains, 612 x.

In the seminiferous tubule, spermatogenic cells are arranged in orderly layers between the basement membrane and the lumen.

**Spermatogonia:** Located directly above the basement membrane. Spherical nucleus. Spermatogonia are the germ cells from which spermatozoa ultimately arise. They are the only sex cells present before onset of puberty. They contain 23 pairs of chromosomes.

**Primary spermatocytes:** Lie in the next layer, deep to the spermatogonia. Largest germ cells. Nuclei are large and vesicular with condensed chromatin. Chromatin may appear as elongated spiremes, *i.e.*, irregularly disposed chromatin filaments. Primary spermatocytes divide by meiosis. Meiosis is nuclear division in which the diploid chromosome number (23 pairs) is halved to the haploid number (23 single set) in the formation of sex cells.

**Spermatids:** Adjacent to the lumen. Small in size. They constitute the last stage in the transformation to spermatozoa.

**Spermatozoa:** Sperm heads are located near Sertoli cells, and tails project into the lumen. Heads are transformed nuclei of spermatids.

**Sertoli cells:** Supporting cells of the testicular epithelium which were first described by the Italian physiologist Enrico Sertoli in 1865. Tall columnar cells extend from the basement membrane to the lumen. Nucleus ovoid in shape with prominent nucleolus. Cell borders are difficult to outline in this preparation.

The process of spermatogenesis from spermatogonia to mature spermatozoa requires 74 days in man.

## INTERSTITIAL CELLS
### Testis

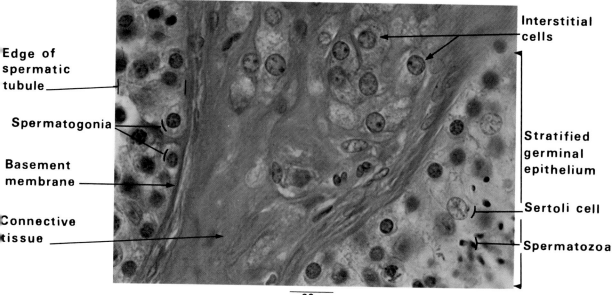

**Interstitial cells**

**Edge of spermatic tubule**

**Spermatogonia**

**Basement membrane**

**Connective tissue**

**Stratified germinal epithelium**

**Sertoli cell**

**Spermatozoa**

$20\,\mu$

**Human, 10% Formalin, H. & E., 612 x.**

    This figure shows parts of two seminiferous tubules separated by a connective tissue sheath. Within this connective tissue sheath are embedded large ovoid cells, the interstitial cells of Leydig. These occur in groups, have a rounded, large eccentric nucleus with a prominent nucleolus and a vacuolated cytoplasm which results from the loss of lipid droplets and crystals during tissue processing. The interstitial cells are believed to be the source of testosterone, the male sex hormone, whose functions include: the development and maintenance of secondary sex characteristics and the structure and function of the male accessory organs, the development of psychosexual behavior (in part) in the mature male, a role in protein metabolism, and the regulation of the output of the pituitary gonadotropic hormone. The seminiferous tubules shown reveal part of their contents, spermatogonia, spermatozoa and Sertoli cells (see Plates 20, 224 and 225).

## TESTIS
### Straight tubules and rete testis

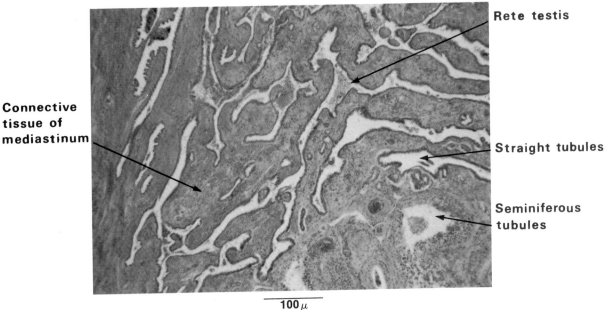

Rete testis

Connective
tissue of
mediastinum

Straight tubules

Seminiferous
tubules

100 μ

Human, 10 % Formalin, H. & E., 50 x.

The seminiferous tubules of the testis join at the apex of the testis lobule and open into the straight tubules. The latter are short, straight tubules lined with a single layer of tall columnar Sertoli cells. The straight tubule passes into a system of irregular, anastomosing epithelial-lined cavernous spaces, the rete testis, located in the dense connective tissue of the mediastinum.

# VAS DEFERENS
## cross section

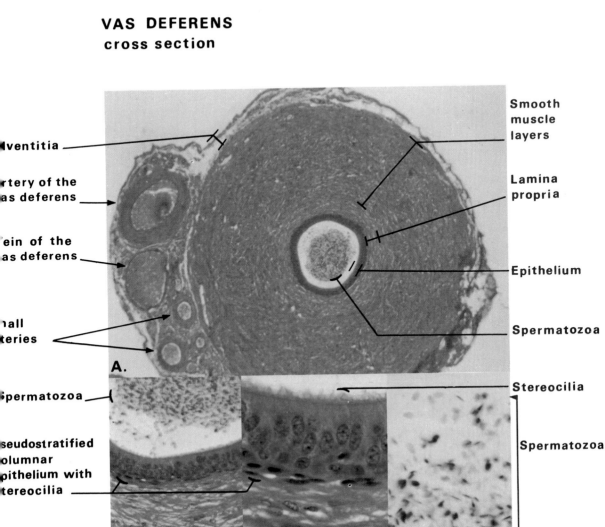

Adventitia

Artery of the vas deferens

Vein of the vas deferens

Small arteries

Spermatozoa

Pseudostratified columnar epithelium with stereocilia

Lamina propria

Smooth muscle layers

Lamina propria

Epithelium

Spermatozoa

Stereocilia

Spermatozoa

A.

B.

C.

D.

A. 0.2mm    B. 100μ    C. & D. 20μ

**Dog, 10% Formalin, H. & E., A.50x., B.162x., C. & D.612x.**

The tail of the epididymis enlarges into the vas deferens. It is characterized by a very thick muscular wall and a relatively narrow lumen filled with spermatozoa.

The epithelial lining is pseudostratified columnar with stereocilia. The lamina propria is rich in elastic fibers and is surrounded by a thick coat of smooth muscle fibers in three different layers.

The whole vas deferens, with its layers, is seen in A. Also seen in A are structures located in the adventitia that accompany the vas in the scrotum and inguinal canal, namely the testicular artery and the pampiniform plexus of veins. The cremaster muscle is not seen in this plate. In B, only a section of the wall and lumen is seen. Stereocilia on the pseudostratified epithelial lining are distinctly seen in C. Stereocilia are large, nonmotile elongated microvilli. In D, only the lumen filled with spermatozoa is seen.

## SEMINAL VESICLE

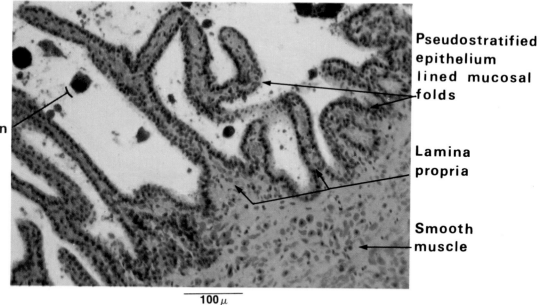

Secretion

Pseudostratified
epithelium
lined mucosal
folds

Lamina
propria

Smooth
muscle

100 μ

## Human, 10% Formalin, H. & E., 162 x.

The seminal vesicle is a diverticulum of the adjacent ductus deferens with a remarkably folded mucosal lining of pseudostratified cuboidal or columnar epithelium projecting into the lumen. The lumen frequently contains acidophilic rounded secretion masses. Underlying the epithelial lining is a thin supporting sheath of connective tissue, the lamina propria, which extends into the mucosal folds. Beneath the lamina propria is a coat of smooth muscle fibers consisting of an inner circular layer and an outer longitudinal layer.

# PROSTATE GLAND

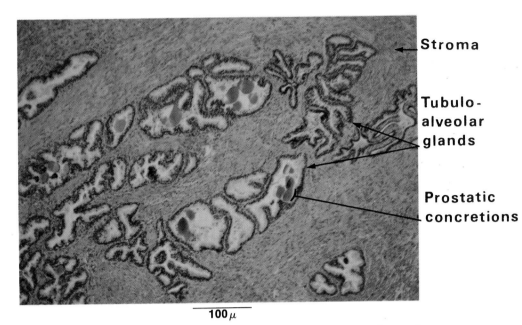

Stroma

Tubulo-
alveolar
glands

Prostatic
concretions

$100\mu$

## Human, 10% Formalin, H. & E., 162 x.

**Stroma:** Abundant and continuous with the gland capsule, it constitutes one-third to one-fourth of the gland volume composed of fibroelastic connective tissue intermixed with smooth muscle fibers. Glands are embedded in the stroma.

**Tubuloalveolar glands:** Irregular, large lumen, widely spaced tubules with alveolar extensions, which vary greatly in shape and size. Epithelial lining in tissue sections is simple cuboidal to columnar in shape.

**Prostatic concretions:** Corpora amylacea, acidophilic condensed secretions of prostatic glands. May be lamellated. Increase in number with advancing age. Source of prostatic calculi.

The prostate is located at the origin of the urethra (which it surrounds), adjacent to the urinary bladder. The prostate secretes a thin, opalescent, slightly acid fluid which contains several enzymes, including diastase and proteases, and citric acid. The smaller prostatic concretions are found in the prostatic fluid.

## PENIS
### Cross section

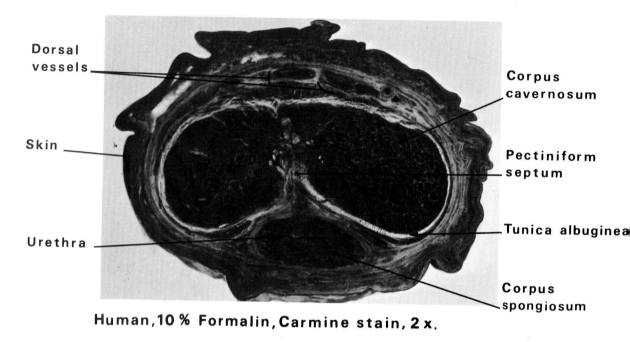

Dorsal vessels

Skin

Urethra

Corpus cavernosum

Pectiniform septum

Tunica albuginea

Corpus spongiosum

**Human, 10 % Formalin, Carmine stain, 2 x.**

The penis is formed primarily of three cylindrical masses of erectile tissue. Note the paired corpora cavernosa and the ventrally placed corpus spongiosum (corpus spongiosum urethrae) containing the urethra. A dense collagenous tissue capsule, the tunica albuginea, surrounds the corpora cavernosa. This capsule fuses in the midline to form the pectinate septum which is thickest and most complete near the root of the penis. The tunica albuginea of the corpus spongiosum is thin. Each corpus consists of a network of cavernous vascular sinuses lined with endothelium, separated by fibromuscular trabeculae composed of connective tissue and smooth muscle fibers.

The three corpora are encompassed by a common, loose connective tissue fascia rich in elastic fibers and a thin skin. Note the dorsal vessels (arteries and veins) of the penis, located in the fascia, which are part of the complicated blood supply of this organ. See also Plate 232.

## PENIS
### Corpus cavernosum

Clotted blood

Trabeculae

Central (deep) artery

Nerve

Tunica albuginea

Cavernous spaces

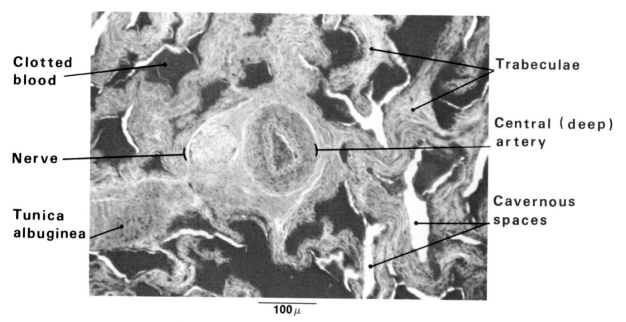

100 μ

**Human, 10 % Formalin, H. & E., 162 x.**

The erectile tissue of the corpus cavernosum of the penis is composed of cavernous spaces separated by fibromuscular septae or trabeculae. The latter are extensions of the tunica albuginea, the fibrous coat that surrounds the corpus. The cavernous spaces are filled with blood and the engorgement of these spaces results in the erection of the penis. Note the central (deep) artery which traverses the corpus cavernosum. This artery gives rise to the spiraling helicine arterioles that open into the sinuses. The central artery is the principal vessel for filling the sinuses during erection.

Adjacent to the central artery, note the nerve cut in cross section. The penis is richly supplied with spinal, sympathetic and parasympathetic fibers. The autonomic fibers innervate the smooth muscle in the arterial wall and trabeculae.

# Section 15    The Endocrine Glands

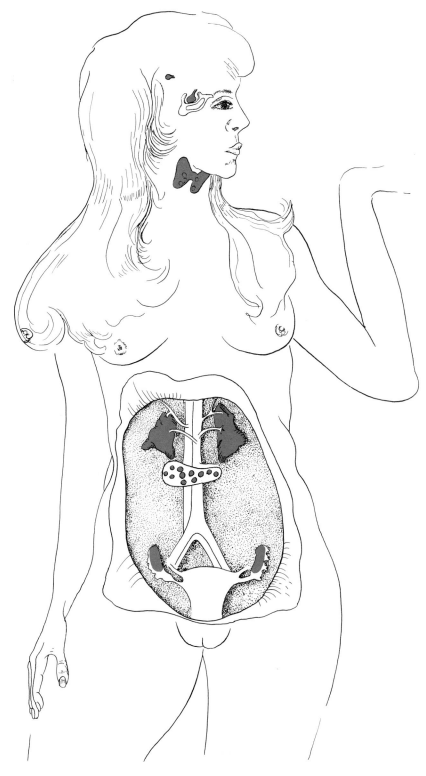

# The Endocrine Glands

These cellular masses, designated as the ductless glands or glands of internal secretion, have during development lost their original connection with the epithelium of the free surface. Their secretions are called hormones. The gland cells produce specific chemical substances which are secreted in a rich capillary bed and carried by the blood to another part, or parts, of the body where they have a distinctive function. The endocrine glands are essentially a vertebrate development, and any one of these hormonal substances has a similar action in all vertebrates with little or no species-specific function.

Endocrine glands may appear as distinct organs (*e.g.,* the hypophysis and adrenal glands), may be found associated with exocrine glands (*e.g.,* pancreatic islets and the interstitial cells of the testis), may appear as mixed endocrine glands (*e.g.,* the thyroid and parathyroid glands), or may have cells so diffusely distributed that they are not usually considered an organ (*e.g.,* argentaffin cells of the digestive system).

Some endocrine glands are essential for life and these include the adrenal cortex, pancreatic islets and the parathyroid glands. The other endocrine glands, while not essential for life, determine to a great extent the quality of one's life and the ability to adapt to stress. The endocrine glands, separately and in conjunction with the nervous system, are coordinators of body functions which maintain the organism in a viable homeostatic state.

The structural-functional organization of the endocrine glands is diverse but distinctive. In general, all endocrine glands store their secretory products either within the cells of origin or within cellular follicles or sacs. The cells of the adrenal cortex contain minimal amounts of stored hormone while in the pancreas and pituitary gland (hypophysis) secretory granules (if preserved) are usually evident. In the thyroid gland the hormone is stored extracellularly in a pool surrounded by epithelial gland cells (a follicle). In this case, the release of the hormone into the blood stream involves the reabsorption and transfer of the hormone through the cells of origin into the extracellular space, where it enters the capillaries.

An essential feature of the endocrine glands is the manner in which the secretory activity is regulated by a feedback mechanism. As an example, the beta cell of the anterior lobe of the hypophysis secretes adrenocorticotropic hormone (ACTH), which stimulates the secretion of some hormones from the adrenal cortex. As the level of adrenal cortical hormones rises in the blood stream the secretion of ACTH is inhibited. Declining levels of the hormones of the adrenal cortex result in an increased secretion of ACTH by the pituitary. In this manner, appropriate levels of adrenal cortical hormones are maintained in the blood stream.

Specific details of structure and function of the endocrine glands will be found in this section and as appropriate in the sections concerned with the digestive, urinary, male reproductive, female reproductive, and nervous systems.

## HYPOPHYSIS
### Anterior, intermediate and posterior lobe

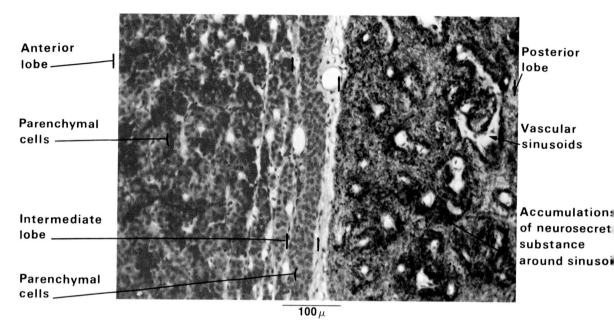

Anterior lobe

Parenchymal cells

Intermediate lobe

Parenchymal cells

Posterior lobe

Vascular sinusoids

Accumulations of neurosecret substance around sinusoi

100 μ

**Rat, 10% Formalin, Gomori's chrom alum hematoxylin and phloxine stains, 162 x.**

This plate shows a portion of the three lobes of the hypophysis.

The anterior lobe is made of anastomosing cords and plates separated by capillaries. Several tropic hormones are produced in this lobe: somatotropin, follicle-stimulating hormone, luteinizing hormone, luteotropic hormone (prolactin), thyrotropic hormone and adrenocorticotropic hormone.

The intermediate lobe is sandwiched between the anterior and posterior lobes. It has colloid-filled cysts. It elaborates melanocyte-stimulating hormone in some species (amphibia). In man and other mammals, the hormone appears to influence melanin synthesis.

The posterior lobe is made of sheets of cells and is rich in neurosecretory material. The latter is concentrated around the sinusoids. Two hormones have been extracted from this neurosecretory material, antidiuretic hormone and oxytocin.

# PITUITARY GLAND
## Anterior lobe

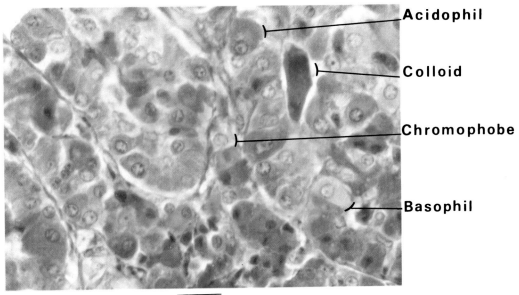

Acidophil

Colloid

Chromophobe

Basophil

20 μ

## Human,10 % Formalin,Masson's stain,612 x.

**Chromophobe:** Small, poorly staining cell. The cytoplasm is scanty and devoid of granules. Cell contours are rounded or polygonal. Also known as reserve or chief cell.

**Acidophil:** Larger than a chromophobe. Cytoplasm rich in granules which stain with acid dyes. Since they also take basic dyes, a better name might be alpha cell. Secrete growth and lactogenic hormones. The lactogenic hormone-producing acidophils increase during pregnancy. Excessive production of growth hormone as occurs in pituitary tumors produces gigantism if it occurs before puberty and acromegaly if it occurs after puberty.

**Basophil:** Beta cell. Larger than the average acidophil and less heavily granulated. Secretes thyroid-stimulating hormone (TSH), adrenocorticotropic hormone (ACTH), follicle-stimulating hormone (FSH) and luteinizing hormone (LH).

**Colloid:** Secretion product. Found in center of some cords.

## PITUITARY GLAND
### Anterior lobe

Colloid

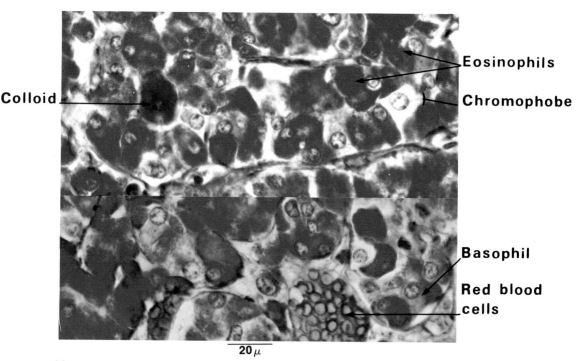

Eosinophils

Chromophobe

Basophil

Red blood cells

20 μ

**Human, 10% Formalin, Masson's stain, 612 x.**

**Colloid:**   Secretion product. Found in the center of some cords.

**Chromophobe:**   Small, faintly staining and less numerous than other cells in the pituitary. Scanty cytoplasm devoid of granules. Tend to cluster near center of cords.

**Eosinophils:**   Alpha cells. Larger than chromophobes. Cytoplasm filled with acidophilic granules. Source of growth and lactogenic hormones.

**Basophil:**   Beta cell. Larger than the average eosinophil and less heavily granulated. Secretes thyroid-stimulating hormone, adrenocorticotropic hormone, follicle-stimulating hormone and luteinizing hormone.

**Red blood cells:**   Filling the sinusoids.

## THYROID GLAND

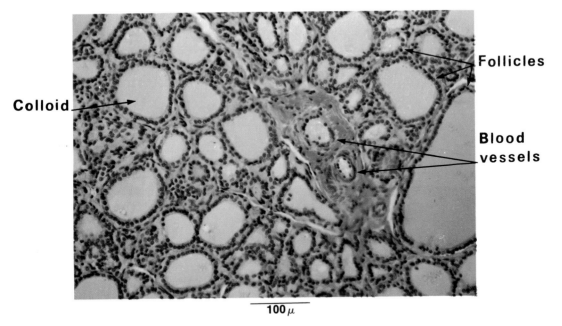

**Colloid**

**Follicles**

**Blood vessels**

100 µ

## Human, 10 % Formalin, H. & E., 162 x.

**Follicles:** Structural units of the thyroid gland. Note variations in shape (rounded or tubular) and size (0.05 to 0.5 mm diameter). Close packing with a thin reticular network in between adjacent follicles. Single layer of cells forms a hollow sphere. Nucleus centrally or basally placed.

**Colloid:** Found in the lumen of follicles. Chemical composition is a glycoprotein-iodine complex (thyroglobulin). Of the several iodinated compounds found in the gland the 3,5,3'-triiodothyronine is hormonally the most active. The follicles release about 100 mg of hormone daily. Normal thyroid function is essential for the normal growth, development and well-being of man and animals. Hypofunction of the thyroid in infants results in cretinism, characterized by dwarfism, mental deficiency, slow heart rate, muscular weakness and gastrointestinal disturbances. Thyroid hormone given to infants at an early stage of cretinism can alleviate the symptoms. In adults, hypothyroidism results in muscular weakness, mental deterioration, reflex and skin changes. When the hormone is produced in excess (hyperthyroidism) excessive appetite and thirst, weight loss, rapid respiration, sweating, muscular weakness, tremor and an increase in heart rate (tachycardia) follow. Emotional disturbance and nervousness are also common symptoms.

**Blood vessels:** The thyroid is richly supplied with blood vessels which are intimately associated with the follicles.

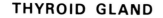

# THYROID GLAND

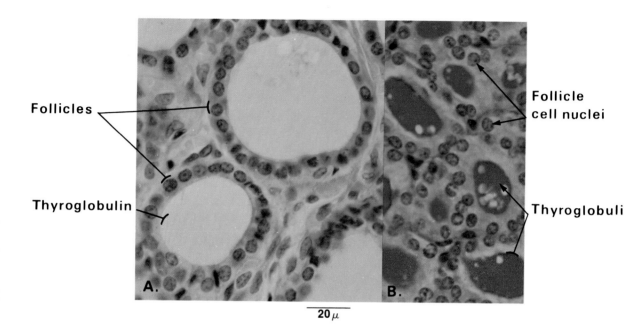

Follicles

Thyroglobulin

Follicle
cell nuclei

Thyroglobuli

A.    B.

20 μ

Human, 10 % Formalin , A.  H.&E.,  B. Periodic acid-
Schiff and hematoxylin stains, 612 x.

**Follicles:**  Structural units of the thyroid gland supported and separated by connective tissue. Note variation in size. A single layer of cells forms the follicle. Shape of cells reflects functional activity. Cells in these
follicles are cuboidal with central, rounded nuclei, indicating normal activity.

In *A*, the colloid in the lumen of the follicle is not stained. In *B*, the colloid is specifically stained red with the
periodic acid-Schiff method because of the chemical composition of colloid, which is a glycoprotein-iodine
complex (thyroglobulin).

## PARATHYROID GLAND

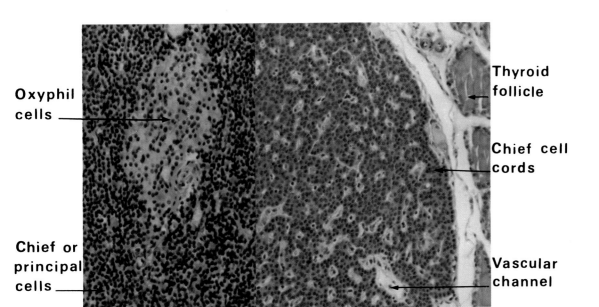

Oxyphil cells

Thyroid follicle

Chief cell cords

Chief or principal cells

Vascular channel

100 μ

### Human, 10% Formalin, H. & E., 162 x.

Parathyroid glands are essential for life. In the absence of parathyroid hormone there is a pronounced decrease in blood calcium resulting in tetany, the intense, involuntary spasm of skeletal muscle.

**Oxyphil cells:** Occur in groups or nests among chief cells. Larger than chief cells, cytoplasm acidophilic. Oxyphils increase with age and are not found in all mammals. Function remains unknown.

**Chief or principal cells:** Much more numerous than oxyphil cells and functionally more important. Nucleus round and centrally located. Cytoplasm homogeneous. Arranged in cords or plates separated by vascular channels. These cells produce parathyroid hormone, which is important in calcium metabolism.

**Thyroid follicle:** Seen adjacent to the capsule of the parathyroid gland.

# PANCREAS
## Islet of Langerhans

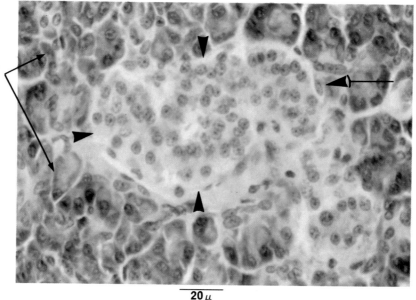

Acinar cells

Islet

20 μ

Rhesus monkey, Helly's fluid, H. & E., 612 x.

**Islet:** Pale-staining area demarcated by arrows. Contains irregular clumps of cells. Separated from the acinar cells by a thin partition of reticular tissue. This endocrine gland elaborates the hormones insulin and glucagon, which are secreted into the rich capillary bed and carried via the portal system of veins into and through the hepatic lobules before reaching the general circulation. Insulin and glucagon constitute an important system for the regulation of blood glucose levels. This endocrine organ is essential for life. Dysfunction results in diabetes mellitus, a common disorder of man, characterized in its uncontrolled and severest form by polyuria (frequent urination), glycosuria (sugar in the urine), ketonuria (ketones in the urine), acidosis (inability to buffer the blood at pH 7.2 to 7.4), wasting of the body and early death in a comatose state.

**Acinar cells:** Darker staining, irregular cells. Rich in cytoplasmic ribonucleic acid (RNA). Elaborate digestive enzymes, which are carried to, and are active in, the duodenum. Pancreatic enzymes break down partially digested food from the stomach into simple compounds. Carbohydrates, fats and proteins are hydrolyzed by the enzymes amylase, lipase and various proteases (including the nucleoproteases) secreted by the acinar cells.

## PANCREAS
### Islet of Langerhans

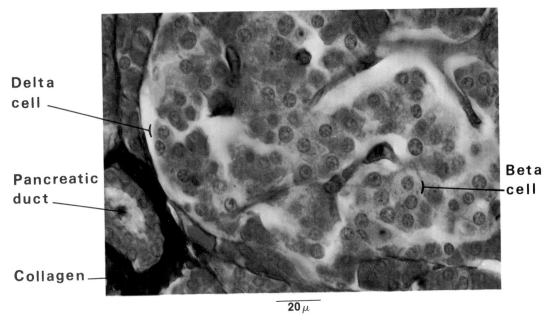

Delta cell

Pancreatic duct

Collagen

Beta cell

20 μ

Human, Helly's fluid, Mallory-azan stain, 612 x.

The islets of Langerhans were described by Paul Langerhans, a German physician, anatomist and pathologist, in 1869. Although in routine histological preparations all of the islet cells appear to be similar, special methods reveal three types, alpha, beta and delta.

**Delta cell:** Few in number compared to alpha or beta cells. Significance not well understood. Cytoplasm stains blue with Mallory's stain.

**Beta cell:** More numerous than alpha or delta cells. Produce insulin. Insulin increases cellular uptake of glucose and its conversion to glycogen. Beta cells may occur outside the islets. Granules are diffusely scattered in cytoplasm.

**Pancreatic duct:** Found in interlobular connective tissue, lined by cuboidal to columnar epithelium. Size varies with that of the territory drained.

**Collagen:** In the interlobular connective tissue. Stains dark blue with Mallory's stain.

Alpha cells (not seen in this preparation) secrete the hormone glucagon, which effects the breakdown of liver glycogen and elevates the blood glucose level.

# ADRENAL GLAND

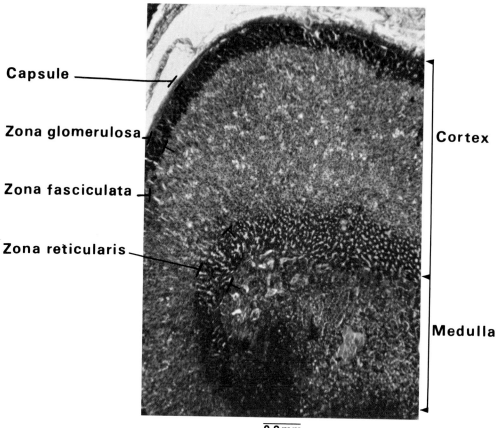

Capsule

Zona glomerulosa

Zona fasciculata

Zona reticularis

Cortex

Medulla

0.2 mm

## Rhesus monkey, Helly's fluid, H. & E., 50 x.

**Capsule:**  A tough fibroelastic covering of the adrenal gland.

**Cortex:**  Three concentric zones, each with a different cell arrangement, are shown. The adrenal cortex is essential to life. It controls the electrolyte and water distribution in the body and maintains proper carbohydrate balance.

**Zona glomerulosa:**  Outermost narrow zone of the adrenal cortex. Deeply staining, densely packed nuclei. Elaborates aldosterone.

**Zona fasciculata:**  The broadest zone of the adrenal cortex. Cells are arranged in long cords. Elaborates cortisol.

**Zona reticularis:**  Innermost layer of adrenal cortex. Cells are arranged in irregular cords separated by sinusoids (clear spaces) giving the appearance of a meshwork. Stains deeper than zona fasciculata.

**Medulla:**  Irregularly arranged mass of cells in cords. Highly vascularized. Rich in chromaffin substance. Produces epinephrine and norepinephrine.

# ADRENAL GLAND
## Cortex and medulla

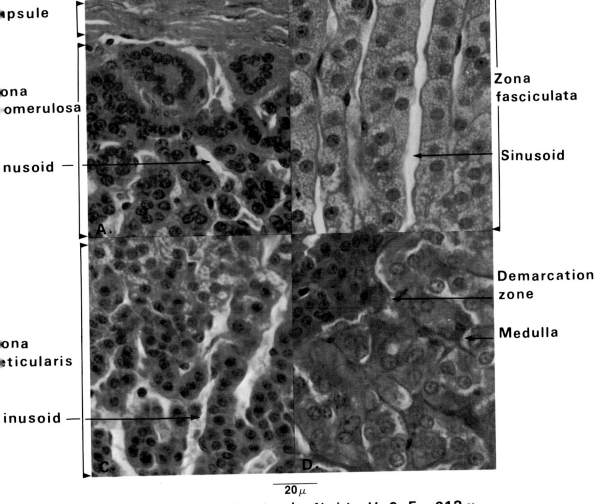

Capsule

Zona glomerulosa

Sinusoid

A.

Zona reticularis

Sinusoid

C.

Zona fasciculata

Sinusoid

Demarcation zone

Medulla

D.

20 μ

Rhesus monkey, Zenker's fluid, H. & E., 612 x.

This plate illustrates the different zones of the adrenal gland, from the capsule to the medulla.

**Capsule:** A tough fibroelastic covering with delicate trabeculae extending into the substance of the gland.

**Zona glomerulosa:** Outermost narrow zone of the adrenal cortex. Cells arranged in ovoid groups without a significant lumen. Component cells are columnar with spherical, deeply staining nuclei. Richly supplied with blood. The zona glomerulosa secretes hormones concerned primarily with mineral metabolism. The mineralocorticoids are deoxycorticosterone and aldosterone.

**Sinusoid:** Sinusoids arise from multiple arterioles in the capsule. Course between cell cords.

**Zona fasciculata:** The middle and broadest zone of the adrenal cortex. Cells are regularly arranged in parallel cords, one to two cells thick. Component cells are cuboidal, frequently containing two vesicular nuclei. Vacuoles seen in some cells represent dissolved lipid droplets. Cholesterol is chiefly present in this zone. Cell cords are surrounded by sinusoids. Secretes the glucocorticoids, cortisone and cortisol.

*Text continued on following page.*

325

**Zona reticularis:** Innermost layer of the adrenal cortex. Cells are arranged in irregular cords, are smaller than those of the zona fasciculata and stain darker. Nuclei stain deeply. Sinusoids separate cell cords. Secretes the same glucocorticoids as the zona fasciculata. These hormones participate in carbohydrate, protein and fat metabolism.

**Demarcation zone:** Shows zone of transition from zona reticularis to medulla.

**Medulla:** Polyhedral cells arranged in anastomosing cords. Prominent nuclei. Contain chromaffin granules, precursors of epinephrine and norepinephrine. Richly supplied with blood.

The adrenal cortex is essential for life and, through its hormones, is involved in numerous body functions. These activities include the maintenance of water and electrolyte balance, carbohydrate metabolism and the normal functioning of connective tissue cells. Destruction or removal of the cortex results in Addison's disease unless cortical hormones are given to the patient.

The adrenal medulla is not essential for life. The hormones of the adrenal medulla influence the metabolic rate and cardiovascular function and induce lipolysis and the release of fatty acids from adipose tissue.

## CHROMAFFIN CELLS
### Heart
### Coronary sulcus

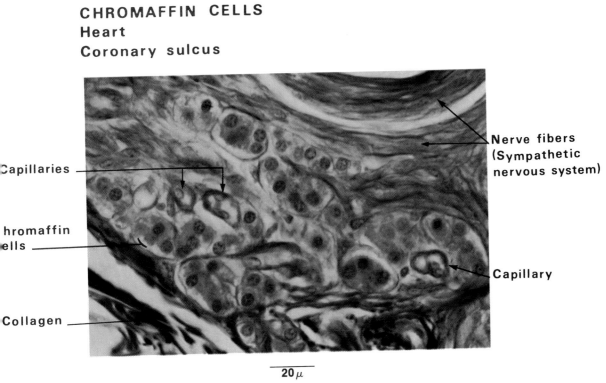

Capillaries

Nerve fibers
(Sympathetic
nervous system)

hromaffin
ells

Capillary

Collagen

20 μ

**Human, Helly's fluid, Mallory-azan stain, 612 x.**

Scattered islands of chromaffin cells are found in the subepicardial connective tissue of the coronary sinus. Note relation to capillaries into which it is believed they pour their secretion of catecholamine. Chromaffin cells are usually closely associated with sympathetic nerve fibers and ganglion cells. The brownish coloration is due to oxidation of chromaffin granules by potassium dichromate in the fixative used in this preparation. Because of their structural similarity to cells of the adrenal medulla, it is assumed that chromaffin cell secretion augments action of the sympathetic nervous system by elevating blood sugar, increasing heart rate, raising blood pressure and generally preparing the organism for emergency situations ("flight or fight").

## PINEAL GLAND

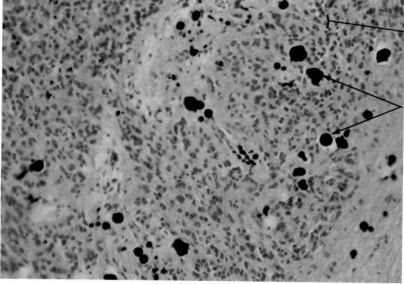

Parenchymal cells

Calcareous granules or brain sand

100μ

**Human, 10% Formalin, H.& E., 162x.**

The pineal gland is made up of plates of cells separated by septa. Two cell types are recognized by special techniques, the more common parenchymal cell and the neuroglial (astrocyte-like) supporting cell. The latter are found between clusters of parenchymal cells. The two cell types cannot be distinguished in ordinary H. & E. preparations. Concretions or brain sand characterize the pineal gland and increase with age. They have a mineralized organic matrix and, at high magnification, appear lamellated.

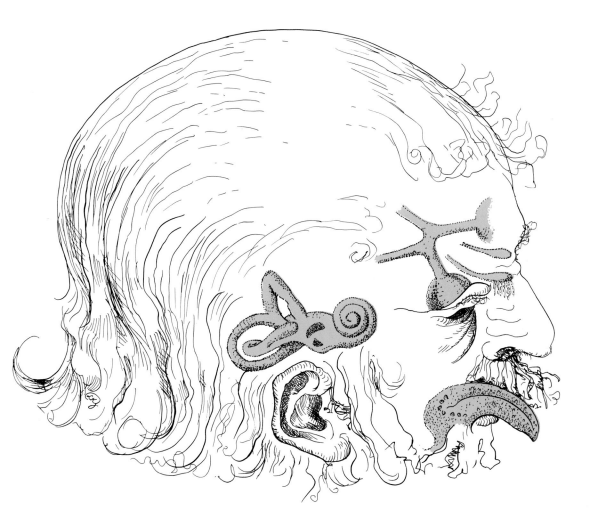

# Special Senses

The different sensations perceived by the human body are grouped into two major categories: those concerned with general sensations (touch, pressure, pain and temperature) and those concerned with special sensations (olfaction, taste, vision, audition and sense of position and movement). Illustrations of nerve endings concerned with general sensibility are found in the section on nervous tissue. This section is devoted to a consideration of the organs of special senses. While endings concerned with general sensibility are widely distributed, those concerned with special sensations are limited to specific areas of the body.

### I. Olfaction

The olfactory organ is located in the mucous membrane lining the uppermost part of the roof of the nasal cavity. From the roof, the olfactory epithelium extends down both sides of the nasal cavity to cover most of the superior concha laterally and 1 cm of nasal septum medially. The specialized nerve cells of the olfactory epithelium are highly sensitive to different odors. The presence of these nerve cells at the surface exposes them unduly to damage; it is estimated that 1 per cent of the fibers of the olfactory nerves (processes of olfactory neurons) is lost each year of life because of injury to the perikarya. The sense of smell thus diminishes in the elderly as a result of the exposure of the olfactory epithelium to repeated infections and trauma in life. The presence of olfactory neurons at the surface represents the only exception to the evolutionary rule by which nerve cell bodies of afferent neurons migrate along their axons to take up more central and well-protected positions. The olfactory neurons (Plate 246) are bipolar nerve cells with short peripheral processes reaching the surface of the epithelium and longer central processes that constitute the olfactory nerves. The peripheral short processes end in sensory receptor hairs. The surface of the epithelium is constantly moistened by secretions of Bowman's glands. The moistening of the epithelium helps dissolve the gaseous substances, facilitating stimulation of the olfactory epithelium. The continuous secretion prevents retention of dissolved odors.

It is believed that different basic odors stimulate different olfactory neurons that are not evenly distributed throughout the olfactory mucosa. Stimulation of different combinations of receptors for basic odors is believed to be the basis for man's ability to recognize all the varieties of odors to which he is exposed.

### II. Taste

The gustatory (taste) sense organs in higher vertebrates are limited to the cavity of the mouth. The sensory organ of taste is the taste bud (Plates 157 and 247), which is a pale, ovoid structure within the stratified squamous epithelium. It is estimated that one vallate papilla of the tongue contains 200 taste buds on its sides and about 50 buds in the wall of the trench opposite the papilla. This number decreases progressively with age. In addition to the vallate and fungiform papillae of the tongue, taste buds are found in the soft palate, pharynx and epiglottis. The taste bud contains neuroepithelial and supporting cells. The neuroepithelial cells are stimulated by substances in solution. Although all taste buds look histologically alike, sensitivity to the four basic taste modalities is different in different regions of the tongue. Some buds may respond only to sweet, sour, salt or bitter. Substances in solution enter the pore of the taste bud and stimulate the hairs of neuroepithelial taste cells.

Taste sensations from the anterior two-thirds of the tongue are mediated to the central nervous system via the chorda tympani of the seventh (facial) cranial nerve, those from the posterior one-third of the tongue via the ninth (glossopharyngeal) cranial nerve and those from the epiglottis and lower pharynx via the tenth (vagus) nerve. These nerves contain the peripheral processes of pseudounipolar sensory nerve cells located in the geniculate ganglion (seventh nerve), petrous ganglion (ninth nerve) and nodose ganglion (tenth nerve). These peripheral processes enter the deep ends of the taste buds and establish intimate contact with the neuroepithelial cells of the buds. The central processes of these sensory neurons project to the nucleus of the tractus solitarius in the brain stem.

## III. Vision

Vision is by far the most important of man's senses. Most of our perception of the environment around us comes through our eyes. Our visual system is capable of adapting to extreme changes in light intensity to allow us to see clearly; it is also capable of color discrimination and depth perception.

The organ of vision is the eye; accessory structures include the eyelids, lacrimal glands and the extrinsic eye muscles. The eye has been compared to a camera. While structurally the two are similar, the camera lacks the intricate nervous mechanism involved in vision. As an optical instrument, the eye has four functional components: a protective coat, a nourishing lightproof coat, a dioptric system and a receptive integrating layer. The protective coat is the tough, opaque sclera which covers the posterior five-sixths of the eyeball; it is continuous with the dura mater around the optic nerve. The anterior one-sixth is covered by the transparent cornea, which belongs to the dioptric system. The nourishing coat is made up of the vascular choroid which supplies nutrients to the retina and, because of its rich content of melanocytes, acts as a light-absorbing layer. It corresponds to the pia-arachnoid layer of the nervous system. Anteriorly, this coat becomes the ciliary body and iris. The iris ends at a circular opening, the pupil. The dioptric system includes the cornea, the lens, the aqueous humor within the anterior eye chamber and the vitreous body. The dioptric system helps focus the image on the retina. The greatest refraction of incoming light takes place at the air-cornea interface. The lens is supported by the suspensory ligament from the ciliary body, and changes in its shape permit change of focus. This is a function of the ciliary muscle, which is supplied by the parasympathetic nervous system. In late middle age, the lens loses its elastic properties and a condition known as presbyopia results wherein accommodative power is diminished, especially to near vision. The amount of light entering the eye is regulated by the size of the pupil. Pupillary size is controlled by the action of the constrictor and dilator smooth muscles of the iris. The constrictor muscle is supplied by the parasympathetic nervous system, and the dilator by the sympathetic nervous system.

The receptive integrating layer is the retina, which is an extension of the brain to which it is connected by the optic nerve. The rods and cones are the sensory retinal receptors. The rods are about four times as numerous as the cones. Rods function best during dim light vision, and cones during bright light vision and in color discrimination. The outer segments of rods and cones contain the visual pigments, rhodopsin and iodopsin, respectively. Light falling on these pigments results in a series of chemical changes leading to depolarization of the receptor cell membrane and the formation of an action potential which is then conducted to the brain.

## IV. Audition

The organ of hearing is the organ of Corti, situated in the inner ear. Sound waves reaching the tympanic membrane will initiate vibrations that are transmitted through the bony ossicles of the middle ear to the oval window. Vibrations of the oval window are transmitted to the perilymph in the scala vestibuli and through the vestibular membrane to the endolymph of the cochlear duct (Plate 260). Such induced pulsations in the endolymph will displace the basilar membrane on which the organ of Corti lies (Plate 260), and alter the relationship of the tectorial membrane, which overlies the organ of Corti, to the hairs of the hair cells. This bending or stretching of the hairs acts as a stimulus to the hair cells. This stimulus is then transmitted to the peripheral processes of bipolar neurons in the spiral ganglion (Plate 96). The central processes comprise the auditory component of the eighth cranial nerve, which projects centrally to the cochlear nuclei. The cochlea and the organ of Corti follow a spiral course of $2\frac{1}{2}$ turns. The lower turns are wider than the apical turns. It is believed that the hair cells in the lower turns respond best to high frequency sounds while those of the upper turns respond best to low frequency sounds.

## V. Position and Movement

The organ of posture and equilibrium is a composite one located in the semicircular canals, the utricle and the saccule of the inner ear. The dilated ends of the semicircular canals contain the cristae, which constitute the neurosensory epithelium that responds to changes in rotational motion. Displacement of endolymph against the cupula overlying a crista disturbs and, therefore, stimulates its hair cells. Each crista is stimulated by movements occurring in the plane of its semicircular canal. The neuroepithelial component of the utricle (macula) provides information regarding static equilibrium and position of the head in space. Gravitational pull acts on the otoconia on the surface of the macula, and the hair tufts of underlying neuroepithelial hair cells are thus stimulated. Stimuli from the vestibular sense organs travel via the peripheral processes of the bipolar neurons of the ganglion of Scarpa. The central processes form the vestibular component of the eighth nerve.

## NASAL MUCOSA

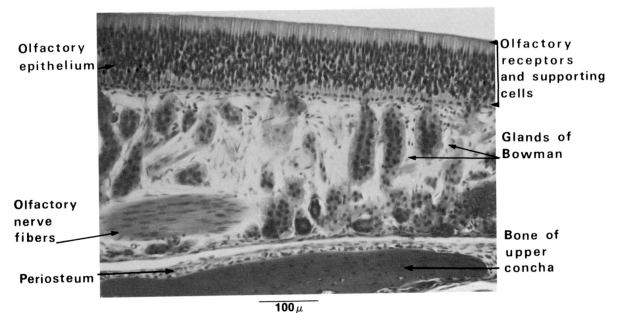

Olfactory epithelium

Olfactory receptors and supporting cells

Glands of Bowman

Olfactory nerve fibers

Bone of upper concha

Periosteum

100 μ

## Human, Müller's fluid, H. & E., 162 x.

**Olfactory epithelium:** Thick pseudostratified epithelium containing bipolar receptor neurons and sustentacular (supporting) cells. Cells are densely packed. No goblet cells are present in this region.

**Glands of Bowman:** Located in the lamina propria. Branched tubuloalveolar glands that secrete a seromucus. Ducts carry the secretion to the surface of the epithelium. The secretion serves to keep the epithelial surface moist and to facilitate solution of substances being smelled.

**Olfactory nerve fibers:** Nonmyelinated axons of bipolar receptor neurons. Located deep in the lamina propria.

**Bone of upper concha:** Olfactory epithelium covers the superior conchae and the adjacent portion of the nasal septum.

**Periosteum:** Fibrous, osteogenic connective tissue covering bone.

# OLFACTORY EPITHELIUM
## Bipolar receptor neurons

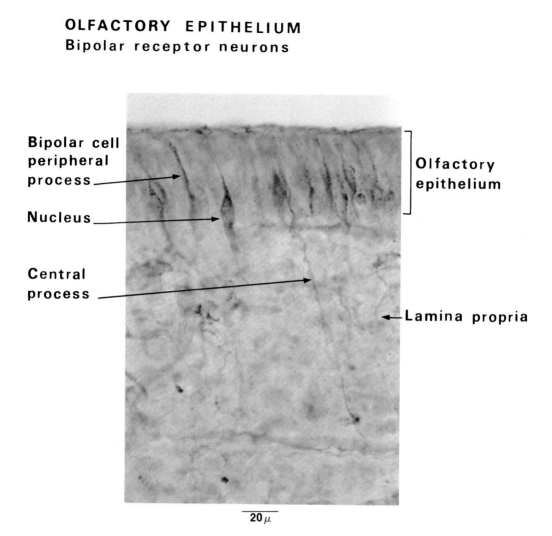

Bipolar cell peripheral process

Nucleus

Central process

Olfactory epithelium

Lamina propria

20 μ

Dog, 10 % Formalin, Silver diammine hydroxide, 500 x.

In this plate, a special staining technique is used to demonstrate the olfactory receptor (bipolar) neurons in the olfactory mucosa.

The nuclei of the receptor cells are usually deeply located in the epithelium. From the nuclear region of the neuron, a delicate peripheral neural process reaches the exposed surface of the epithelium. At the opposite pole of the cell, an unmyelinated axon extends centrally. The axons of receptor cells are gathered together to form the olfactory nerve (cranial nerve I). The olfactory nerve terminates in the olfactory bulb, where synaptic contacts are established with neurons which form the olfactory tract.

The olfactory bipolar neurons are located between the more numerous sustentacular cells which are seen in Plate 245.

# TASTE BUD
## Tongue
### vallate papilla

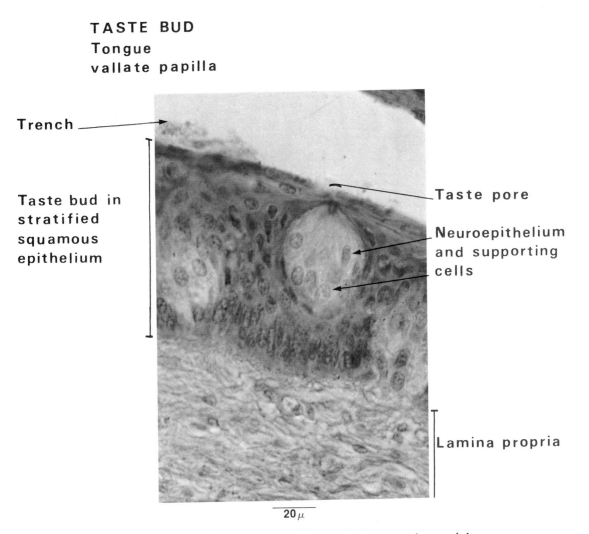

Trench

Taste bud in stratified squamous epithelium

Taste pore

Neuroepithelium and supporting cells

Lamina propria

20 μ

## Human, Zenker's fluid, Phosphotungstic acid hematoxylin stain, 612 x.

Taste buds are located in the tongue epithelium of vallate (circumvallate) papillae, and occasionally in the fungiform papillae and in the surface epithelium around them. A few taste buds are also present in the palate and epiglottis.

**Trench:**  Surrounds vallate papillae. Covered by nonkeratinized stratified squamous epithelium.

**Taste bud in stratified squamous epithelium:**  Barrel-shaped. Extends from the basement membrane to the free surface of the stratified squamous epithelium covering the papilla. Taste buds are the receptor organs of taste.

**Taste pore:**  The opening of the taste canal at the surface of the epithelium.

**Neuroepithelial and supporting cells:**  The two types of cells are packed within the concavity of the taste bud. The neuroepithelial cells are slender, dense and spindle-shaped. They constitute the taste receptor cells. Supporting cells or sustentacular cells are stouter and lighter.

**Lamina propria:**  Connective tissue core of the papilla.

See also Plate 157.

# CONJUNCTIVA AND CORNEA

Lamina
propria

Stratified
columnar
epithelium
and Goblet
cells

Corneal
stroma

Corneal
epithelium

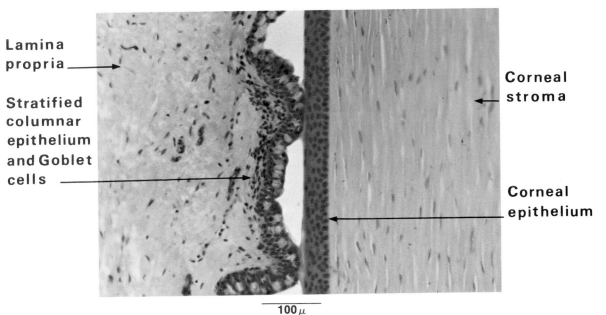

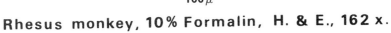

100 μ

**Rhesus monkey, 10% Formalin, H. & E., 162 x.**

This plate includes part of the cornea (right) and the covering bulbar conjunctiva (left). The conjunctiva at this site is composed of the following elements.

**Lamina propria:** A loose, superficial fibroelastic connective tissue stroma which becomes increasingly dense at deeper levels. Rich in blood vessels.

**Stratified columnar epithelium:** Eight to ten cells thick. Superficial layers near the cornea rich in goblet cells.

**Corneal epithelium and stroma:** See Plate 249.

# CORNEA

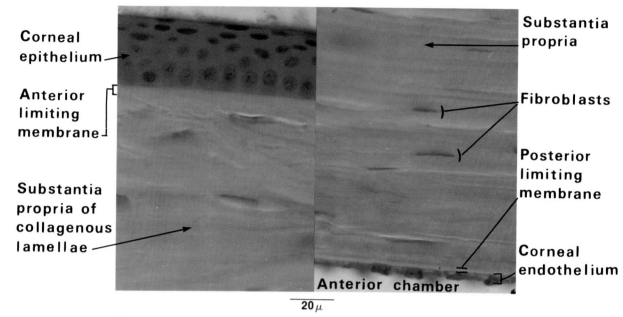

Corneal epithelium

Anterior limiting membrane

Substantia propria of collagenous lamellae

Substantia propria

Fibroblasts

Posterior limiting membrane

Corneal endothelium

Anterior chamber

20 μ

**Rhesus monkey, 10 % Formalin, H. & E., 612 x.**

The cornea is the bulging front portion of the eye. It is nonvascular and transparent. Microscopically five distinct layers can be recognized.

**Corneal epithelium:** Nonkeratinized stratified squamous type of epithelium. Note that the basal layer of cells is columnar and the most superficial are flattened.

**Anterior limiting membrane:** The second layer of the cornea was described by Sir William Bowman, an English surgeon, and therefore is called Bowman's membrane. This membrane appears homogeneous and structureless by light microscopy. By electron microscopy it is shown to be composed of fine collagenous fibrils.

**Substantia propria:** Comprises nine-tenths of the thickness of the cornea. Composed of collagen fibrils, fibroblasts and cementing substance. The fibrils are arranged in lamellae that run parallel to the surface of the cornea. The fibroblasts are flattened and lie between the fibrous lamellae. A mucopolysaccharide cements the different lamellae and the collagenous fibrils within lamellae together. The metachromatic protein polysaccharide ground substance and the arrangement of fibrils within the substantia propria contribute to the transparency of the cornea.

**Posterior limiting membrane:** The posterior limiting membrane of the cornea was described by the French surgeon Descemet in 1758 and is known by his name. English anatomists state that it was first described by Benedict Duddell, an English oculist. This membrane appears homogeneous in the light microscope. Electron microscopy reveals a wide basement membrane made of atypical collagen.

**Corneal endothelium:** Low cuboidal epithelium. The term "endothelium" is a misnomer since this epithelium is bathed by aqueous humor of the anterior chamber and not blood or lymph.

## EYE

Suspensory ligament

Lens

Ciliary processes

Ciliary body

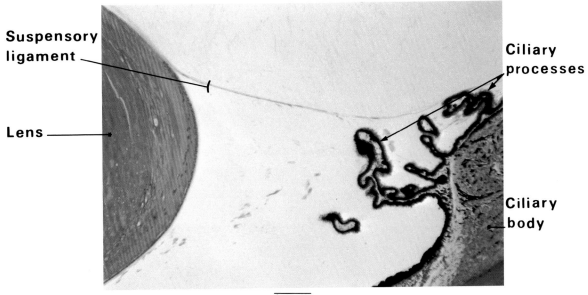

0.2 mm

Rhesus monkey, 10 % Formalin, H. & E., 50 x.

**Ciliary body:** A ring of muscle and vascular tissue, part of the vascular and pigmented tunic of the eye which includes, in addition, the choroid and iris. The ciliary body is attached to the lens by the suspensory ligament. Contraction of muscle of the ciliary body results in lens accommodation.

**Ciliary processes:** Ridges of the ciliary body as it approaches the iris. Run in a meridional plane. Provide an anchor for the suspensory ligaments of the lens. Produce aqueous humor.

**Suspensory ligament:** Made up of delicate collagenous fibers that stretch between the lens capsule and ciliary processes from which the lens is suspended. The suspensory ligament is under tension when the eye is at rest and relaxes when the lens accommodates, as in near vision.

**Lens:** Transparent biconvex disc enclosed in a homogeneous elastic capsule and located behind the iris. Made up of concentric layers of lens fibers and a cement substance. Changes in configuration of the lens are important in accommodation. The lens, cornea and the vitreous are the important refractive media of the eye.

# CILIARY MUSCLE AND CILIARY PROCESSES

Circular portion of the ciliary muscle

Ciliary processes

Zonular fibers of suspensory ligaments

Melanocyte

Columnar epithelium

Posterior chamber

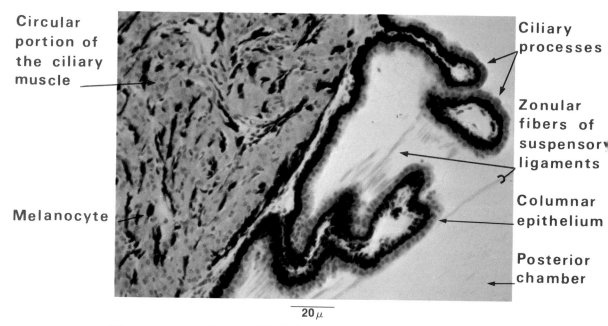

$\overline{20\,\mu}$

Rhesus monkey, 10% Formalin, H. & E., 612 x.

**Ciliary processes:** Ridges of the ciliary body as it approaches the iris run in a meridional plane. They provide an anchor for the suspensory ligaments of the lens.

**Zonular fibers of suspensory ligament:** Seen attached to the ciliary processes. Inelastic and radially arranged fibers from which the lens is suspended. Extend from ciliary processes to the lens capsule. When the eye is at rest, zonular fibers under tension from elastic fibers in the choroid stretch the lens. Tension in zonular fibers is reduced when ciliary muscles contract. This results in a change in the shape of the lens (accommodation). The lens becomes more spherical due to its inherent elasticity.

**Columnar epithelium:** Columnar or cuboidal epithelium which covers the ciliary processes. Indistinct cell borders. Elaborates aqueous humor.

**Posterior chamber:** The space between the iris and suspensory ligament of the lens. Contains aqueous humor.

**Ciliary muscle:** Smooth muscle fibers intermixed with melanocytes. Runs in three directions: circular, radial and meridional. Circular fibers lie at the inner edge of the ciliary body. Contraction of ciliary muscles releases tension in suspensory ligament of the lens and of the lens capsule, thus allowing the lens to change shape to accommodate for near vision. The ciliary muscle is a continuation of the suprachoroid layer.

**Melanocytes:** Pigment-laden cells scattered in the connective tissue elements between muscle fibers.

# IRIS AND LENS

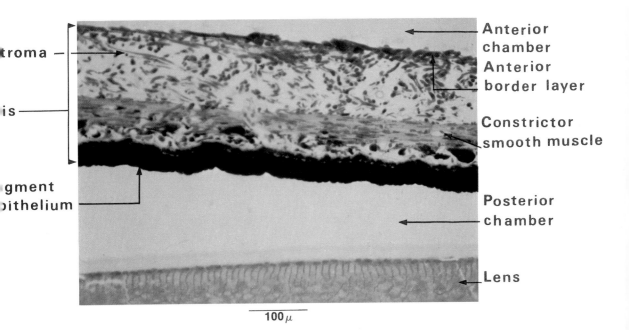

Stroma —

Iris —

Pigment
epithelium —

Anterior
chamber

Anterior
border layer

Constrictor
smooth muscle

Posterior
chamber

Lens

100 μ

**Rhesus monkey, 10% Formalin, H. & E., 162 x.**

The iris, like the ciliary body, is a continuation of the retina and choroid. It is attached to the ciliary body and extends in front of the lens. All the layers of the iris are shown in this figure except the endothelial cell layer which outlines the anterior boundary of the iris. This is a thin and delicate layer which is difficult to see in ordinary light microscopic preparations.

**Anterior chamber:** Located anterior to the iris and communicates with the posterior chamber through the pupil. Contains aqueous humor.

**Anterior border layer:** A condensation of the stroma of the iris. Formed principally of pigment cells containing a variable amount of yellowish-brown pigment. Thickness of this layer determines the color of the iris. It is thin in blue-eyed individuals and thick in brown-eyed individuals.

**Stroma:** Consists of loose connective tissue, in which is found a large number of blood vessels. Pigment connective tissue cells are scattered in this loose connective tissue stroma.

**Sphincter smooth muscle fibers:** Constricts the pupil. Supplied by the parasympathetic postganglionic neurons located in the ciliary ganglion.

**Pigment epithelium:** Continuation of the ciliary epithelium. Vast amounts of melanin pigment obscure cell boundaries and nuclei.

**Posterior chamber:** Between the iris and the lens. Communicates with anterior chamber through the pupil. Contains aqueous humor.

**Lens:** See Plate 250.

## IRIS

Blood vessel

Melanophores

Pigmented
epithelium

Constrictor
smooth musci

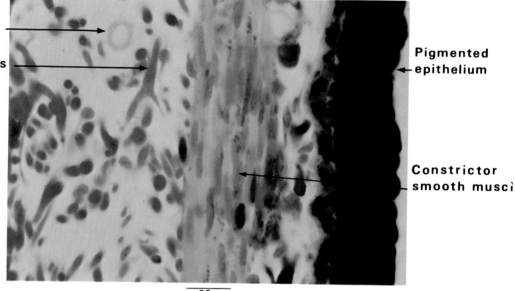

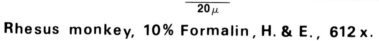

20 μ

### Rhesus monkey, 10% Formalin, H. & E., 612 x.

**Pigmented epithelium:** On the posterior surface of the iris. A layer of cuboidal cells whose outlines are masked by the heavy pigment.

**Sphincter smooth muscle:** The fibers are arranged circumferentially at the margin of the pupils. Contraction will constrict the pupil. Supplied by parasympathetic postganglionic neurons located in the ciliary ganglion.

**Blood vessels:** In the iris stroma. Have a thick adventitial layer forming a unique fibrous acellular wall.

**Melanocytes:** Spindle-shaped connective tissue cells, with long processes containing yellow-brown pigment, scattered in the loose stroma of the iris. Most commonly seen along the anterior border of the iris. The number of pigment cells varies with the individual's complexion.

PLATE 254

# RETINA

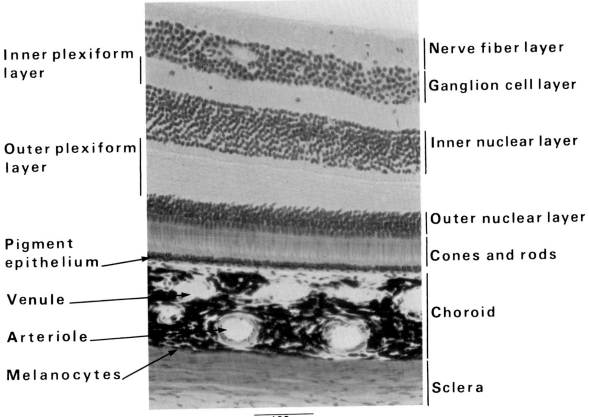

| Inner plexiform layer | | Nerve fiber layer |
| Outer plexiform layer | | Ganglion cell layer |
| Pigment epithelium | | Inner nuclear layer |
| Venule | | Outer nuclear layer |
| Arteriole | | Cones and rods |
| Melanocytes | | Choroid |
| | | Sclera |

100 μ

Rhesus monkey, Helly's fluid, H. & E., 162 x.

**Nerve fiber layer:** Consists of nonmyelinated axons of ganglion cells. They converge at the optic disc to form the optic nerve. Fibrous neuroglial cells are scattered among nerve fibers.

**Ganglion cell layer:** Composed of multipolar ganglion cells. Only nuclei are seen by this method of staining.

**Inner plexiform layer:** Contains processes of amacrine cells, axons of bipolar cells and dendrites of ganglion cells.

**Inner nuclear layer:** Contains the nuclei of bipolar neurons and association neurons (horizontal and amacrine cells), as well as the nuclei of supporting (Müller's) cells.

**Outer plexiform layer:** Contains axons of rod and cone cells, dendrites of bipolar cells and processes of the horizontal cells.

**Outer nuclear layer:** Contains rod and cone cell bodies and nuclei. Cone nuclei are ovoid and limited to a single row (compare with fovea in Plate 255). Rod nuclei are rounded and distributed in several layers.

**Cones and rods:** Light-sensitive end portions of rod and cone cells. Contain an unstable, light-sensitive substance (rhodopsin in rods and iodopsin in cones). Both pigments play an important role in the visual process.

*Text continued on following page.*

Rhodopsin and iodopsin consist of vitamin $A_1$ aldehyde conjugated to a specific protein (rod opsin and cone opsin).

**Pigment epithelium:** Single layer of pigmented cuboidal cells firmly bound to the choroid layer. Contains melanin pigment.

**Choroid:** Heavily pigmented layer of loose connective tissue characterized by extreme vascularity. Provides nourishment for the outer portions of the retina.

**Sclera:** Firm external coat of the eye. Composed of dense collagenous connective tissue. A narrow pigmented zone near its internal surface merges with the choroid. The tendons of the six extraocular striated muscles insert on the sclera.

PLATE 255

# RETINA
## Fovea centralis

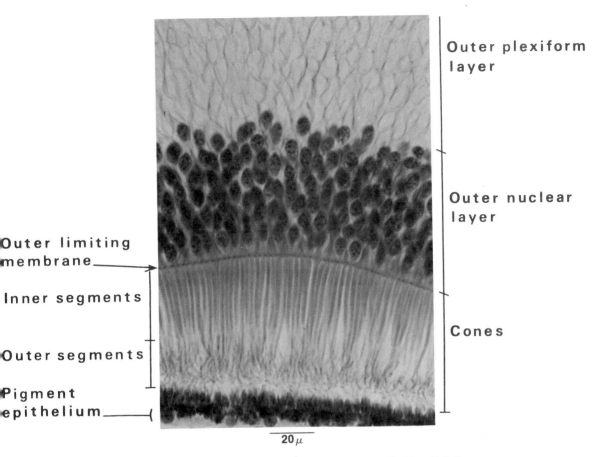

Outer plexiform layer

Outer nuclear layer

Outer limiting membrane

Inner segments

Cones

Outer segments

Pigment epithelium

20 μ

Rhesus monkey, Helly's fluid, H. & E., 612 x.

**Outer plexiform layer:** Contains axons of cone cells, dendrites of bipolar neurons and processes of horizontal cells.

**Outer nuclear layer:** Nuclei of visual receptor cells. Note ovoid nuclei of the cones. Multiple rows of nuclei are characteristic of the fovea.

**Outer limiting membrane:** Sievelike sheet. Region of junctional complexes between the outer ends of the tall supporting Müller cells and the adjoining photoreceptor cells. Not an actual membrane. The visual cells pass through perforations in this so-called membrane.

**Cones:** Light-sensitive end portions of cone cells. Respond to light of high intensity. Function is visual acuity and color perception. Compare cones in fovea with those seen in other regions of the retina (Plate 256).

**Inner segments:** Thicker proximal segments of the cones. Rich in mitochondria.

**Outer segments:** Slender distal segments of cones. Consist largely of stacked discs 0.014 μ thick. Contain iodopsin, an unstable, light-sensitive visual pigment, which chemically is composed of vitamin $A_1$ aldehyde conjugated to a specific protein (cone opsin).

**Pigment epithelium:** Single layer of pigmented cuboidal cells firmly bound to the choroid layer. Cells contain melanin pigment. The cytoplasmic processes of the pigment cells interdigitate with the outer segment of cones.

## EYE
## Cone and Rod vision

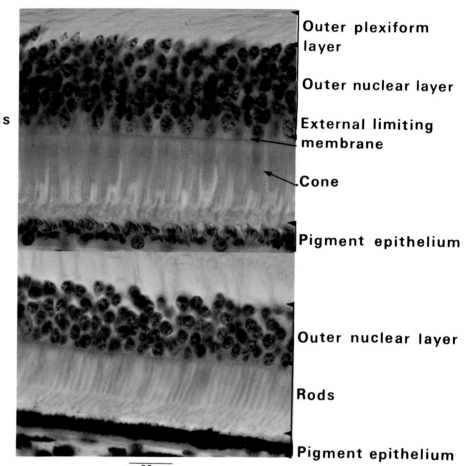

Retinal cones
near the
fovea centralis

Retinal rods
near the
ora serrata

Outer plexiform
layer

Outer nuclear layer

External limiting
membrane

Cone

Pigment epithelium

Outer nuclear layer

Rods

Pigment epithelium

20 μ

Rhesus monkey, 10% Formalin, H. & E., 612 x.

This figure shows variation in retinal structure near the fovea centralis and at the periphery of the retina (ora serrata). In both sites the layers of the retina are diminished. Absent are the ganglion cell layer, the inner plexiform layer and the bipolar cell layer. The fovea constitutes the zone of greatest visual acuity. At the fovea, the photoreceptors are thin, slender elements (cones). They resemble rods more than cones. See Plate 255. The thinning of the retina at the fovea reduces to a minimum tissue through which light passes, and hence improves visual acuity. Note ovoid nuclei of cones in the outer nuclear layer. Multiple rows of these nuclei are characteristic of this region. Typical cones, which predominate here, function for sharp vision and color perception. It is estimated that there are 6 to 7 million cones in the retina.

Near the ora serrata, rods increase in number and in thickness, and become shorter. The cones decrease in number, and also become shorter at the periphery of the retina. Rods number approximately 100 million and function for night vision and black and white discrimination. Note the multiple rows of rounded rod nuclei in the outer nuclear layer. The pigmented epithelium layer is similar in both fovea and ora serrata. It is firmly bound to the choroid layer and contains melanin pigment.

## EYELID

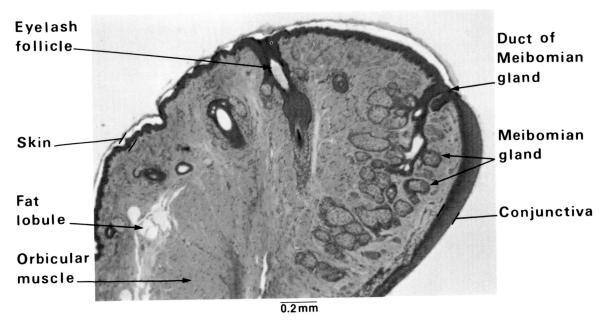

Eyelash follicle

Skin

Fat lobule

Orbicular muscle

Duct of Meibomian gland

Meibomian gland

Conjunctiva

0.2 mm

**Rhesus monkey, 10% Formalin, H.& E., 50 x.**

The eyelid is a fold of skin; superficially, the keratinized epidermis blends internally with a mucous membrane (the conjunctiva). These layers are supported by a dermal core of connective tissue in which striated and smooth muscle, glands and hair follicles are located.

**Eyelash follicle:** A row of short stout hairs are found at the free margin of the lid. Penetrate deep into the dermis. Their follicles are similar to those found elsewhere in the body but lack the arrector pili smooth muscle.

**Skin:** Thin layer of epidermis continuous with the conjunctiva.

**Fat lobule:** Scattered in the connective tissue core of the eyelid.

**Orbicular muscle:** Skeletal muscle bundles that lower the eyelids.

**Conjunctiva:** Mucous membrane lining the inside of the eyelid. The epithelium is stratified columnar with goblet cells scattered among the superficial cells.

**Meibomian gland:** The tarsal glands of the eyelids, first noted by Casserius in 1609 and described by Heinrich Meibom, a German anatomist, in 1666. These are simple, branched alveolar sebaceous glands disposed in a plane perpendicular to the lid margin. The glandular alveoli are connected by short lateral ducts to a long central excretory duct lined with stratified squamous epithelium. The glands open at the inner free margin of the lid at the junction of the skin and conjunctiva. Secretion of the glands serves to lubricate the surface of the lids.

## LACRIMAL GLAND

Serous
acini

Intercalated
duct

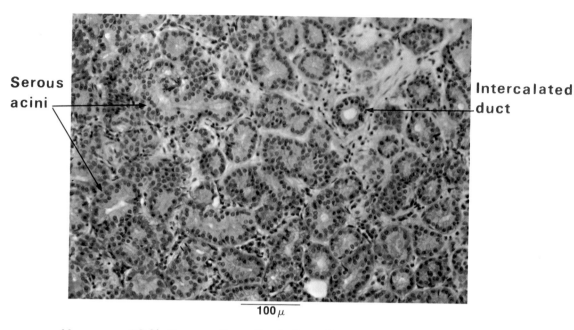

100 μ

Human, 10% Formalin, H. & E., 126 x.

The lacrimal gland is composed of a number of compound tubuloalveolar serous glands. The serous acini are made up of tall cells with basal nuclei. The secretory product fills the apical cytoplasm. The acini are separated by a thin connective tissue stroma. The aqueous secretion (tears), after flushing the conjunctival-corneal surfaces, drains into ducts that carry it, via the nasolacrimal duct, to the anterior portion of the inferior meatus of the nose.

## ORGAN OF CORTI

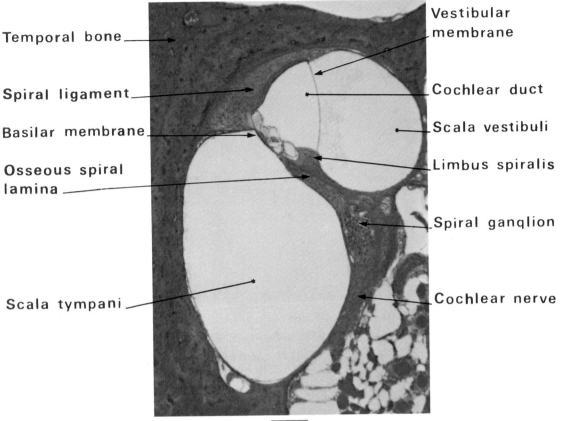

Temporal bone

Spiral ligament

Basilar membrane

Osseous spiral lamina

Scala tympani

Vestibular membrane

Cochlear duct

Scala vestibuli

Limbus spiralis

Spiral ganglion

Cochlear nerve

0.2 mm

Cat, Müller's fluid, H. & E., 50 x.

**Temporal bone:** The bone in which the cochlea is located.

**Spiral ligament:** A projection of thickened periosteum along the outer wall of the osseous canal of the cochlea.

**Osseous spiral lamina:** A bony shelf projecting from the modiolus across the osseous canal of the cochlea. Follows the spiral turns of the cochlea. Divides the osseous canal of the cochlea into an upper scala vestibuli and a lower scala tympani. The former is continuous with the oval window; the latter ends at the round window. The two scalae are continuous at the helicotrema.

**Vestibular membrane:** Also called Reissner's membrane. A thin membrane extending from the upper surface of the limbus spiralis to the upper part of the spiral ligament. It forms the roof of the cochlear duct, which is a part of the membranous labyrinth, and houses the organ of hearing.

**Limbus spiralis:** A thickening of periosteal connective tissue at the outer border of the osseous spiral lamina. The vestibular membrane attaches to the upper surface of the limbus.

**Basilar membrane:** Forms the base of the cochlear duct. Gives support to the organ of Corti.

**Spiral ganglion:** Ganglion of the bipolar cells. Peripheral processes contact the hair cells of the organ of Corti and the longer central processes form the cochlear nerve.

**Cochlear nerve:** Formed by the central processes of the bipolar cells of the spiral ganglion, these nerve fibers, upon entering the brain stem, terminate in the dorsal and ventral cochlear nuclei (see Plate 276).

# ORGAN OF CORTI
## Cochlea

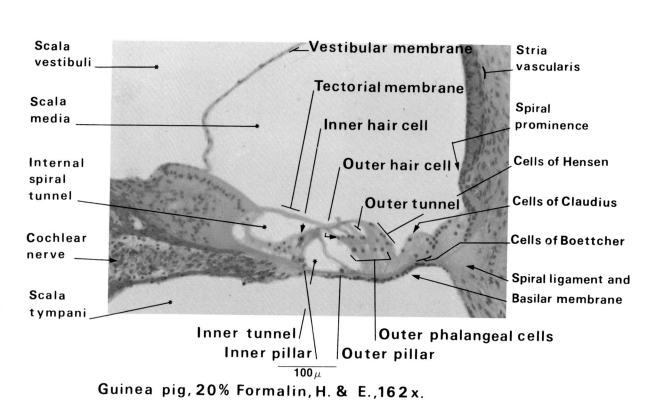

Scala vestibuli

Scala media

Internal spiral tunnel

Cochlear nerve

Scala tympani

Vestibular membrane

Tectorial membrane

Inner hair cell

Outer hair cell

Outer tunnel

Stria vascularis

Spiral prominence

Cells of Hensen

Cells of Claudius

Cells of Boettcher

Spiral ligament and Basilar membrane

Inner tunnel

Inner pillar

Outer phalangeal cells

Outer pillar

100 μ

**Guinea pig, 20% Formalin, H. & E., 162 x.**

This plate is a cross section of the bony cochlea, and shows three compartments: the upper, scala vestibuli; the lower, scala tympani; and the middle, scala media. The scala vestibuli and scala tympani are perilymphatic spaces. The scala vestibuli reaches the inner surface of the oval window. The scala tympani reaches the inner surface of the round window. Both scalae communicate at the helicotrema at the apex of the cochlea. The scala media or cochlear duct is part of the endolymphatic system and contains the organ of Corti. The vestibular membrane or Reissner's membrane forms the roof of the cochlear duct. The basilar membrane forms the base of the cochlear duct and gives support to the organ of Corti. The outer wall of the cochlear duct is made up of the spiral ligament, which is a thickening of the periosteum. The crest of the spiral ligament forms the spiral prominence. The part of the spiral ligament between the spiral prominence and the vestibular membrane is the stria vascularis. The epithelium here is thick and pseudostratified. The subepithelial connective tissue is rich in capillaries. The stria vascularis is believed to be active in the production of endolymph and the regulation of its ion content. The epithelium of the spiral prominence continues onto the basilar membrane. Cells here become cuboidal. Those cells continuing onto the pars pectinata of the basilar membrane are known as cells of Claudius. In parts of the cochlea, polyhedral cells separate the Claudius cells and the basilar membrane and are known as cells of Boettcher. The organ of Corti is composed of two types of cells, hair and supporting cells. The supporting cells are tall, slender cells extending from the basilar membrane to the free surface of the organ of Corti. The supporting cells include the outer and inner pillars, inner and outer phalangeal cells and cells of Hensen. The inner tunnel within the organ of Corti is bounded below by the basilar membrane and above by the outer and inner pillar cells. The outer phalangeal cells act as supporting elements for the three to four rows of outer hair cells. The cells of Hansen are located adjacent to the last row of outer phalangeal cells. They constitute the outer border of the organ of Corti. The hair cells are of two types: the inner and outer hair cells. The inner hair cells are in a single row. The outer hair cells form three rows lodged between the outer pillar and outer phalangeal cells. The tectorial membrane is in contact with the hairs of hair cells, and transmits to them endolymph vibrations. The cochlear nerve is formed by central processes of the bipolar cells of the spiral ganglion. In the inner angle of the scala media, the periosteal connective tissue of the spiral lamina bulges into the scala media overhanging the internal spiral tunnel.

## SEMICIRCULAR  CANAL
### Temporal  bone

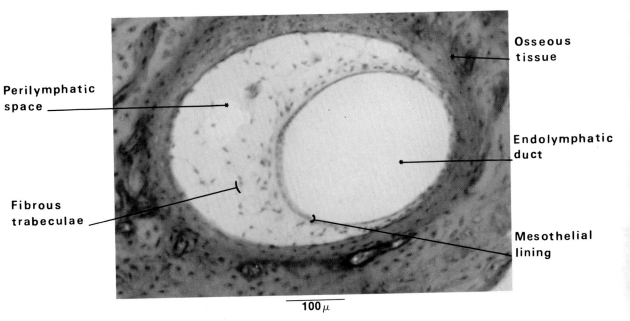

Osseous
tissue

Perilymphatic
space

Endolymphatic
duct

Fibrous
trabeculae

Mesothelial
lining

$\overline{100\,\mu}$

### Cat, Müller's  fluid, H. & E., 162 x.

**Perilymphatic space:**  Intervenes between the osseous labyrinth and the membranous labyrinth. Traversed by fibrous trabeculae. Contains the fluid, perilymph.

**Osseous tissue:**  Compact bone forming the osseous labyrinth. The surface facing the perilymph has a periosteum covered by mesenchymal tissue.

**Endolymphatic space:**  The stimulation of the vestibular receptors (the crista ampullaris and the two maculae) depends upon the movement of endolymph, the fluid contained within the endolymphatic space in the semicircular canals, saccule and utricle. See Plates 262 and 263. Note the mesothelial lining enclosing the endolymphatic space.

# SEMICIRCULAR CANAL
## Crista ampullaris

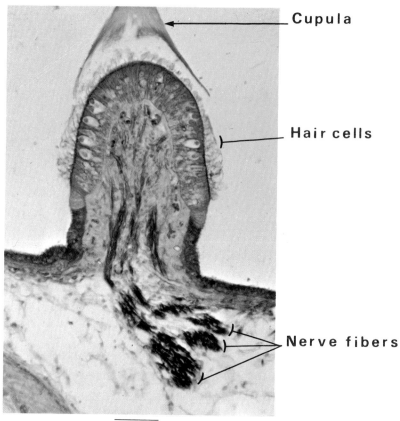

Cupula

Hair cells

Nerve fibers

20 μ

Guinea pig, Müller's fluid, Iron hematoxylin stain, 612x.

**Cupula:** Gelatinous dome-shaped mass in which the hairs of the hair cells are embedded. Similar to the cells of the otolithic membrane but lacks otoconia. Movements of the cupula are transmitted to the hairs of the receptor cells.

**Hair cells:** Flask-shaped cells that occupy the outer part of the epithelium but do not reach the basement membrane. Nuclei close to the lumen. A tuft of hairs is found in the apex of each cell. Compare hair cells to the adjacent tall, columnar sustentacular cells with basal nuclei that reach the basement membrane.

**Nerve fibers:** Myelinated processes of the vestibular nerve lose their myelin close to the hair cells of the crista. Naked fibers ramify among the hair cells of the crista, forming a dense arborization.

## MACULA UTRICULI
### Membranous Labyrinth

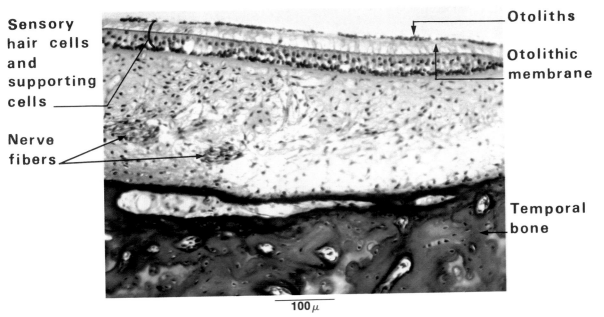

Sensory hair cells and supporting cells

Nerve fibers

Otoliths

Otolithic membrane

Temporal bone

100 μ

**Cat, Müller's fluid, Iron hematoxylin, 162 x.**

Sensory area of the utricle. The sensory epithelium is composed of two types of cells.

**Hair cells:** Flask-shaped. Nuclei occupy the upper part of the epithelial sheet. These receptors of the macula utriculi are concerned with the orientation of the body with regard to gravity. The receptor cells of the macula sacculi however appear to respond primarily to vibratory stimuli.

**Supporting cells:** Slender. Nuclei are lined up near the basement membrane of the epithelium.

The surface of the macula is covered by a gelatinous material, the otolithic membrane, through which hairs of the hair cells project. The upper surface of the membrane contains densely packed crystals of a calcium carbonate-protein mixture, the otoliths. The utricle and saccule which are similar in appearance constitute the "otolith organ."

**Nerve fibers:** Afferent components of the vestibular portion of the eighth cranial nerve, *i.e.,* the vestibulo-cochlear nerve.

**Temporal bone:** Forming the osseous labyrinth.

# Section 17

# The Central Nervous System

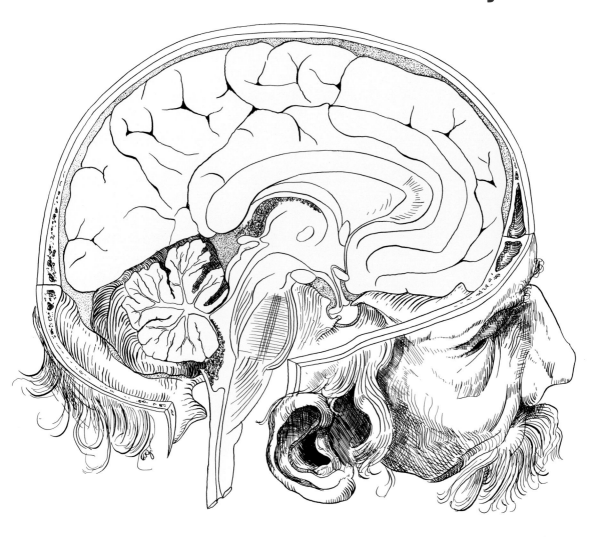

# The Central Nervous System

Knowledge of the structural organization of the nervous system is essential to the proper understanding of its normal as well as altered function.

For didactic purposes, the nervous system is generally divided into central and peripheral components. The central nervous system includes the brain and the spinal cord. The peripheral nervous system includes cranial and peripheral nerves and associated ganglia. The autonomic nervous system includes parts of the central and peripheral nervous systems.

The brain includes the cerebral hemispheres, the cerebellum and the brain stem. The latter includes the diencephalon, the mesencephalon or midbrain, the pons and the medulla oblongata. Each of these components is made up of cell groups and fibers, arranged in a manner that characterizes the particular component. Bundles of nerve fibers serving a common function and sharing a common origin and destination are grouped together in tracts or fasciculi. A group of neurons serving a common function forms a nucleus.

Knowledge of the existence and location of tracts has come through years of clinical observation and experimentation in both animals and man. Some of the methods used in the study of tracts are outlined below.

1. *Study of normal preparations:* many aspects of fiber connectivity of the nervous system have been elucidated by early studies utilizing normal material and methods that demonstrate myelin sheaths (Weigert and Weil methods) or that impregnate cell bodies and their processes (Golgi method). The disadvantage of these methods is the difficulty of determining the site of termination of these fibers.

2. *Myelinogenesis:* this method, introduced by Flechsig, makes use of the fact that different fiber tracts become myelinated at different times in their development. Thus, study of the nervous system in embryos and in early neonatal life often affords information about the existence and locality of the different fiber tracts. This method is infrequently used today.

3. *Study of pathological conditions in humans and experimental lesions in animals:* this method accounts for most of our present knowledge of neural connectivity. Although human material has been of use, experimentally produced lesions in animals have the major advantage of selectivity of site and size. Caution, however, should be exercised in applying to humans results achieved in experimental animals.

After a lesion has been produced in animal or man, and sufficient time has elapsed for degeneration to set in, the brains and spinal cords can be studied, and degenerated tracts localized by one of the following methods:

a. Methods that stain normal myelin (Weigert, Weil): in such preparations the degenerated tracts will be conspicuous by their failure to pick up the stain.

357

b. Methods that stain degenerating myelin (Marchi): in such preparations only degenerating tracts pick up the stain and can be followed from origin to termination. The disadvantage of this method is that thinly myelinated or unmyelinated tracts will not stain.

A neuroanatomist is interested not only in the location and course of fiber tracts but also in their site of termination. To determine the latter, methods that stain the terminal boutons (Glees, Bodian) are utilized. Recently, electron microscopy has also been used for this purpose.

4. *Retrograde cell changes:* by this method the position of neurons giving rise to the tract is determined. Such neurons undergo chromatolytic changes of their Nissl substance or disappear completely (retrograde degeneration) if the tract is severed. These changes can be demonstrated by any of the Nissl methods.

5. *Physiological exploration:* by this method electrodes inserted into the brain or spinal cord can pick up action potentials generated by stimulation of the tract or nerve ending to which it is connected.

The above methods used to study neural connectivity are based on the principle of the neuron as a trophic unit. If an axon is transected, its peripheral parts, including its termination, undergo degeneration. This is referred to as anterograde degeneration. The methods described under 3 are utilized to show this type of degeneration. Simultaneously with anterograde degeneration, changes occur in the proximal components of the neuron, namely in the proximal axon, the cell body and dendrites. These changes are known as retrograde changes.

When considered together anterograde and retrograde methods allow a detailed mapping of neural connectivity.

## SPINAL CORD
### Cervical region

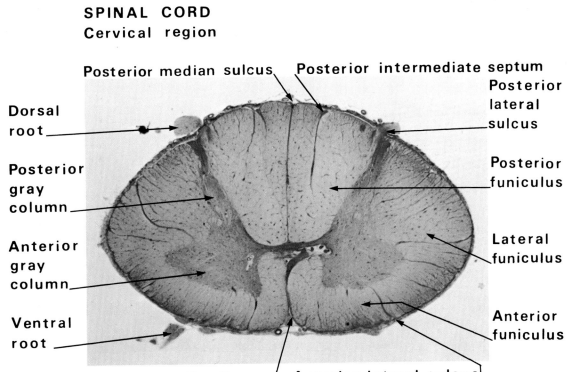

Posterior median sulcus

Posterior intermediate septum

Posterior lateral sulcus

Dorsal root

Posterior gray column

Anterior gray column

Ventral root

Posterior funiculus

Lateral funiculus

Anterior funiculus

Anterior median fissure

Anterior lateral sulcus

**Human, Müller's fluid, Carmine stain, 8x.**

**Dorsal root:** The dorsal root carries both myelinated and unmyelinated afferent fibers to the spinal cord. Each fiber is the central process of a dorsal root ganglion cell.

**Posterior gray column:** Long and narrow columns of gray matter reach almost to the surface of the spinal cord. Primarily concerned with sensory input.

**Anterior gray column:** Short and broad columns of gray matter. Concerned with motor function. Both posterior and anterior gray columns are sites where sensory and motor cell bodies, respectively, are found.

**Ventral root:** Bundle of somatic motor fibers (axons of somatic motor neurons) and preganglionic fibers of the autonomic system. Constitute the efferent outflow of the spinal cord.

**Anterior median fissure:** About 3 mm deep. Contains blood vessels supplying the anterior half of the cord.

**Anterior lateral sulcus:** Site of exit of ventral root. Hardly distinguishable in this preparation.

**Anterior funiculus:** Between the anterior median fissure and anterolateral sulcus (ventral root). Merges with the lateral funiculus. Contains ascending and descending tracts.

**Lateral funiculus:** Between the dorsal and ventral roots. Merges with the anterior funiculus. Contains ascending and descending tracts.

**Posterior lateral sulcus:** Site of entry of dorsal root.

**Posterior funiculus:** Between posterior median sulcus and dorsal root. Contains ascending tracts.

**Posterior intermediate septum:** Found only in cervical and upper thoracic segments.

**Posterior median sulcus:** About 5 mm deep, reaches the deep-lying gray matter.

# SPINAL CORD
## Cervical level

Dorsal root

Spino-cerebellar tracts

Reticular process

Anterior gray horn

Posterior column

Substantia gelatinosa

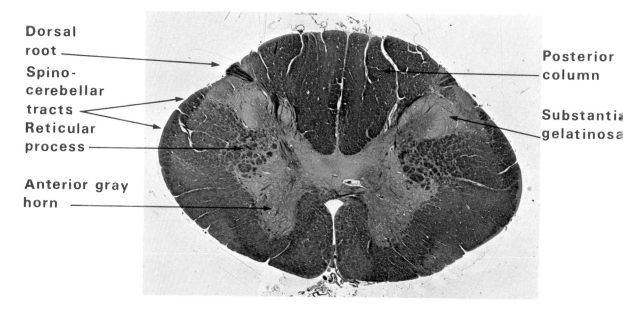

Human, 10% Formalin, Weigert-carmine, 11 x.

**Posterior column:** The white matter located between the posterior central septum and the medial border of the posterior horn. Contains heavily myelinated nerve fibers that form the ascending gracile and cuneate tracts. These tracts carry impulses from proprioceptive and tactile receptors (Pacinian corpuscles, Golgi tendon organs, neuromuscular spindles and Meissner's corpuscles) which give rise to sensations of position, movement and tactile localization. These receptors are seen in Plates 108, 110, 111 and 112.

**Substantia gelatinosa:** Appears as a caplike structure at the head of the posterior horn. It is largest in the first cervical and in the lumbosacral segments but extends the whole length of the cord. This nucleus contains small cells about 6 to 20 $\mu$ in diameter and is the primary associative center of the posterior horn for incoming impulses carried by the dorsal root. This nucleus is an important part of the pathway for pain, temperature and some tactile impulses.

**Dorsal root:** Sensory nerve fibers entering the spinal cord. Follow some of these fibers to the anterior horn where they terminate on motor neurons.

**Spinocerebellar tracts:** The spinocerebellar tracts convey impulses to the cerebellum from the muscle, tendon and joint proprioceptors, thus enabling the cerebellum to coordinate skeletal muscle activity (posture and movement).

**Reticular process:** Contains small- and medium-sized cells which send their axons to the adjacent as well as to the opposite anterolateral white column. Also known as the nucleus reticularis.

**Anterior gray horn:** Contains cells whose axons pass to the extrafusal fibers of striated skeletal muscle. The cells are the largest found in the spinal cord. These multipolar neurons have as many as 20 dendrites, and axons approximately 12 $\mu$ in diameter. Smaller neurons with thin axons (gamma efferent fibers) supply the motor endings for the small intrafusal muscle fibers of the neuromuscular spindle (Plates 108 and 109).

# SPINAL CORD
## Thoracic region

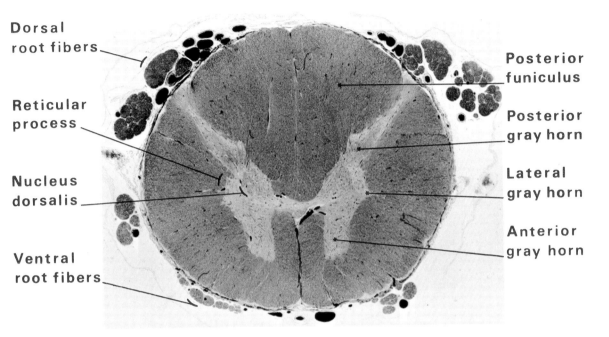

Dorsal root fibers

Reticular process

Nucleus dorsalis

Ventral root fibers

Posterior funiculus

Posterior gray horn

Lateral gray horn

Anterior gray horn

Human, Müller's fluid, Weigert's method, 10 x.

**Dorsal root fibers:** See Plates 264, 265, 268, 269 and 270.

**Reticular process:** Characteristic of cervical levels of the spinal cord. Located between the posterior and anterior horns and produced by an extension of gray matter into the adjacent white substance. Constitutes the lateral zone of lamina V of Rexed. See also Plate 265.

**Nucleus dorsalis:** Distinct nuclear mass located in the medial part of the base of the posterior horn. In this nucleus, dorsal root fibers synapse with neurons destined to form the dorsal (posterior) spinocerebellar tract. The nucleus extends between $C_8$ and $L_2$ spinal segments. Also known as the column of Clark.

**Ventral root fibers:** See Plates 102, 268, 269 and 270.

**Posterior funiculus:** The white matter of the cord located between the posterior central septum and the medial border of the posterior horn. Contains heavily myelinated fibers that form the gracile and cuneate tracts. Note the large size of this funiculus compared to lower levels of the spinal cord. See also Plates 264, 265 and 267.

**Posterior gray horn:** A mass of neurons in the posterolateral part of the spinal cord. Receive collaterals or terminals of dorsal root fibers. Sends axons to anterior horn cells, interneurons or to ascending tracts. See also Plates 264 and 270.

**Lateral gray horn:** Characteristic of thoracic level, this projection is formed by the intermediolateral nucleus. Contains visceral efferent neurons of the sympathetic nervous system. Extends from $C_8$ to $L_{2-4}$. Axons of neurons here exit with the ventral horn fibers to terminate in the chain of ganglia (sympathetic), where they synapse with ganglion cells whose axons are widely distributed to the iris (dilator smooth muscle); lacrimal, salivary and sweat glands; bronchi; heart; smooth muscle of the gastrointestinal tract; sex organs; urinary bladder; adrenal medulla; and blood vessels.

**Anterior gray horn:** A mass of large neurons in the anterolateral part of the spinal cord. Contains somatic efferent neurons. Compare the size of the horn at this level with those seen at higher and lower levels. See also Plates 264, 265 and 270.

## SPINAL CORD LESION
Thoracic level
dorsal funiculus

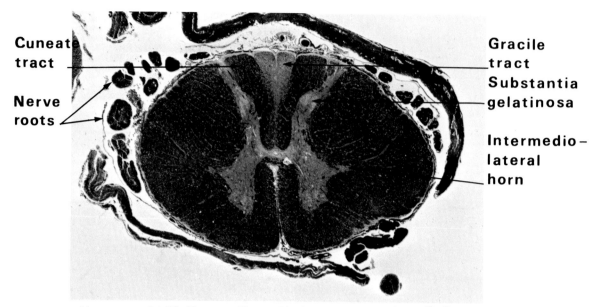

Cuneate tract

Nerve roots

Gracile tract

Substantia gelatinosa

Intermedio-lateral horn

**Human, 10% Formalin, Weigert-carmine, 9.4 x.**

**Gracile tract:** Note that the gracile tract stains lighter than the adjacent cuneate tract. See Plates 265 and 269. This is due to the degenerating myelinated fibers in the gracile tract, which are not stained by this method. This slide was taken from a human with a spinal cord lesion in the dorsal (posterior) funiculus below the sixth thoracic segment. Fibers entering the spinal cord below this level form the gracile tract. The fibers entering above $T_6$ form the cuneate tract and therefore escape degeneration.

**Substantia gelatinosa:** See Plates 265, 269 and 270.

**Intermediolateral horn:** Lateral gray horn. See Plates 266 and 270.

**Nerve roots:** Incoming dorsal roots.

## SPINAL CORD
### Lumbar region

Dorsal roots

White matter

Substantia gelatinosa

Ventral roots

Gray matter

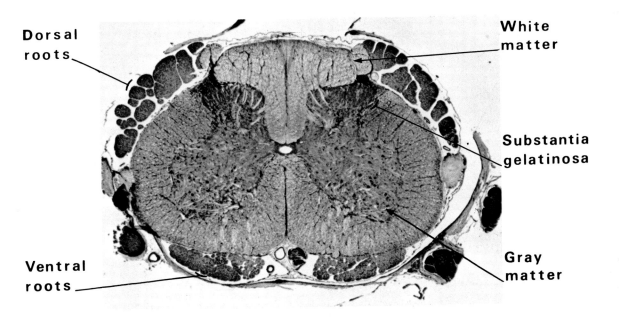

## Human, Müller's fluid, Hematoxylin stain, 8 x.

**White matter:** Less abundant than at higher levels. Plates 264, 265, 266 and 267.

**Gray matter:** Massive gray matter characterizes this level of the spinal cord. H-shaped. Note nuclei of motor neurons in anterior gray column, which is widened laterally to accommodate cells whose axons form the lumbar plexus. Note the prominent cap of the posterior gray column, the substantia gelatinosa.

**Dorsal roots:** Represent central processes of dorsal root ganglion cells. Convey afferent (sensory) impulses to the spinal cord from peripheral organs. Plates 264, 265, 266, 269 and 270.

**Ventral roots:** Axons of somatic and visceral motor neurons in the anterior (ventral) and lateral gray column. Plates 264, 266, 269 and 270.

Note the arachnoid mémbrane enclosing the dorsal and ventral roots.

363

# SPINAL CORD
## Sacral region

Dorsal
root fibers

Zone of
Lissauer

Collaterals
and termi-
nals of
dorsal root
fibers

Ventral
root fibers

Fasciculus
gracilis

Substantia
gelatinosa

Central
canal

Ventral
white
commissure

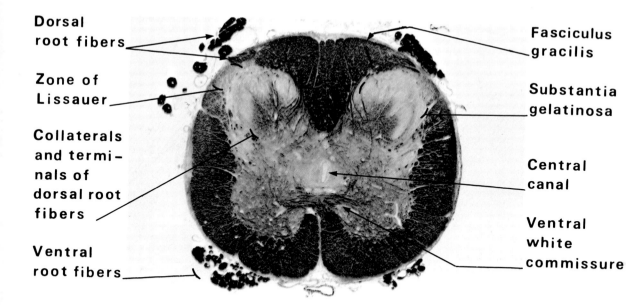

## Human, Müller's fluid, Weigert's method with carmalum stain, 14 x.

**Dorsal root fibers:** Bundles of heavily myelinated nerve fibers entering the spinal cord. Represent central processes of dorsal root ganglion neurons. Convey afferent impulses from peripheral organs to the spinal cord. Some of these fibers go directly to form tracts (fasciculus gracilis), others give collaterals or terminate on neurons in the spinal cord. Plates 264, 265, 266, 268 and 270.

**Zone of Lissauer:** Also known as fasciculus dorsolateralis. Composed of fine myelinated and nonmyelinated fibers that carry pain, thermal and light touch impulses or that interconnect different levels of the substantia gelatinosa.

**Ventral root fibers:** Axons of somatic and visceral motor neurons in the anterior (ventral) and lateral gray columns. Heavily myelinated.

**Fasciculus gracilis:** Heavily myelinated ascending fiber system. Conveys kinesthetic sense and discriminative touch. Note the absence of the fasciculus cuneatus, which appears at spinal cord levels above $T_6$. Plates 267, 271 and 274.

**Substantia gelatinosa:** An expanded cell mass that forms the cap of the posterior gray horn of the spinal cord. Its size is related to that of the dorsal root. This area functions as an association region for incoming impulses. This region corresponds to lamina II of Rexed. Plates 265, 267 and 270.

**Central canal:** Runs throughout the length of the cord. Partially obliterated in the adult. Plate 117.

**Ventral white commissure:** Bundle of myelinated fibers crossing from one side of the spinal cord to the other.

## SPINAL CORD
### Dorsal root collaterals

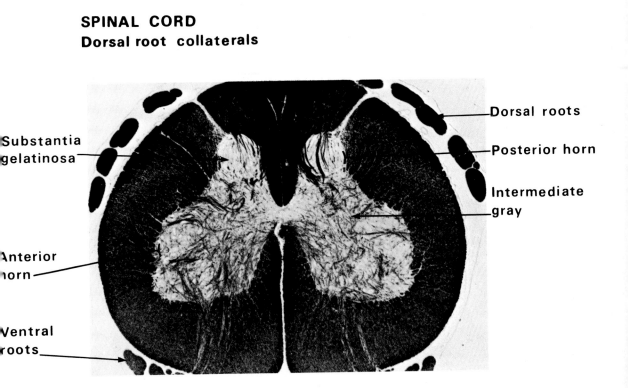

Dorsal roots

Posterior horn

Intermediate gray

Substantia gelatinosa

Anterior horn

Ventral roots

**Dog, Müller's fluid, Weigert's method, 3.75 x.**

This is a section of the spinal cord showing the distribution of dorsal root collaterals. Note that the coarser, heavily myelinated collaterals are medially located. They are seen passing to the posterior horn, intermediate gray and anterior horn. Many fibers of this bundle enter the posterior funiculus. Finer, poorly myelinated collaterals are more laterally located and are seen entering the substantia gelatinosa. Some heavily myelinated fibers also enter the substantia gelatinosa. The medial bundle is the larger of the two. Collaterals that pass directly to the anterior horn constitute components of monosynaptic reflex arcs. Their number is relatively small since most of the collaterals to the anterior horn terminate on at least one interneuron before reaching the final efferent neuron. Note the bundle of somatic motor fibers (axons of somatic motor neurons) leaving the anterior horn to form the ventral roots.

# MEDULLA OBLONGATA
## Motor decussation

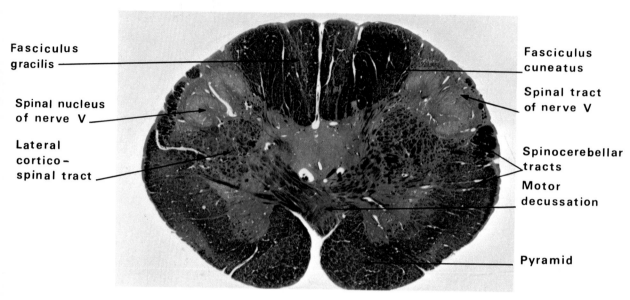

Fasciculus gracilis

Spinal nucleus of nerve V

Lateral cortico- spinal tract

Fasciculus cuneatus

Spinal tract of nerve V

Spinocerebellar tracts

Motor decussation

Pyramid

## Human, 10% Formalin, Pal-Weigert and carmine stains, 11x.

**Fasciculus gracilis:**  Rostral continuation of the same tract seen at several spinal cord levels (see Plates 267 and 269). The lightly stained islands within the fasciculus represent neurons of the nucleus gracilis. This nucleus is larger at more rostral levels.

**Fasciculus cuneatus:**  Rostral continuation of the same tract seen at spinal cord levels (Plate 267).

**Spinal nucleus of nerve V:**  Functionally analogous to and structurally a continuation of the substantia gelatinosa seen at several spinal cord levels. In it terminate fibers of the descending (spinal) tract of cranial nerve V (trigeminal) which enters the neuraxis at a rostral level (see Plate 278). The nucleus is primarily concerned with the perception of pain and thermal sense from the homolateral face.

**Spinal tract of nerve V:**  Thinly myelinated fibers, hence less densely stained than the heavily myelinated fibers of the fasciculi gracilis and cuneatus or the spinocerebellar tracts. This tract is composed of descending trigeminal fibers and extends from the site of entry of the trigeminal nerve in the pons down to the second cervical spinal segment. Primarily concerned with pain and thermal sense. Synapse in the spinal nucleus of nerve V. See Plate 278.

**Spinocerebellar tracts:**  Heavily myelinated. Continuation of the same tracts seen at several spinal cord levels on their way to the cerebellum.

**Motor decussation:**  Constitutes one of the most conspicuous features of sections at this level. Site of crossing of the pyramids to form the lateral corticospinal tracts. Approximately 90 per cent of descending pyramidal fibers cross at this level. The motor decussation forms the basis for voluntary motor control of one-half of the body by the contralateral cerebral hemisphere.

**Lateral corticospinal tract:**  Formed by decussation of the pyramidal tracts. Descends throughout the extent of the cord (see Plates 272 and 277).

**Pyramid:**  Heavily myelinated motor fiber system. Represents descending fibers from the cerebral cortex that pass through the internal capsule, cerebral peduncle and pons before reaching the medullary pyramids. Fibers in the pyramid undergo partial crossing in the motor decussation to give rise to the lateral corticospinal tracts.

## MEDULLA OBLONGATA
### Motor decussation

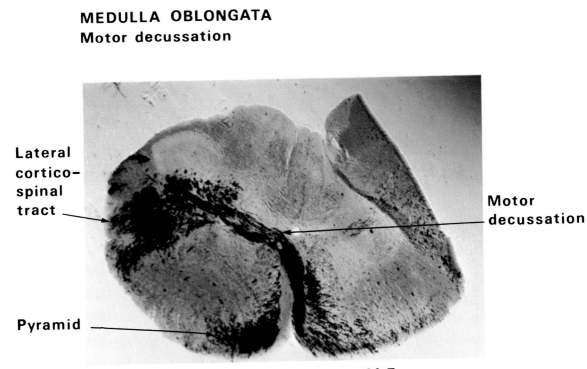

**Lateral cortico-spinal tract**

**Motor decussation**

**Pyramid**

**Cat, 10 % Formalin, Marchi stain,11.5 x.**

This is a section of the medulla oblongata, stained by the Marchi method, which reveals degenerated myelin. Note the degenerated fibers (black) in the pyramid and the crossing of these fibers to form the lateral corticospinal tract. An artifact of tissue preparation is seen in the upper right hand corner of the section. The tissue became folded during handling.

## SPINAL CORD
### Spinocerebellar tract

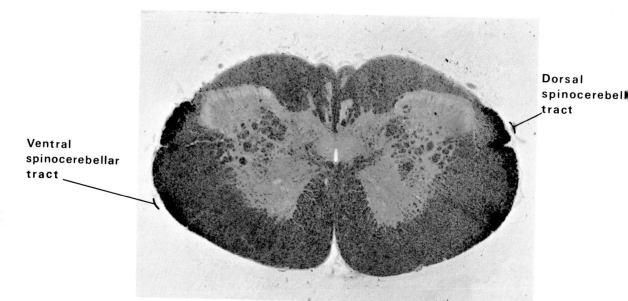

**Ventral spinocerebellar tract**

**Dorsal spinocerebellar tract**

## Dog, Müller's fluid, Marchi method, 12 x.

This cross section of the lower medulla is stained with the Marchi method, which selectively stains degenerated myelinated tracts black. In this section black staining outlines the dorsal and ventral spinocerebellar tracts. These are fiber tracts that convey proprioceptive impulses to the cerebellum. They are concerned with unconscious proprioception. Three types of end organs are associated with proprioception: Pacinian corpuscles, muscle spindles and Golgi tendon organs (see Plates 108, 109, 110 and 112). These receptors detect movements of joints and changes in stretch and tension in muscles and tendons.

# MEDULLA OBLONGATA
## Sensory decussation

Fasciculus and nucleus gracilis

Spinal nucleus of V

Spinocerebellar tract

Sensory decussation

Pyramid

Fasciculus and nucleus cuneatus

Internal arcuate fibers

Medial longitudinal fasciculus

**Human, 10% Formalin, Pal—Weigert and carmine stains, 7x.**

**Fasciculus and nucleus gracilis:**   Note the reduction in size of the fasciculus gracilis as the nucleus gracilis develops. Fibers of the fasciculus synapse on neurons of the nucleus gracilis. The nucleus gracilis appears and terminates caudal to the nucleus cuneatus (Plates 271, 273 and 275).

**Fasciculus and nucleus cuneatus:**   Note that the nucleus cuneatus is not as well developed at this level as the nucleus gracilis.

**Internal arcuate fibers:**   Second order fibers arise from gracile and cuneate nuclei, course in the tegmentum of the medulla and cross in the sensory decussation to form the medial lemniscus. They convey the same modalities of sensation as the gracile and cuneate tracts (proprioception, touch and vibratory sense).

**Medial longitudinal fasciculus:**   Descending portion of a fiber system with ascending and descending components. Arise from various brain stem nuclei, but with a major vestibular component. This system is concerned with eye movements.

**Spinal nucleus of V:**   Trigeminal nerve. Continuation of same nucleus seen at more caudal levels (see Plate 271).

**Spinocerebellar tract:**   Continuation of the same tract seen at several caudal levels (see Plates 265, 271 and 273).

**Sensory decussation:**   Also known as decussation of the medial lemniscus. Internal arcuate fibers cross here to form the contralateral medial lemniscus. Provides an anatomical basis for sensory representation of one half of the body in the contralateral cerebral cortex.

**Pyramid:**   Same system as described in Plates 271 and 273.

# MEDULLA OBLONGATA
## Inferior olive

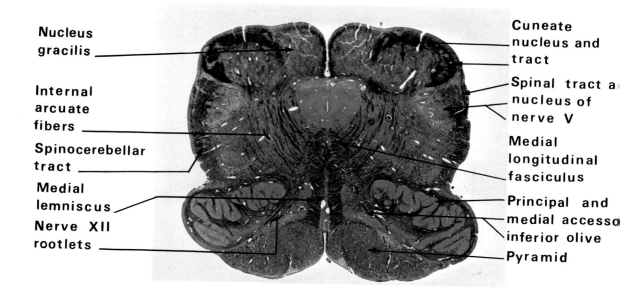

Nucleus gracilis

Internal arcuate fibers

Spinocerebellar tract

Medial lemniscus

Nerve XII rootlets

Cuneate nucleus and tract

Spinal tract a nucleus of nerve V

Medial longitudinal fasciculus

Principal and medial accesso inferior olive

Pyramid

## Human, 10% Formalin, Pal-Weigert and carmine stains, 7x.

**Nucleus gracilis:**  Fully developed at this level. Only a small remnant of the fasciculus gracilis caps the nucleus.

**Cuneate nucleus and tract:**  Note that a definite portion of the fasciculus cuneatus caps the nucleus cuneatus as compared to that seen on the adjacent nucleus gracilis. The lightly stained island in the fasciculus cuneatus represents neurons of the accessory cuneate nucleus.

**Spinal tract and nucleus of nerve V:**  Continuation of similar structures seen at more caudal levels (Plates 271 and 274).

**Medial longitudinal fasciculus:**  Note the change of position of the fasciculus in this figure as compared to a more caudal level (Plate 274). This is a result of the formation of the medial lemniscus, which displaces the medial longitudinal fasciculus to a more dorsal location.

**Principal and medial accessory inferior olive:**  This nuclear group distinguishes sections of the medulla at this level. The principal olive is the larger component with its hilum directed medially. The medial accessory olive is found along the border of the medial lemniscus. Neurons here give rise to the olivocerebellar fibers that project into the cerebellum.

**Pyramid:**  See the same structure at more caudal levels. Plates 271, 272 and 274.

**Internal arcuate fibers:**  See Plate 274.

**Spinocerebellar tract:**  See Plates 265, 271, 273 and 274.

**Medial lemniscus:**  Formed by the decussating internal arcuate fibers. Constitutes the second order neurons of the posterior column pathways (fasciculi gracilis and cuneatus and their nuclei) conveying kinesthetic sense and discriminative touch to higher levels of the neuraxis.

**Nerve XII rootlets:**  Hypoglossal cranial nerve. Note their characteristic location medial to the inferior olive and lateral to the pyramid. This proximity to the pyramid is the anatomical basis for the inferior or hypoglossal alternating hemiplegia resulting from lesions in this area. This syndrome consists of lower motor neuron paralysis of the ipsilateral half of the tongue and contralateral hemiplegia. The hypoglossal nerve supplies all the intrinsic and extrinsic muscles of the tongue except the palatoglossus muscle.

## MEDULLA OBLONGATA
### Cochlear nuclei and ninth nerve

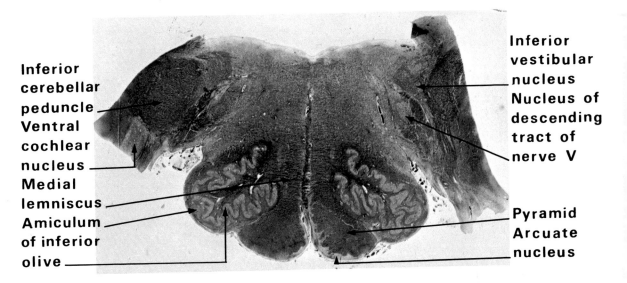

Inferior
cerebellar
peduncle
Ventral
cochlear
nucleus
Medial
lemniscus
Amiculum
of inferior
olive

Inferior
vestibular
nucleus
Nucleus of
descending
tract of
nerve V

Pyramid
Arcuate
nucleus

### Human, 10% Formalin, Pal–Weigert and carmine stains, 4.5 x.

**Inferior cerebellar peduncle:** Also known as restiform body (L. *restis*, rope; L. *forme*, shape; thus, a structure shaped like a rope). A compact bundle of nerve fibers connecting the medulla with the cerebellum. Described first in 1695 and named by Humphrey Ridley, an English anatomist. Tracts and fibers forming this bundle originate in the medulla and the spinal cord.

**Ventral cochlear nucleus:** Located lateral and ventral to the inferior cerebellar peduncle. Receives fibers of the cochlear division of the 8th cranial nerve. Cochlear fibers terminating in this nucleus originate in the upper coils of the cochlea.

**Medial lemniscus:** Continuation of the same fiber system described at a more caudal level (see Plate 275). Occupies the same paramedian location.

**Amiculum of inferior olive:** Band of myelinated fibers surrounding the inferior olive. Contains descending fibers terminating on cells of the inferior olive and arising from cortical and subcortical areas.

**Inferior vestibular nucleus:** Characteristic location medial to the inferior cerebellar peduncle and traversed by myelinated fibers of vestibular origin. One of the four vestibular nuclei located in the floor of the fourth ventricle.

**Nucleus of descending tract of nerve V:** Continuation of the same structure described at caudal levels (see Plates 271, 274 and 275).

**Pyramid:** Note the lighter area medial to the pyramid. This is the beginning of the arcuate nucleus. See Plates 271, 272, 274 and 275.

**Arcuate nucleus:** (L. *arcuatus*, arched or bowed.) The position of this nucleus varies somewhat in different levels. Rostrally it enlarges considerably and becomes continuous with the pontine nuclei.

## PONS
### Sixth and seventh nerves

Brachium conjunctivum

Genu of nerve VII

Sixth nerve rootlets

Brachium pontis

Cortico-ponto-cerebellar fibers

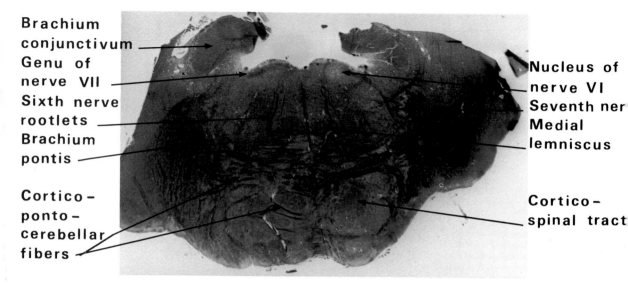

Nucleus of nerve VI

Seventh ner

Medial lemniscus

Cortico-spinal tract

### Human, 10% Formalin, Pal-Weigert and carmine stains, 3.7x.

**Brachium conjunctivum:** (L. *brachium*, arm; L. *conjunctivum*, connecting.) Also known as the superior cerebellar peduncle. Most important efferent fiber system of the deep cerebellar nuclei. Located dorsolateral to the fourth ventricle. Later it dips into the tegmentum of the pons and midbrain (see Plates 279, 280 and 281). The nerve fibers are destined to reach the red nucleus and ventrolateral nucleus of the thalamus.

**Genu of nerve VII:** (Skr. *janu*; L. *genu*, knee.) Refers to the bundle of seventh cranial nerve (facial) motor root fibers located over the dorsal surface of the sixth nerve (abducens) nucleus at the cranial border of the nucleus. Facial genu and underlying sixth nerve nucleus form a rounded prominence in the floor of the fourth ventricle known as the facial colliculus.

**Sixth nerve rootlets:** Emerge from the medial aspect of the sixth cranial nerve (abducens) nucleus and course through the pontine tegmentum to emerge at the caudal border of the pons. Supply the lateral rectus (extraocular) muscle.

**Brachium pontis:** Massive bundle of fibers connecting the basal portion of the pons with the cerebellum. Also known as the middle cerebellar peduncle.

**Corticopontocerebellar fibers:** An important two-neuron fiber system arising from wide areas of the cerebral cortex, synapsing on pontine nuclei and crossing to reach the contralateral cerebellar hemisphere via the brachium pontis.

**Nucleus of nerve VI:** Paramedian location similar to other somatic motor cranial nerve nuclei. The nucleus is capped by the genu of cranial nerve VII (facial). Rootlets of the sixth cranial nerve (abducens) emerge from the medial aspect of the nucleus.

**Nerve VII:** Facial nerve. Coursing ventrolaterally to emerge at the caudal border of the pons.

**Medial lemniscus:** Note change in orientation from the previously vertical to the horizontal. Carries kinesthetic sense and discriminative touch.

**Corticospinal tract:** The long descending fiber system passes through the medulla (pyramid) at caudal levels, and through the spinal cord as the lateral and anterior corticospinal tracts. Note that the descending corticospinal fibers are sectioned transversely while the horizontally oriented corticopontocerebellar fibers are sectioned longitudinally.

## PONS
### Fifth nerve and deep cerebellar nuclei

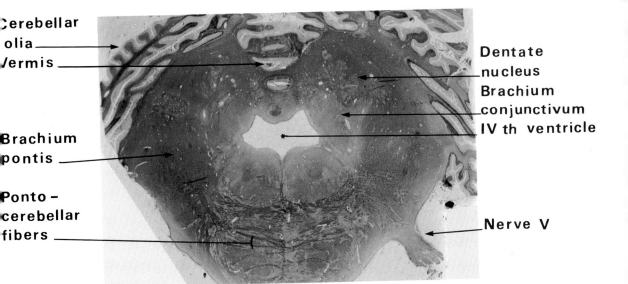

Cerebellar folia

Vermis

Brachium pontis

Ponto – cerebellar fibers

Dentate nucleus

Brachium conjunctivum

IV th ventricle

Nerve V

### Human, 10 % Formalin, Pal-Weigert and carmine stains, 2 x.

**Dentate nucleus:** (L. *dentatus*, toothed.) The largest of the deep cerebellar nuclei. Embedded in the deep white matter of the cerebellar hemisphere in close proximity to the vermis. Afferent input from Purkinje cells of the cerebellum. Efferent output forms part of the brachium conjunctivum.

**Brachium conjunctivum:** Forms dorsolateral wall of the fourth ventricle. Also see Plates 277, 279, 280 and 281.

**IVth ventricle:** Floor formed by the pontine tegmentum, roof by the cerebellum and dorsolateral wall by the brachium conjunctivum.

**Nerve V:** The largest cranial nerve (the trigeminal) in this section is seen entering the lateral part of the pons and coursing through the tegmentum. See also Plates 271, 274, 275 and 276.

**Cerebellar folia:** Narrow laminae of the cerebellar cortex. Possess secondary and tertiary infoldings.

**Vermis:** The vermis of the cerebellum was likened to a worm by Galen (L. *vermis*, worm). It is the median portion of the cerebellum between the two expanded cerebellar hemispheres.

**Brachium pontis:** See Plate 277.

**Pontocerebellar fibers:** Traversing the pons to enter the brachium pontis. See also Plates 277 and 280.

# PONS MESENCEPHALIC JUNCTION

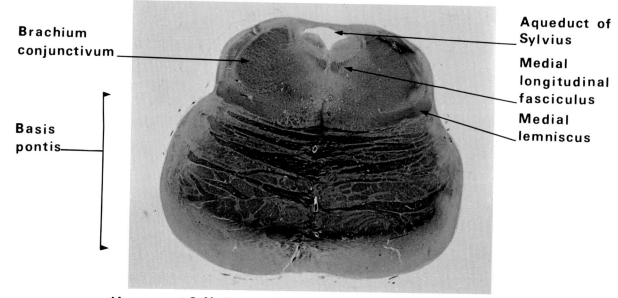

Brachium conjunctivum

Basis pontis

Aqueduct of Sylvius

Medial longitudinal fasciculus

Medial lemniscus

**Human, 10 % Formalin, Weigert-carmine, 3.4 x.**

**Aqueduct of Sylvius:** Named after the French anatomist Jacobus Sylvius (1478–1555). Connects the third and fourth ventricles.

**Medial longitudinal fasciculus:** See Plates 274, 275, 280 and 281.

**Medial lemniscus:** See Plates 275, 276, 277, 280, 281, 282 and 283.

**Basis pontis:** Contains corticopontocerebellar fibers (running horizontally) and corticospinal fibers (running vertically), as well as pontine nuclei.

**Brachium conjunctivum:** Massive outflow tract from the cerebellum seen at this level prior to decussation. Lesions in this area will result in a disorder of coordinated movement.

## MESENCEPHALON
### Level of nerve IV

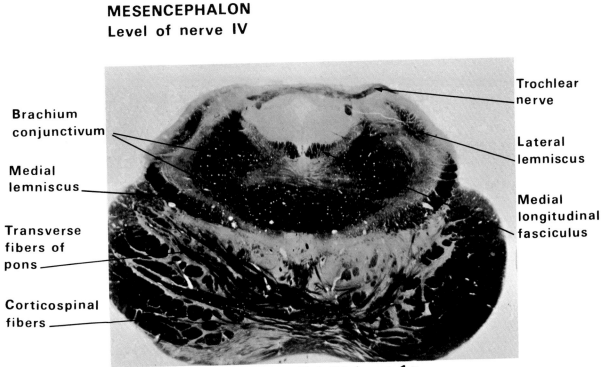

Brachium conjunctivum

Medial lemniscus

Transverse fibers of pons

Corticospinal fibers

Trochlear nerve

Lateral lemniscus

Medial longitudinal fasciculus

Human, 10% Formalin, Pal Weigert, 1x.

**Brachium conjunctivum:** Massive outflow tract of the cerebellum is seen at this level. Fibers are seen prior to and in decussation. Fibers project, after decussation, into the red nucleus and ventrolateral nucleus of the thalamus. Lesions in this region result in a disorder of coordinated movement.

**Medial lemniscus:** See Plates 275, 276, 277, 279, 281, 282 and 283.

**Transverse fibers of the pons:** On their way to the brachium pontis and cerebellum.

**Corticospinal fibers:** Cut in cross section descending to lower levels.

**Trochlear nerve:** Seen decussating before exit from the midbrain. The fourth cranial nerve supplies the superior oblique muscle, which serves to intort the eye when the eye is in the abducted position and to depress the eye when it is in the adducted position. Lesions affecting this nerve produce vertical diplopia. The only cranial nerve to decussate or cross completely.

**Lateral lemniscus:** Located laterally and dorsally on its way to the inferior colliculus and medial geniculate body. Concerned with audition.

**Medial longitudinal fasciculus:** See Plates 274, 275, 279 and 281.

## MESENCEPHALON
### Inferior colliculus

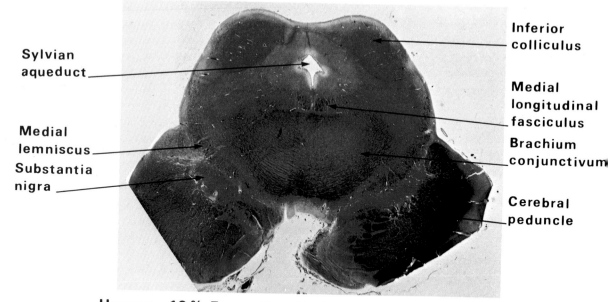

Sylvian aqueduct

Inferior colliculus

Medial longitudinal fasciculus

Medial lemniscus
Substantia nigra

Brachium conjunctivum

Cerebral peduncle

**Human, 10% Formalin, Weigert-carmine, 4x.**

**Inferior colliculus:** Ovoid cellular mass belonging to the auditory system.

**Medial longitudinal fasciculus:** See Plates 274, 275, 279 and 280.

**Brachium conjunctivum:** Efferent outflow of the cerebellum. Fibers in this system decussate at this level on their way to the red nucleus and thalamus.

**Cerebral peduncle:** Descending corticofugal fiber system. Lesions here interrupt corticospinal fibers and result in weakness or paralysis of the contralateral half of the body including the face.

**Sylvian aqueduct:** See Plate 279.

**Medial lemniscus:** See Plates 275, 276, 277, 279, 280, 282 and 283.

**Substantia nigra:** Sandwiched between the medial lemniscus and cerebral peduncle. A mass of pigmented cells (melanin). This area is invariably the site of pathological changes associated with Parkinson's disease.

## MESENCEPHALON
## Level of nerve III

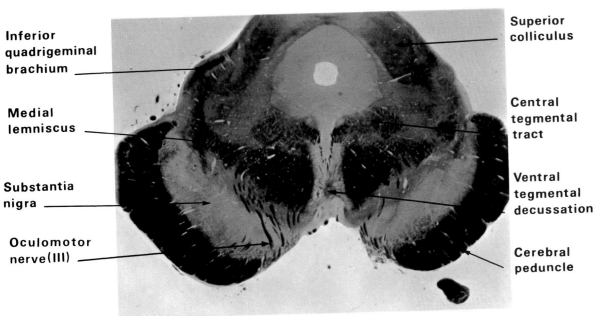

Inferior
quadrigeminal
brachium

Medial
lemniscus

Substantia
nigra

Oculomotor
nerve(III)

Superior
colliculus

Central
tegmental
tract

Ventral
tegmental
decussation

Cerebral
peduncle

Human, 10% Formalin, Pal Weigert, 1x.

**Inferior quadrigeminal brachium:** Bundle of nerve fibers arising from the lateral lemniscus and the inferior colliculus on their way to the medial geniculate body. This fiber bundle conveys auditory impulses from the midbrain to the thalamus.

**Medial lemniscus:** Occupies here a location dorsal to the substantia nigra. Note that it is displaced laterally by the red nucleus and brachium conjunctivum. For modalities conveyed by the medial lemniscus, see Plates 275 and 277.

**Substantia nigra:** See Plates 281 and 283.

**Oculomotor nerve:** Rootlets of the third cranial nerve leaving the midbrain. Supplies the levator palpebrae superioris, the superior rectus, inferior rectus, medial rectus and inferior oblique muscles. Note their relation to the cerebral peduncle. Combined lesions of the third nerve and the cerebral peduncle at this site give a characteristic clinical syndrome. The signs are an ipsilateral paralysis of the eye muscles supplied by the third nerve combined with a contralateral hemiplegia of the body and extremities. Clinically known as oculomotor alternating hemiplegia.

**Superior colliculus:** Cellular mass concerned with reflex eye movement.

**Central tegmental tract:** Compact fiber bundle located dorsal to the lateral part of the medial lemniscus. Carries fibers from midbrain tegmentum, red nucleus and periaqueductal gray matter to the inferior olivary complex.

**Ventral tegmental decussation:** Decussating fibers of the rubrospinal tract. Fibers arise from the red nucleus, cross at this level and descend in the neuraxis to the spinal cord.

# MESENCEPHALON
## Junction with diencephalon

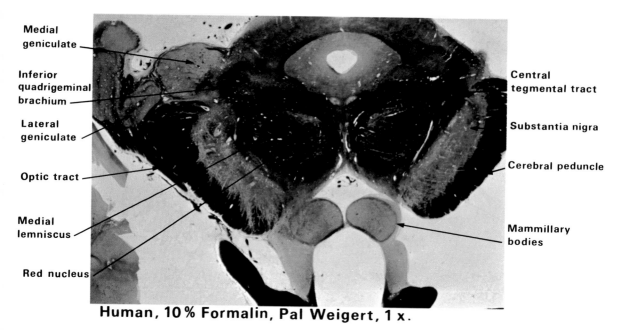

Medial geniculate

Inferior quadrigeminal brachium

Lateral geniculate

Optic tract

Medial lemniscus

Red nucleus

Central tegmental tract

Substantia nigra

Cerebral peduncle

Mammillary bodies

**Human, 10 % Formalin, Pal Weigert, 1 x.**

**Medial geniculate body:** A thalamic nucleus concerned with audition. Receives auditory fibers from the inferior quadrigeminal brachium located medial to it.

**Lateral geniculate:** A thalamic nucleus concerned with vision. Receives fibers of the optic tract.

**Medial lemniscus:** Occupies a position lateral to the red nucleus at this level.

**Red nucleus:** So called because of a pinkish color in the fresh state due to its high vascularity. This nucleus links the cerebellum, motor cortex and spinal cord. Major input is from the brachium conjunctivum. Projects into the motor area and the spinal cord.

**Central tegmental tract:** See Plate 282.

**Substantia nigra:** See Plates 281 and 282.

**Cerebral peduncle:** See Plates 281 and 282.

**Mammillary bodies:** A pair of nuclear masses located in the interpeduncular fossa. Form part of the posterior floor of the third ventricle. Receive fibers from the hippocampus and project fibers into the anterior thalamic nucleus.

# DIENCEPHALON
## Mammillary body

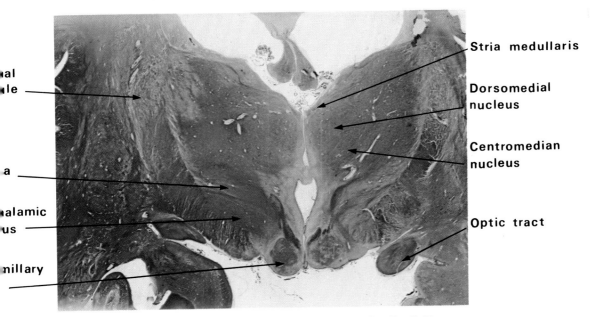

Stria medullaris

Dorsomedial nucleus

Centromedian nucleus

Optic tract

al le

a

alamic us

millary

## Human, 10% Formalin, Luxol fast blue–PAS, 2.7x.

**Stria medullaris:** A bundle of myelinated fibers connecting the septal nuclei with the habenular complex. Characteristically located dorsomedial to the diencephalon.

**Dorsomedial nucleus:** One of a group of thalamic nuclei located medial to the internal medullary lamina. Has reciprocal connections with the prefrontal cortex and hypothalamus. Concerned with emotional behavior.

**Centromedian nucleus:** Belongs to the intralaminar group of thalamic nuclei. Located between the dorsomedial and ventral posterior nucleus. Almost completely surrounded by fibers of the internal medullary lamina. Projects mainly to the putamen and plays an important role in intrathalamic regulating mechanisms.

**Optic tract:** Containing crossed visual fibers from the contralateral nasal retina and uncrossed fibers from the homolateral temporal retina.

**Internal capsule:** Heavily myelinated fiber bundle arising from many areas of the cerebral cortex, and descending to lower levels of the neuraxis. Considered the single most important descending tract in the brain. Lesions here result in paralysis of muscles in the contralateral half of the body.

**Zona incerta:** An area of gray matter located dorsal to the subthalamic nucleus. Receives fibers from the precentral cortex.

**Subthalamic nucleus:** Also known as corpus Luysi, shaped like a biconcave lens. Receives fibers from and projects to the globus pallidus. Discrete lesions here result in an abnormal type of movement known as ballism. These unusually violent involuntary movements involve primarily the proximal muscles of the upper and lower extremities. Facial and cervical muscles may also be involved.

**Mammillary body:** A pair of nuclear masses located in the interpeduncular fossa and forming part of the floor of the third ventricle posteriorly. Receives fibers from the hippocampus and projects to the anterior thalamic nucleus.

# DIENCEPHALON
## Posteroventral nucleus

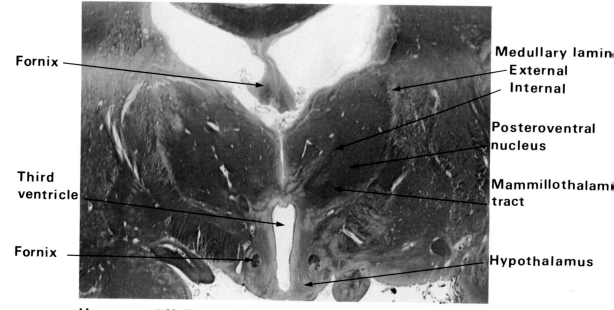

Fornix

Medullary lamin
External
Internal

Posteroventral
nucleus

Third
ventricle

Mammillothalami
tract

Fornix

Hypothalamus

**Human, 10% Formalin, Luxol fast blue—PAS, 2.7x.**

**Fornix:** Cut in cross section here, it is an arched, paired fiber tract connecting the hippocampus and the mammillary bodies.

**Third ventricle:** Sandwiched between the two diencephalons.

**Medullary lamina:** A band of white matter separating the medial and lateral groups of thalamic nuclei (internal) and delimiting the lateral boundary of the thalamus (external).

**Posteroventral nucleus:** One of the lateral group of thalamic nuclei. A major station in the pathway of exteroceptive and proprioceptive impulses to the cerebral cortex. Receives fibers from the medial lemniscus, the spinothalamic tract and the trigeminal system. Projects fibers to the primary sensory (somesthetic) cortex.

**Mammillothalamic tract:** Seen in cross section. A fiber system that connects the mammillary bodies with the anterior thalamic nuclei. Also called tract of Vicq d'Azyr after Felix Vicq d'Azyr, the French anatomist who described this bundle in 1781.

**Hypothalamus:** Ventral to the thalamus forming part of the lateral wall of the third ventricle.

## DIENCEPHALON
### Ansa lenticularis

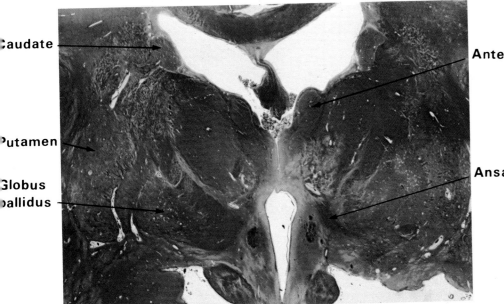

Caudate ⟶

Anterior nucleus

Putamen ⟶

Ansa lenticularis

Globus
pallidus ⟶

**Human, 10% Formalin, Luxol fast blue–PAS, 2.7x.**

**Caudate:** One of the basal ganglia. Note how it bulges into the cavity of the lateral ventricle.

**Putamen:** The largest part of the basal ganglia. Traversed by myelinated bundles of fibers. Similar in cytological structure to the caudate.

**Globus pallidus:** Belongs to the basal ganglia group of nuclei. Traversed by many bundles of myelinated fibers. Comprises the principal efferent nucleus of the basal ganglia. Receives fibers from the caudate and putamen and projects to the thalamus and subthalamus.

**Anterior nucleus:** Located in rostral levels of the thalamus. Receives the mammillothalamic tract and projects fibers to the cingulate gyrus of the cerebral cortex. See also Plates 287 and 288.

**Ansa lenticularis:** Efferent fiber bundle from the globus pallidus en route to the thalamus. Sweeps around the internal capsule on its way to the thalamus.

## DIENCEPHALON
### Ventrolateral nucleus

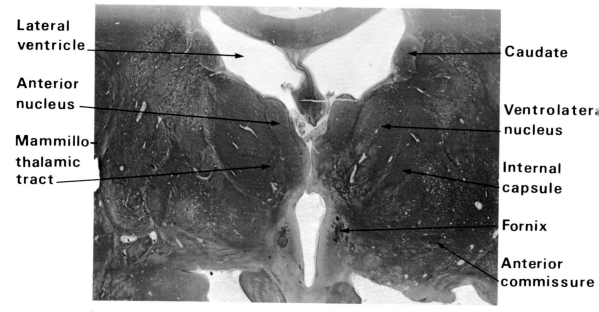

Lateral ventricle

Anterior nucleus

Mammillo-thalamic tract

Caudate

Ventrolateral nucleus

Internal capsule

Fornix

Anterior commissure

Human, 10% Formalin, Luxol fast blue–PAS, 2.7x.

**Lateral ventricle:** Anterior horn. Note the projections of the caudate which bulge into the cavity of the ventricle.

**Anterior nucleus:** See Plates 286 and 288. Note the mammillothalamic tract approaching the nucleus.

**Mammillothalamic tract:** See Plates 285, 288 and 289.

**Caudate:** See Plates 286, 290, 297 and 298.

**Ventrolateral nucleus:** Traversed by a heavy bundle of myelinated fibers. Receives fibers from the dentatorubrothalamic system and projects to the motor cortex. A common site for stereotaxic surgical lesions to relieve abnormal movements.

**Internal capsule:** See Plates 284, 288, 289, 290 and 298.

**Fornix:** See Plates 285, 288, 289, 296 and 297.

**Anterior commissure:** A compact fiber bundle containing the larger, posterior portion of the anterior commissure is seen here. This bundle courses inferior to the globus pallidus and putamen. This bundle interconnects the middle temporal gyri and the inferior temporal gyri. See also Plates 289, 296 and 299.

# DIENCEPHALON
## Ventral anterior nucleus

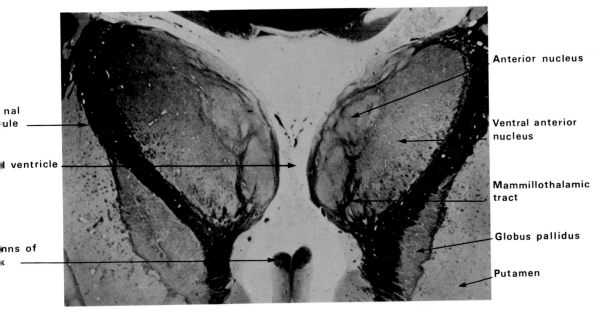

nal
ule

4 ventricle

nns of
k

Anterior nucleus

Ventral anterior
nucleus

Mammillothalamic
tract

Globus pallidus

Putamen

## Human, 10% Formalin, Weigert method, 2x.

**Mammillothalamic tract:** Seen entering the anterior thalamic nucleus.

**Putamen:** One of the nuclei of the basal ganglia. Similar in structure and connections to the caudate. Lies ventral and lateral to the internal capsule. See Plates 286 and 299.

**Globus pallidus:** Another of the basal ganglia nuclei. Receives fibers from the caudate and putamen and projects information from the basal ganglia to the thalamus (nucleus ventralis anterior). Has reciprocal connections with the subthalamic nucleus. Microscopic structure differs from that of the caudate and putamen. Plates 286, 289 and 298.

**Anterior nucleus thalamic:** Located in the most rostral level of the diencephalon. Receives the mammillothalamic tract from the mammillary body and projects fibers to the cingulate gyrus of the cerebral cortex. The heavily myelinated mammillothalamic tract is seen entering the nucleus.

**Ventral anterior nucleus:** One of the lateral group of thalamic nuclei located rostrally. Receives fibers from the globus pallidus and projects fibers to the cerebral cortex. Important in the genesis of movement disorders.

**Internal capsule:** See Plates 284, 287, 289, 290 and 298.

**Third ventricle:** Sandwiched between the two thalami.

**Columns of the fornix:** Rostrally the fornix bundles separate as the columns of the fornix (seen here in cross section) and arch ventrally and caudally enroute to the mammillary bodies.

# DIENCEPHALON
## Anterior commissure

Dorsomedial nucleus

Internal capsule

Globus pallidus
outer segment
inner segment

Inferior thalamic peduncle

Third ventricle

Ventrolateral nucleus

Internal medullary lamina

Mammillothalamic tract

Fornix

Anterior commissure

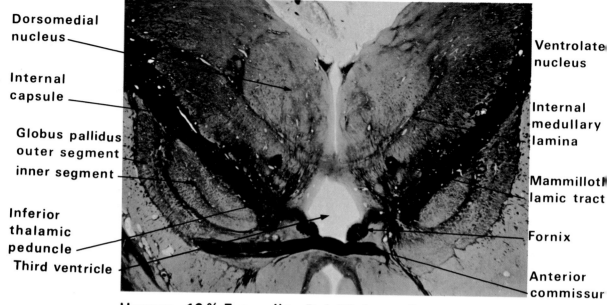

**Human, 10% Formalin, Pal Weigert, 1x.**

**Dorsomedial nucleus:** Located medial to the internal medullary lamina. Has reciprocal connections with the prefrontal cortex and hypothalamus. Concerned with emotional behavior. See Plate 284.

**Internal capsule:** Separates the diencephalon and basal ganglia. Heavily myelinated fiber system arising from wide areas of the cerebral cortex and descending to the spinal cord. Lesions here result in paralysis of muscles in the contralateral half of the body. Plates 284, 287, 288, 290 and 298.

**Globus pallidus:** Belongs to the basal ganglia group of nuclei. Outer and inner segments are separated by a medullated lamina. The nucleus is traversed by many bundles of myelinated fibers. Comprises the principal efferent system of the basal ganglia. Receives fibers from the caudate and putamen, and projects fibers to the thalamus and subthalamus. Plates 286, 288, 289 and 298.

**Inferior thalamic peduncle:** Myelinated fiber bundle connecting the thalamus, hypothalamus and amygdaloid nucleus.

**Third ventricle:** The space between the two diencephalons. Filled with cerebrospinal fluid.

**Ventrolateral nucleus:** Lateral to the internal medullary lamina. Traversed by a heavy bundle of myelinated fibers. Receives fibers from the deep cerebellar nuclei and projects to the motor cortex. A common site for stereotaxic surgical lesions for the relief of abnormal movements. Plate 287.

**Internal medullary lamina:** A band of myelinated fibers that separate the medial from the lateral groups of thalamic nuclei. Splits rostrally to enclose the anterior thalamic nucleus.

**Mammillothalamic tract:** Cut in cross section. A fiber system connecting the mammillary bodies with the anterior thalamic nucleus. Also called tract of Vicq d'Azyr, after the French anatomist who described this bundle in 1781. Plates 285, 287 and 288.

**Fornix:** Cut in cross section before it dips behind the anterior commissure to reach the mammillary bodies. The fornix is a C-shaped, paired fiber system that connects the hippocampus with the mammillary bodies. Plates 285, 287, 288, 296, 297 and 299.

**Anterior commissure:** A compact fiber bundle in close proximity to the fornix. Interconnects the olfactory nuclei and the temporal cortex.

## BASAL GANGLIA
### Caudate nucleus

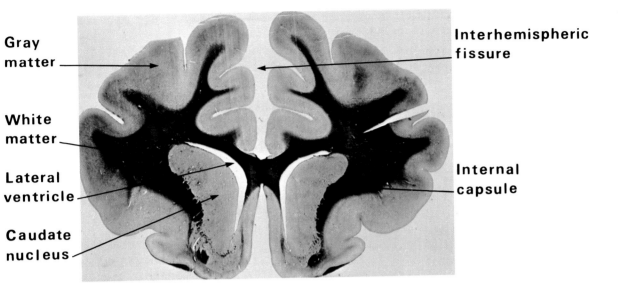

Gray matter

Interhemispheric fissure

White matter

Lateral ventricle

Internal capsule

Caudate nucleus

**Cat, 10% Formalin, Weil, 3.4x.**

**Interhemispheric fissure:** Separates the two cerebral hemispheres. Filled with a dural fold, the falx cerebri, which has been stripped away in this preparation.

**Internal capsule:** Heavily myelinated broad band of white substance that arises from wide areas of the cerebral hemispheres and descends to lower levels. Lesions of the internal capsule result in paralysis of the contralateral half of the body. Maintains a characteristic location lateral to the caudate nucleus. Plates 284, 287, 288, 289 and 298.

**Gray matter:** Varies in thickness from 1.5 to 4.5 mm throughout the cerebral cortex, depending on function and location. Thickest in the motor cortex.

**White matter:** Lies deep to the gray matter. Contains association, commissural as well as corticofugal and corticopetal fiber systems.

**Caudate nucleus:** C-shaped mass of gray matter closely related to the lateral ventricle. The part seen in this figure is the head of the nucleus which characteristically bulges into the lateral ventricle. Rich in catecholamines. Concerned with the regulation of movement.

## CEREBELLUM
### Deep cerebellar nuclei

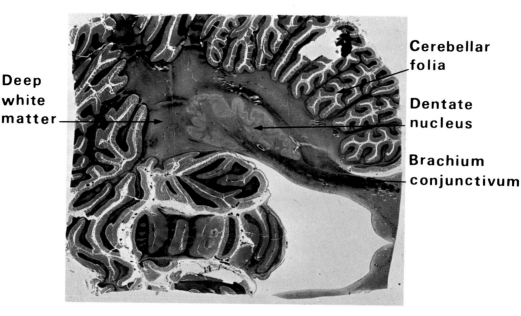

Deep white matter

Cerebellar folia

Dentate nucleus

Brachium conjunctivum

**Human, 10% Formalin, Weigert-carmine, 2.5 x.**

**Cerebellar folia:**   Leaflike folds of the cerebellar cortex separated from each other by sulci and supported by a core of white matter.

**Dentate nucleus:**   One of the deep cerebellar nuclei embedded in the deep white matter. Resembles the inferior olive in its purselike appearance. Receives axons of Purkinje cells of the cerebellum and projects through the brachium conjunctivum to the red nucleus and ventrolateral nucleus of the thalamus. Lesions of the dentate nucleus result in homolateral volitional tremor. See plates 278 and 298.

**Brachium conjunctivum:**   Outflow tract of the cerebellum. Heavily myelinated. Projects to the red nucleus and ventrolateral nucleus of the thalamus. Lesions of this tract result in homolateral volitional tremor.

**Deep white matter:**   A compact mass of white matter which is continuous between cerebellar hemispheres. In it are embedded the deep cerebellar nuclei. Extends into the folia as a core of white matter.

# CEREBELLUM

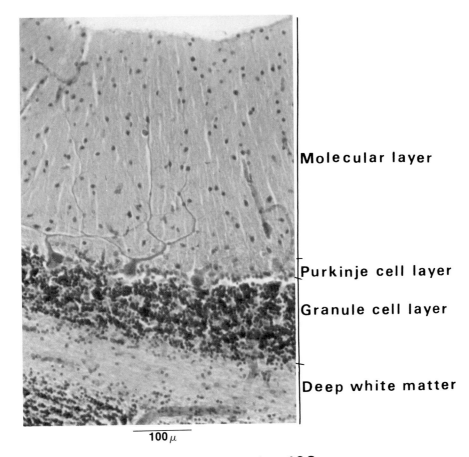

Molecular layer

Purkinje cell layer

Granule cell layer

Deep white matter

100 μ

**Human, Müller's fluid, Carmine stain, 162 x.**

**Molecular layer:** Most superficial layer. Sparsely cellular. Primarily composed of nonmyelinated fibers. Dendrites of Purkinje cells are seen arborizing in this layer. Plates 293, 294 and 295.

**Purkinje cell layer:** Single row of flask-shaped large neurons. Largest neurons in the cerebellum. Dendrites arborize richly in molecular layer. Axons enter medullary core.

**Granule cell layer:** Closely packed with chromatic nuclei of small granule cell neurons. Lighter islands in this layer represent glomeruli where synapses are established.

**Deep white matter:** Contains afferent and efferent fibers of the cerebellum. Also known as medullary core.

See also Plates 88, 89, 90, 91, 293, 294 and 295.

## CEREBELLUM
### Nerve cell processes

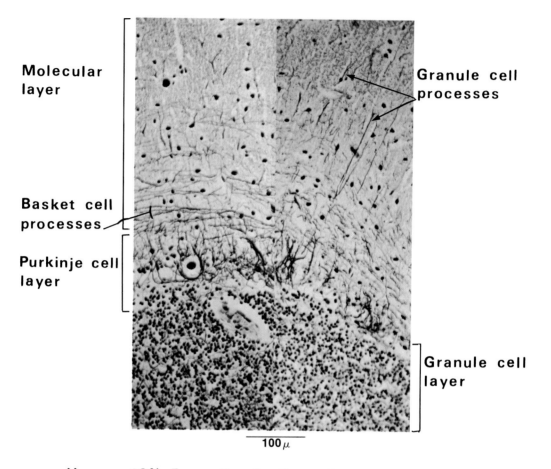

Molecular layer

Granule cell processes

Basket cell processes

Purkinje cell layer

Granule cell layer

100 μ

**Human, 10% Formalin, Bodian silver, 162 x.**

**Molecular layer:** Outermost layer of the cerebellum. Plates 88, 89, 90, 292 and 295.

**Purkinje cell layer:** Single row of large flask-shaped cells. Plates 88, 89, 90, 91, 292, 294 and 295.

**Granule cell layer:** Deep to the Purkinje cell layer. Contains small closely packed granule cells.

**Granule cell processes:** Axons of granule cells reach the molecular layer where they bifurcate (parallel fibers) to establish synapses.

**Basket cell processes:** Axons of basket cells. So named because they form a basket-like arborization around Purkinje cells.

# CEREBELLUM
## Cortex

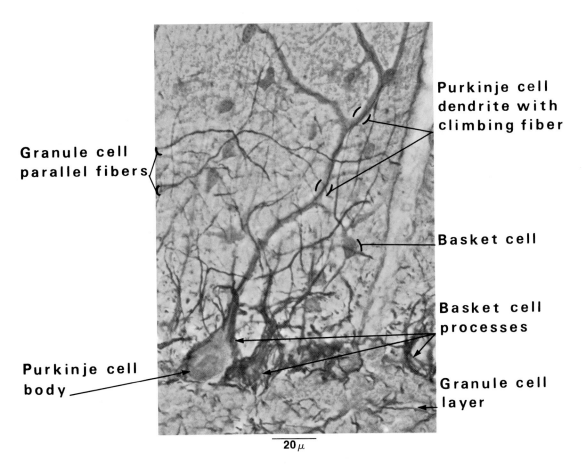

Granule cell parallel fibers

Purkinje cell dendrite with climbing fiber

Basket cell

Basket cell processes

Purkinje cell body

Granule cell layer

20 μ

**Dog, Ranson's method, 612 x.**

**Granule cell parallel fibers:** Axons of granule cells ascend from the granule cell layer to the molecular layer, where each divides into two branches which run horizontally across the layer establishing synapses with dendrites of several Purkinje cells.

**Purkinje cell body:** Large flask-shaped cell.

**Purkinje cell dendrite with climbing fiber:** Purkinje cell dendrites and climbing fibers run parallel to each other. The latter have an excitatory influence on Purkinje cells and may be a part of an extensive intracortical or nucleocortical feedback system.

**Basket cell:** A special variety of stellate cell in the molecular layer close to the Purkinje cells. Axons of basket cells run transversely in the molecular layer, giving off collaterals that form a "basket" arborization around Purkinje cells.

**Granule cell layer:** A layer of small granule cells under the Purkinje cell layer. Receives the major input to the cerebellum.

See also Plates 88, 89, 90, 91, 292, 293, 294 and 295.

# CEREBELLUM

Granular layer

Molecular layer

Purkinje cells

Basket cell processes

Medullary core

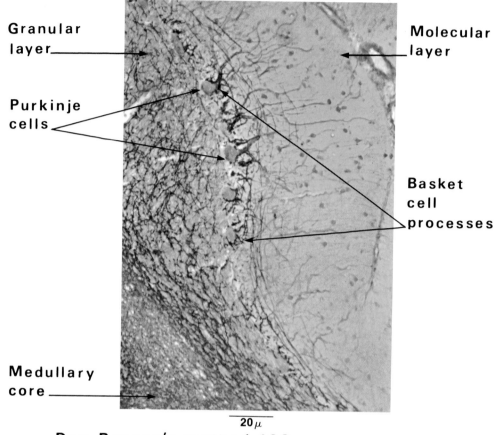

20 μ

Dog, Ranson's method, 162 x.

**Molecular layer:** Most superficial layer, containing few neurons. Composed mainly of unmyelinated fibers from the granule cell layer and dendritic processes from Purkinje cells. A few myelinated fibers are found in deeper portions.

**Basket cell processes:** Axons of basket cells run transversely in the folium giving off collaterals that form a basket-like arborization around Purkinje cell bodies.

**Medullary core:** Deep white matter. Contains the entire afferent and efferent axons of the cerebellum.

**Granule cell layer:** A plexus or network composed of processes of granule cells and Golgi Type II cells (Plate 90) as well as mossy fiber input. Mossy fibers are the terminations of fibers entering the cerebellum from the spinocerebellar, olivocerebellar and pontocerebellar tracts. Other sources have not been fully determined.

**Purkinje cells:** Single row of large flask-shaped cells. Dendrites arborize richly in the molecular layer. Note black arborization of basket cell axons around the Purkinje cells.

## BRAIN
## Midsagittal section

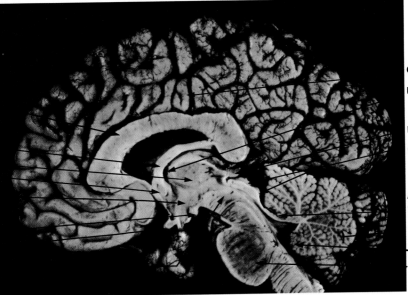

us callosum

ix

amus

rior commissure

othalamus

nmillary body

c chiasma

sencephalon

Cingulate gyrus

Foramen of Monro

Pineal gland

Corpora quadrigemina

Anterior medullary velum

Cerebellum

Fourth ventricle

Pons

## Human, 10% Formalin, 0.25x.

In this section, structures located on the medial surface of the brain are seen. Note the cingulate gyrus above the corpus collosum. This gyrus receives fibers from the anterior nucleus of the thalamus. Note the massive myelinated fiber bundles, the C-shaped corpus callosum and fornix. The first is important in interhemispheric transfer of information and the latter links the hippocampus and mammillary bodies. The dark space between them represents the depth of the lateral ventricles and in appropriate sections is traversed by the septum pellucidum. Note the fornix dipping into the depth of the hypothalamus on its way to the mammillary bodies. Rostral to it at this point is the anterior commissure, cut in cross section. Underneath the fornix, note the thalamus, a major sensory and motor integrating center. Below the thalamus, the hypothalamus. The two are separated by the hypothalamic sulcus. Note the mammillary body at the caudal extremity of the hypothalamus. The mammillary bodies receive fibers from the fornix and project fibers to the anterior nucleus of the thalamus. The optic chiasma is seen anterior and inferior to the hypothalamus. Tumors of the hypothalamus in this region compress the optic chiasma and result in characteristic visual field defects.

Dorsal to the rostral extremity of the thalamus note the foramen of Monro. It connects the lateral and third ventricles. The latter is the space between the two thalami and hypothalami. Caudal to the thalamus is the mesencephalon, capped by the corpora quadrigemina. The latter represent the two superior and two inferior colliculi. The former belong to the visual system and the latter to the auditory system. Rostral to the corpora quadrigemina is the pineal gland. Note the anterior medullary velum extending from the cerebellum to the midbrain. It forms the roof of the fourth ventricle anteriorly and contains the superior cerebellar peduncle (brachium conjunctivum). The pons is seen ventral to the cerebellum.

## BRAIN
### Sagittal section

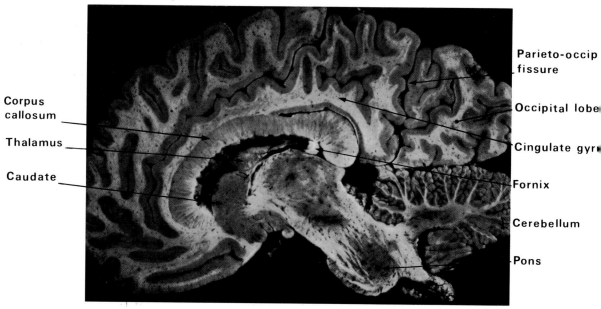

Parieto-occip
fissure

Occipital lobe

Cingulate gyr

Fornix

Cerebellum

Pons

Corpus
callosum

Thalamus

Caudate

**Human, 10% Formalin, 0.25x.**

This is a parasagittal section of the brain close to the midline. The C-configuration of the corpus callosum and its relation to the lateral ventricle are seen in this section. The position of the fornix inferior to the corpus callosum is also seen. The cingulate gyrus follows the contour of the corpus callosum. This gyrus receives fibers from the anterior thalamic nucleus. Note the caudate and thalamic projection into the lateral ventricles. The parieto-occipital fissure is best seen on the medial surface of the hemisphere separating the parietal from the occipital lobes. Note the relationship of the cerebellum beneath the occipital lobe and dorsal to the pons, and the heavily myelinated bundle (brachium pontis) connecting the cerebellum with the pons.

## BRAIN
## Sagittal section

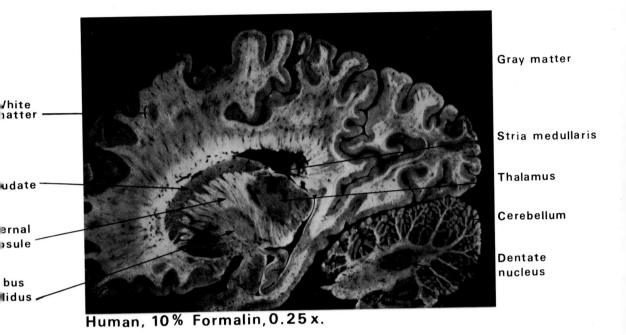

Gray matter

White matter

Stria medullaris

Caudate

Thalamus

Internal capsule

Cerebellum

Globus pallidus

Dentate nucleus

Human, 10% Formalin, 0.25x.

This parasagittal section is away from the midline. Note the gray and white matter of the hemisphere and the varying thickness of gray matter in the different parts of the hemisphere. The head of the caudate nucleus is seen above the internal capsule. Note the internal capsule separating the thalamus and globus pallidus. The thalamus is capped by a white bundle of fibers, the stria medullaris (thalami). The latter connects the septal nuclei and the habenula. In the deep white matter of the cerebellum, note the dentate nucleus.

## BRAIN
### Sagittal section

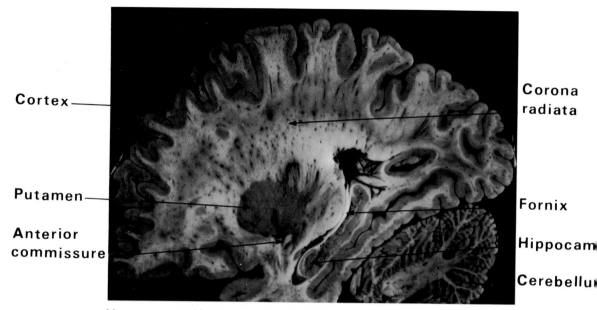

Cortex

Corona radiata

Putamen

Fornix

Anterior commissure

Hippocam

Cerebellu

Human, 10% Formalin, 0.25 x.

This is a parasagittal section showing some cortical and subcortical structures. Note the gray matter (cortex) capping the white matter (corona radiata) of the cerebral hemisphere. The gray mass deep in the white matter is the putamen. Below that is a bundle of white fibers representing the anterior commissure (Plates 287, 289 and 296). Also seen to good advantage in this cut are the hippocampus and the emerging fibers of the fornix. The cerebellum is seen underneath the cerebral hemisphere.

PLATE 300

## CEREBRAL CORTEX
Post central gyrus
cell layering

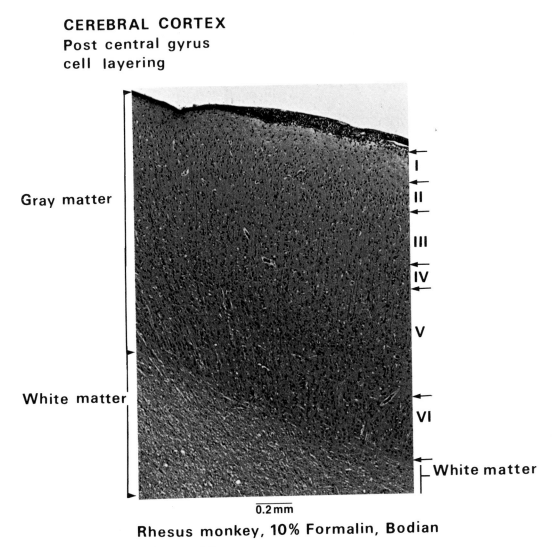

Gray matter

White matter

I
II
III
IV
V
VI

White matter

0.2 mm

Rhesus monkey, 10% Formalin, Bodian silver, 49 x.

Lamination is a major characteristic of cortical structure. Six horizontal laminae distinguish the neocortex. Laminae are differentiated by the type, density and arrangement of cells. The six laminae seen in this plate are, from the surface of the cortex to the white matter, as follows.

**I—Molecular layer or plexiform layer:** Contains few cells and a rich nerve fiber plexus made up of axons and dendrites of cells in other laminae as well as cells in this lamina.

**II—External granular layer:** Closely packed small neurons.

**III—External pyramidal layer:** Composed mainly of pyramidal neurons and many granule cells and cells of Martinotti.

**IV—Internal granular layer:** Composed chiefly of stellate cells which are closely packed.

**V—Internal pyramidal or ganglionic layer:** Consists of medium-sized and large pyramidal cells intermingled with granule cells.

**VI—Multiform layer or layer of fusiform cells:** Contains a variety of cell types.

**White matter:** Contains incoming and outgoing nerve fibers.

# Section 18

# Appendices

## Appendix I: How to Study a Microscope Slide

In studying a histological preparation you should acquaint yourself with the following: (a) the name of the organ or tissue; (b) the animal from which it was prepared; (c) the method of fixation (or preservative) employed; (d) the thickness of the tissue slice; and (e) the stain or stain combination utilized. A sample slide label containing all of the above information is shown below.

| | |
|---|---|
| (a) | Duodenum |
| (b) | Human |
| (c) | Helly's Fluid |
| (d) | 6 $\mu$ |
| (e) | Hematoxylin and Eosin |

It is essential to understand the meaning of each of these notations if you are to gain the maximum amount of information from your subsequent study of the slide.

(a) First, familiarize yourself with the over-all function of the tissue to be examined. In our example above, one should know that the duodenum is the first segment of the tubular small intestine which receives: (1) partially digested food from the stomach; (2) digestive enzymes from the pancreas; (3) bile from the liver; and (4) its own secretion, the intestinal juices. In the small intestine, the digestion of food, which begins in the mouth and stomach, is completed. The end products of the digestive process (*i.e.,* monosaccharides, amino acids and fatty acids), as well as vitamins, salts and water, are absorbed and transported through the columnar epithelium into the capillaries or lymphatic vessels in the wall of the intestine. Any undigested food is carried along through the digestive tube until digestion and assimilation are complete or the undigestible contents are eliminated at the anal orifice.

You should, therefore, examine each of the component parts of this organ. Those parts beginning at the inner or luminal surface include: (1) the *epithelium*, with its four cell types (the simple columnar absorptive cells, goblet cells, Paneth cells and argentaffin cells); (2) the *lamina propria*, which contains the capillaries, both blood vascular and lymphatic, arteries and veins, connective tissue fibers and a variety of important, protective migratory cells, strands of smooth muscle, and nodules or collections of lymphocytes; (3) the *muscularis mucosa*, a thin layer of smooth muscle fibers; (4) the *submucosa*, in which specific duodenal tubular glands (Brunner's mucous glands) and ducts are found leading to the intestinal lumen, autonomic nerve fibers and cell bodies (Meissner's plexus), as well as loose connective tissue supporting the vascular elements; and (5) the *muscularis,* composed of an inner circular layer and an outer longitudinal layer. Between these two smooth muscle layers, autonomic nerve fibers and nerve cell bodies (Auerbach's plexus) may be found; and (6) the outermost loose connective tissue layer which may or may not be covered with mesothelium.

The basic tissues represented in each slide should be identified and their structure and function reviewed.

(b) The animal from which the tissue sections are prepared is important. Although the cells and tissues in most mammals bear marked similarity, subtle to gross differences do occur.

(c) The method of fixation employed in the preparation of cells and tissues will determine the type and quality of tissue preservation as well as the subsequent choice of stains which may be employed.

(d) The notation of section thickness on a microscope slide informs the observer of the approximate level of magnification most suitable for examination of the tissue section. The thinner the tissue section, the higher the magnification and resolution of structural detail possible. In general, cytologists prefer sections 1 to 3 $\mu$ (microns) in thickness, whereas histologists and neuroanatomists may employ sections up to 50 $\mu$ or more.*

(e) The stain notation is most valuable and is an indication of the particular emphasis for which the slide was prepared. This should receive the most careful attention by the student. As will become evident in your reading, a vast array of tissue stains are available to visualize specific cellular and tissue components. Many of the commonly employed stains and stain combinations are represented in this book. Their potential use extends beyond the educational into the very important realm of biomedical research. The student or researcher in any of the basic or applied biomedical sciences can profit from the use of staining techniques which detail each of the component parts of any tissue under investigation regardless of the specific approach, which may be primarily physiological, chemical or anatomical.

After a careful reading of the slide label and preparation for study of the microscope slide, examine the slide with the naked eye and/or the microscope ocular and note any gross features of the section which indicate distinctive structural arrangements to be studied with the microscope. These features include size, color, shape and component parts. If the section is composed of different parts, note their relationship and staining differences if any.

Examine the section to determine whether the tissue was cut from a larger piece and if any natural surfaces are present. This will aid your subsequent study at higher magnification. This should be followed by a systematic scanning of the section by the lowest power objective to identify further and locate the components of the tissue. With the low power (10 × objective) continue the study, paying particular attention to smaller and more subtle staining and structural details. The high dry lens (~43 ×) will allow the study of most of the details found in routine histological sections. Switching the lenses frequently from the lowest to the highest magnification will facilitate the study and prevent missing important component parts of the section.

The oil immersion lens (100 ×) should be employed for the study of cytological and other minute tissue components and is best saved for the final stages of study. The oil should be used sparingly; it may interfere with the study of a slide at low magnifications and may come in contact with the high dry objective lens. If contaminated, the lenses should be carefully wiped only with a high quality, clean lens paper. The use of solvents such as xylol can severely damage or ruin a fine microscope lens. If it is necessary to use a lens cleaner, caution should be exercised.

With practice, most microscopic anatomists find that additional details can

---

*1 $\mu$ = 1/25,400 inch = 1/1000 mm = 10,000 Å.

be seen by making continuous fine adjustments of the focus at higher magnifications in order to visualize structures more superficial or deep in their histological sections. This method of continual fine focus adjustment permits the tracing of structures and their relationships through the full thickness of the tissue section. The three-dimensional effect gained adds a richness which is lost if this technique is not employed.

Simple sketches of the important features of the tissue section are valuable aids to subsequent review of the major features of the tissue studied. The development of this skill is a valuable technique in the learning process, as it requires attention to detail in translating the visual image to a drawing which will have lasting value in forming a permanent mental image.

When your study of the microscope slide is complete, carefully clean again with lens paper any oil or fingerprints from the section cover glass and slide.

The preparation of microscope slides is very costly and in some instances the sections may be, for other reasons, irreplaceable. Use one slide at a time, replacing it in the slide container before removing another for study.

# Appendix II: The Preparation of Cells and Tissue for Microscopic Study

The photographs which comprise this atlas were prepared from tissues obtained either from animals that were sacrificed for the purpose or, in the case of human tissues, from surgical or autopsy specimens.

The tissues were first placed in a solution called a fixative, which ideally preserves and hardens them with minimal distortion of the physical features, chemical characteristics and staining properties. No matter how successful this fixation process, the death of the cells and tissues will ultimately result in artifacts which must be recognized, understood and controlled. As a consequence of this, the histologist is always modifying existing methods and experimenting with new fixatives in order to preserve the essential features of living cells for his microscopic study.

In general the stepwise procedures which follow are employed to prepare stained tissue sections or slices of fixed tissues for microscopic study. The procedure to be outlined relates to paraffin (wax)-embedded tissues, the most commonly used method, but, in principle, similar to those employed with other embedding media. Specific details for the wide range of techniques developed by anatomists can be found in the cited references (Appendix V).

The paraffin or wax method includes the following steps:

1. Fixation (as in 10% formalin, Zenker's fluid, etc.);
2. Rinsing (excess fixative removed with water);
3. Dehydration (in graded ethanol from 70 to 100%);
4. Clearing (to replace ethanol with a solvent miscible with both ethanol and paraffin). Cedar wood oil, xylene or others may be employed;
5. Embedding (impregnation of tissue in molten paraffin and subsequent hardening by cooling);
6. Sectioning (slicing the wax-impregnated tissue on a microtome);
7. Affixing sections on glass slides (usually with egg albumin);
8. Dewaxing sections in xylene and hydrating the tissue with decreasing grades of ethanol and distilled water;
9. Staining or dyeing the tissue;
10. Rinsing (to remove excess dye);
11. Dehydration in graded ethanol and clearing the tissue sections in xylene;
12. Covering the sections with Canada balsam or a synthetic medium and a thin glass coverslip.

These procedures can and do in many instances result in the loss of cellular constituents and inclusions and thereby alter the microscopic appearances of cells and tissues. Because of this, a variety of fixatives are employed to preserve and stabilize certain structures and inclusions to withstand the procedures outlined above. In addition, the choice of fixative must be compatible with the dyes or stains to be employed. Appendix III provides comments about the fixatives and stains employed on tissues which were photographed for this atlas.

# Appendix III: Methods of Fixation and Staining

The following alphabetical listing and brief comments pertain to fixatives and stains which have been employed on the cells and tissues photographed for this atlas. Detailed procedures for their use can be found in Appendix V.

### Aceto-Orcein Method

A staining method for sex chromatin bodies in smears of oral mucosa. This technique has two advantages over other methods for nuclear sexing: both the smear and dye are easy to prepare and the method is just as accurate as other methods but much more rapid. Nuclei stain reddish purple. See Plate 2.

### Acetylcholinesterase Histochemical Method (Seligman)

A method useful for demonstrating enzymatic activity by light and electron microscopy utilizing osmiophilic organic compounds as substrates. Enzyme sites appear black. See Plate 70.

### Ethyl Alcohol

Among the earliest fixing solutions used by histologists, it is not frequently employed as a primary fixative except in Best's carmine method, periodic acid-Schiff reaction and Ranson's method. Alcohol (70 to 100%) is valuable for the preservation of the cellular polysaccharide glycogen for routine light microscopic study. Alcohol fixation can produce distortions and shrinkage unless used at a low temperature.

### Best's Carmine Stain

The rationale for this stain for glycogen is unknown. The carmine is used in an aqueous solution with potassium carbonate and potassium chloride. Glycogen stains bright red. A nuclear stain such as hematoxylin is commonly used with Best's carmine. The periodic acid-Schiff method is another stain for glycogen and other polysaccharides. See Plate 8.

### Bielchowsky's Method

This method consists of silver salt impregnation of blocks of tissue, and the subsequent reduction of the silver. As a result there is silver impregnation of neurofibrils, axons and dendrites. Other structures, such as connective tissue fibers and neuroglia, may be impregnated. This method is valuable for the study of motor and sensory nerve endings. Nerve fibers appear black. See Plate 108.

### Bodian's Silver Method

This is a silver method for the impregnation of nerve fibers in paraffin sections. It was developed by Bodian in 1937. Sections are saturated with an aqueous solution of protargol in the presence of metallic copper. The colloidal silver proteinate is then reduced in hydroquinone and the silver is replaced by gold chloride (toning with gold). Excess silver is removed by sodium thiosulfate. This method gives uniform, sharp and specific staining of neural elements, including axons, neurofibrils and synaptic end feet. Axons appear black or deep blue. See Plates 101 and 106.

### Bouin's Fluid

A commonly used fixative composed of a saturated aqueous solution of picric acid (75 cc), formalin (25 cc) and glacial acetic acid (5 cc). Almost any stain can be used after fixation in Bouin's. The picric acid also enhances cellular and tissue staining reactions. This fixative was described by Bouin in 1897.

### Brilliant Cresyl Blue Stain

A basic dye of the oxazine group used chiefly for staining blood to demonstrate platelets and reticulocytes. The dye has a strong affinity for nucleic acid. See Plate 53.

### Cajal's Gold Sublimate Method

A delicate technique developed by Cajal in 1913 to demonstrate neuroglia astrocytes, using mercuric bichloride and gold chloride. This method is considered the first highly selective neuroglial stain to be developed. It is usually used on frozen sections of material fixed in formalin-ammonium bromide mixture. The chemicals and water used must be of exceptional purity for best results. Protoplasmic and fibrous astrocytes appear reddish purple to near black. See Plate 115.

### Carmine

This dye is of great historic interest, having been used in microscopic work in the Eighteenth Century, considerably before the days of modern histology. It is still of great use for staining embryos, small animals and large blocks of tissue *in toto,* and as a specific stain for glycogen and mucus. The active principle is carminic acid, which is extracted from cochineal (dried female insects, *Coccus cacti*). See Plates 8 and 164.

### Formalin

A 37% solution of formaldehyde. Formaldehyde is a gas soluble to about 55% in water. Solutions employed as fixatives are prepared in terms of the percentage of formalin, not formaldehyde. The commonly used 10% formalin (formol) is 10 cc of formalin and 90 cc of water. Formalin is also employed with other reagents (as in Helley's, Bouin's and Regaud's fluids). Because formalin is a strong reducing agent, it is only mixed with other ingredients immediately before use.

### Formic Acid

A recommended fixative for Ranvier's gold chloride method, as a substitute for undiluted fresh lemon juice.

### Gallocyanin Stain

This method was popularized by Einarson in 1932. It utilizes a basic oxazine dye (gallocyanin) in combination with chrome alum. It was considered by some to be a specific stain for nucleic acids. Nuclear DNA and RNA and cytoplasmic RNA stain blue. Acidic mucopolysaccharides may also be stained. Compared with other basic dyes, gallocyanin binds strongly with nucleic acids. See Plate 86.

### Giemsa Stain

This is a widely used stain for blood, spleen and bone marrow cells, as well as for the identification of protozoan parasites. The stain is composed of methylene blue eosinate, azure A eosinate, azure B eosinate and methylene blue chloride. The stain was employed here because it is technically simple to use and because of its affinity for nuclei and chromosomes. The stained nuclei and chromosomes may vary in color from reddish-blue to purple. See Plate 3.

### Glees' Method

This silver method was developed by Glees in 1946 for the study of normal and degenerating synaptic boutons. It also demonstrates neurofibrils. Although Glees' method has produced valuable results in the hands of experienced investigators, it has not come into general use. One reason for this is that this method has so far been effective only in certain regions of the central nervous system. A factor limiting its usefulness is the concomitant impregnation of normal axons and axon terminals which obscure degenerating axons and terminals. Nerve fibers appear black. See Plates 85 and 87.

### Glutaraldehyde

This five-carbon dialdehyde of relatively simple structure is the most commonly used fixative in electron microscopy, and it is becoming increasingly useful for light microscopy of thin sections of plastic-embedded tissues. It gives superb images of cellular structure and can be used as a fixative in histochemical enzyme localization by light and electron microscopy. Used as a 1 to 6.5% solution in isotonic buffer at 1 to 4°C. Glutaraldehyde and osmium tetroxide are considered the finest fixatives available to the histologist. One of the advantages of glutaraldehyde compared to osmium is that it does not "stain" or alter the staining characteristics of the tissue during fixation. Glutaraldehyde and osmium tetroxide are sequentially employed, in that order, in preparing tissue for electron microscopy. One-micron sections of plastic-embedded tissue permit very high resolution light microscopy. Ultrathin sections of the same material can also be used for electron microscopy.

### Golgi-Cox Method

Golgi silver methods for nerve cells depend upon preliminary fixation in a potassium dichromate solution. The silver is selective, tending to impregnate a few nerve cells completely, which then become blackened when the silver is reduced. Although these methods do not reveal details of the internal structure of nerve cells, they do provide, very importantly, a unique view of the entire cell and its processes. They also demonstrate specific details of non-nervous cells and tissue components such as the parietal cells of the stomach and bile canaliculi of the liver. The Golgi-Cox method is one of the simplest of the complex and time-consuming Golgi methods for demonstrating the relations of dendrites and axons to the nerve cell body. Cell bodies and processes are stained black on a light yellowish or colorless background. Blood vessels may also be impregnated. See Plate 83.

### Gomori's Aldehyde Fuchsin Stain

This is a valuable stain that is compatible with a number of rather striking staining procedures. Aldehyde fuchsin has a poorly understood affinity for elastic tissue, beta granules in pancreatic islets, neurosecretory material, mast cell granules and beta cells in the pituitary. The principal ingredients are basic fuchsin and paraldehyde. Several counterstains may be used. A counterstain is one which enhances the appearance of another primary stain, but in actual practice usually provides additional specific information. Hyaline cartilage, elastic fibers, mucin, mast cell granules, and beta cells stain purple. Other tissues are stained according to the counterstain used. See Plate 45.

### Gomori's Chrome Alum Hematoxylin Stain

Primary fixation should be Bouin's or Helly's fluids, although secondary treatment by these fluids of formalin-fixed material is satisfactory. This method employs chrome alum hematoxylin stain with phloxine as a counterstain. Basophils stain blue and acidophils appear red. In the posterior pituitary gland, neurosecretory substances stain deep blue. See Plate 104.

### Helly's Fluid

Also known as Zenker-formol, this is a modification of Zenker's fluid in which formalin is substituted for acetic acid. The concentration of formalin used varies between 5 and 10%. This is an excellent cytological and tissue fixative.

### H. & E. (Hematoxylin and Eosin Stain)

Most widely used and important general purpose stain combination. May be used after any fixation except osmium tetroxide. Nuclear stain is the basic hematoxylin, while eosin is the cytoplasmic counterstain. Nuclear heterochromatin stains blue and the cytoplasm of cells rich in ribonucleoprotein also stains blue. The cytoplasm of cells with minimal amounts of ribonucleoprotein tends to be lavender in color while the mature red blood cell and muscle contractile protein, which are devoid of RNA, stain red. While it is an esthetically pleasing combination and widely used, it is limited in its ability to differentiate cytoplasmic organelles and many other tissue components. See Plate 13.

### Iron Hematoxylin (Heidenhain)

One of the standard stains which is capable of excellent results after any good fixation. Tissues are stained in aqueous hematoxylin after mordanting in iron ammonium sulfate (iron alum). Many counterstains can be used. It is not specific for any structure but it is particularly useful for demonstrating cell membranes, terminal bars (tight junctions or junctional complexes), secretory granules, nuclear heterochromatin, mitochondria (if preserved) and the cross striations of voluntary muscle. All these structures stain black. See Plate 15.

### Kopsch's Method

One of several methods used to demonstrate the Golgi apparatus. Small pieces of tissue are immersed in 2% osmic acid for 8 to 16 days. The Golgi apparatus stains black. If stained, mitochondria and ground substance appear reddish brown. Several modifications of this method have been developed. See Plate 7.

### Luxol Fast Blue-PAS Method

This method, employing luxol fast blue, has become popular for staining myelin because it can be used with other stains, allowing combinations that are not possible with the older hematoxylin methods. Myelin nerve sheaths stain blue-green. PAS-positive substances stain pink to violet. The method consists of staining in 0.1% alcoholic solution of luxol fast blue, differentiation in lithium carbonate and counterstaining with periodic acid-Schiff. The method was introduced by Klüver and Barrera in 1953. See Plate 284.

### Mallory's Connective Tissue Stain

One of the most beautiful and widely used of all stains. Several modifications of the original method have been developed. Basic ingredients are acid fuchsin, aniline blue, orange G and phosphotungstic acid. Collagen and reticular fibers stain blue; elastic fibers yellow or pink; nuclei, fibrin and neuroglial fibrils red. Heidenhain's azan stain (see below) employs azocarmine instead of acid fuchsin and is a widely used substitute. See Plate 16.

### Mallory-Azan (Heidenhain's Azan) Stain

This connective tissue stain is a modification of Mallory's original connective tissue stain, in which azocarmine is used along with the aniline blue-orange G mixture. Collagen and basophil granules stain blue, muscle and acidophil granules orange to red, and nuclei and cytoplasm stain red. Elastic fibers are unstained or, if stained, yellow or pink. Mallory-azan is an extremely useful and beautiful stain combination. Heidenhain was the first histologist to use the azan modification of Mallory's stain. See Plate 243.

### Marchi Method and Modifications (Swank and Davenport)

Normal adult myelin contains no hydrophobic neutral lipids (triglycerides and cholesterol esters), while degenerating myelin does. All ethylenic (double) bonds, such as those found in fatty acids of all lipids, will reduce osmium tetroxide to the lower oxides and black metallic osmium. They cannot do this, however, if previously or simultaneously oxidized. Thus, if degenerating (hydrophobic) and normal (hydrophilic) myelin lipids are exposed to aqueous potassium chlorate, only normal myelin ethylene bonds will be attacked. Unaffected bonds of degenerating myelin are thus the only ones still free to reduce osmium tetroxide. Nervous tissue in which degenerating myelin is present is fixed for 2 to 3 days in either formalin or a magnesium sulfate–potassium dichromate mixture followed by formalin. The tissue is then placed for 8 to 10 days in a solution containing potassium chlorate, osmium tetroxide, formaldehyde and glacial acetic acid. After a thorough wash, the tissue is embedded in celloidin (nitrocellulose), sectioned and mounted. Degenerating myelin and neutral lipids elsewhere will be black. Normal myelin is unstained. See Plate 273.

### Masson's Trichrome Method

This method was first described by Pierre Masson in 1951. Although Bouin's is the recommended fixative, Orth's (formalin-Müller), Zenker's or 10% formalin in alcohol may be used. Dyes and solutions employed are hematoxylin, acid fuchsin, phosphotungstic acid and light green. Several modifications of this method are available. Nuclei stain dark blue, cytoplasm and neuroglial fibers red, collagen green. See Plate 234.

### Methylene Blue and Erythrocin

A frequently used combination to stain tissues. Methylene blue stains basophilic constituents of the tissue while erythrocin stains the acidophilic elements. See Plate 1.

## Modified Aldehyde Fuchsin Stain

Halmi's modification of Gomori's method employs aldehyde fuchsin with light green or orange G as the counterstain. Nuclei can be stained with celestine blue or haemalum (alum hematoxylin). Depending on the concentration of organelles found in different cell types they may appear yellow, purple or green. Collagen and the basement membrane are green; and mast cells, elastic fibers and goblet cell mucus are purple. See Plate 19.

## Müller's Fluid

Potassium dichromate (2.0 to 2.5%)-sodium sulfate (1%) mixture in distilled water. Formerly much used for prolonged fixation and mordanting of nervous tissue. It is now largely replaced by Orth's fluid which is composed of potassium dichromate (2.0 to 2.5%)-formalin (10%) in distilled water. The sodium sulfate is omitted. Fixatives of this type do not store well and must be prepared immediately before use.

## Nassar-Shanklin Method

A good silver method for staining neuroglia in formalin sections. Formalin-fixed paraffin sections are impregnated with silver diamminohydroxide or with strong Hortega silver carbonate dissolved with strong ammonia after sensitizing with sodium sulfite. Microglia, oligodendroglia, and fibrous and protoplasmic astrocytes can be successfully impregnated by this method. Sensitization with sodium sulfite is essential for good results. See Plates 114 and 116.

## Osmium Tetroxide (OsO$_4$)

Commonly but incorrectly referred to as osmic acid, this is considered an excellent fixative for most cytological morphology. Used either as a primary fixative or secondarily after aldehyde fixation. Cannot be used for histochemical studies. Osmium blackens lipids and stains the Golgi apparatus in light microscopic preparations. A severe limitation of osmium-fixed material is that most routine and special stains cannot be utilized. Its primary use is in electron microscopy. See Plate 9.

## Pal-Weigert Method

First described in 1887, this is a modification of the Weigert method for myelin sheaths in which the differentiation between the myelinated fibers and the surrounding tissues may be carried to a greater degree than in the original method. Originally Müller's fluid was used as the fixative; later formalin was used. Several modifications of the original Pal-Weigert method are available. Normal myelin sheaths are stained deep blue. Degenerative myelin does not stain (see also Weigert method). See Plate 271.

## Periodic Acid-Schiff Method

Principally used to demonstrate structures rich in polysaccharides (glycogen), mucopolysaccharides (e.g., ground substance of connective tissues, basement membrane and mucus), glycoproteins (thyroglobulin) and glycolipids. This method depends on the selective oxidation by periodic acid of 1,2-glycols and 2,2-amino alcohols to aldehydes. The aldehydes are then detected by the Schiff reagent, which stains them reddish purple. Schiff reagent is formed by the reaction of basic fuchsin with sulfurous acid. See Plate 75.

### Phosphotungstic Acid Hematoxylin (PTAH)

This stain was developed by Mallory. It is an ideal stain for the demonstration of astroglial fibers, which stain blue as do striated muscle fibers and mitochondria. Collagen, reticular fibers and ground substance of bone and cartilage stain in varying shades of yellow to brownish red. Coarse elastic fibers stain purple. Nuclei are blue. See Plate 64.

### Pinkus' Acid Orcein-Giemsa Method

This is a modification of the original Unna-Taenzer procedure by Hermann Pinkus in 1944, which has been further modified and simplified by Pinkus and Hunter. A good method to demonstrate connective tissue elements. Material is fixed in 10% formalin, formol-alcohol or absolute alcohol. Paraffin sections are used. Nuclei deep blue, cytoplasm light blue, collagen rose pink, elastic fibers dark brown. See Plate 119.

### Ranson's Method

This is a pyridine silver method described by Ranson in 1911 for impregnating unmyelinated nerve fibers. The largest myelinated axis cylinders are usually yellow surrounded by a colorless ring of myelin, and there is a gradation to black in the small myelinated fibers. Unmyelinated fibers are typically dark brown or black. Nerve cells are yellow to brown, with dark brown to black neurofibrils. End bulbs, when stained, appear black or as small black rings. See Plate 294.

### Ranvier's Gold Chloride Method

Described by Ranvier in 1880. Demonstrates nerve endings in muscle. Nerve fibers are variably stained red to purple-black. The tissue is fixed in formic acid or undiluted fresh lemon juice before immersion in an aqueous solution of gold chloride. See Plate 107.

### Regaud's Method

Described in 1910 by Regaud, this is a modification of Heidenhain's iron hematoxylin method for mitochondria which consists of prolonged mordanting of tissues in potassium dichromate. Stains mitochondria blue-black. It is the most permanent and simplest of all mitochondrial stains. See Plate 6.

### Rossman's Fluid

A fixative capable of preserving cellular glycogen. This fixative consists of absolute ethyl alcohol (90 cc) saturated with picric acid (approximately 9%) and neutral formalin (10 cc). After overnight fixation the excess picric acid is removed by rinsing in 95% alcohol for several days.

### Silver Diammine Hydroxide Method

See Nassar-Shanklin method.

### Tetrazolium Method

Tetrazolium salts have low oxidation-reduction potentials and are thus capable of intercepting electrons in many biological oxidation-reduction reactions including those facilitated enzymatically by dehydrogenases. The reduced, colored end product (blue diformazan) of these reactions is insoluble and thereby demonstrates the sites of such activity. Localization of the site of enzymatic activity is an important contribution to our understanding of cellular function. The methods of Nachlas, Walker and Seligman are outstanding examples of this technique. See Plate 69.

### Toluidine Blue Stain

Toluidine blue O is a basic dye of the thiazine series closely related to methylene blue. In routine preparations, toluidine blue stains nucleic and cytoplasmic ribonucleic acid ortho- or normochromatically (blue) and cartilage matrix and mast cell granules metachromatically (reddish purple). This is thus a metachromatic stain and is very useful for $1-\mu$ sections of plastic-embedded tissue. See Plates 27 and 123.

### Van Gieson's Stain

A good stain for connective tissue. Consists of staining by acid fuchsin and picric acid. Stain fades in time and is therefore not used as frequently as the Mallory connective tissue stain. Collagen stains bright red, muscle and cytoplasm yellow, and nuclei blue to black. Delicate collagen fibrils and reticulum stain very faintly or not at all. It is valuable as a counterstain in techniques which stain elastic fibers a contrasting color (e.g., the methods of Verhoeff and Weigert). Combined with Verhoeff's stain, it is one of the most valuable stains for the study of blood vessels. See Plate 65.

### Van Gehuchten's Fluid

This is a modified mixture of Carnoy's fluid containing absolute alcohol, chloroform and glacial acetic acid. A very fast acting fixative.

### Weigert's Elastic Fiber Stain

This technique is an excellent method for staining elastic fibers. The procedure consists of staining with a ferric chloride-hematoxylin mixture. Several counterstains may be used. Elastic fibers stain blue-black to black. Other tissue elements depend on the counterstain used. Commonly used counterstains are phloxine or van Gieson's. See Plate 135.

### Verhoeff and Van Gieson's Stain

See Van Gieson's stain.

### Weigert's Method

This method was described by Weigert in 1885 for normal myelin sheaths. It is used principally on formol-fixed tissue of the central nervous system to demonstrate fiber tracts and to show the arrangement of gray and white matter. The basic procedure requires the use of a mordant, potassium dichromate, a hematoxylin stain and a differentiating fluid. Normal but not degenerating or degenerated myelin sheaths stain black. See Plate 267.

### Weil's Method

Weil's hematoxylin method for myelin does not depend upon a specific method of fixation, although mordanting of formalin-fixed material by Weigert's potassium dichromate and chromium fluoride is advisable. The stain is composed of equal parts of iron alum (4%) and hematoxylin (1%). Myelin sheaths stain black or dark gray. See Plate 290.

### Wilder's Method

Silver impregnation method for reticular fibers. Reticular fibers stain black, collagen rose color, and other tissue elements depend on the counterstain used. See Plate 36.

### Wright's Stain

A differential stain for blood cells named after the American pathologist James Wright (1869–1928), who described this method in 1902. Main constituents of his stain are methylene blue and eosin. Erythrocytes bind eosin and appear red or pink; nuclei deep blue or purple; basophilic granules deep purple; eosinophilic granules red to red-orange; neutrophilic granules reddish-brown to lilac; platelets violet to purple; and lymphocyte cytoplasm pale blue. See Plates 50, 51 and 52.

### Zenker's Fluid

This excellent fixative is a mixture of potassium dichromate and bichloride of mercury to which glacial acetic acid is added. A mercury precipitate is left in the tissues and is troublesome to the inexperienced microscopist unless removed by an iodine solution.

# Appendix IV: Comments on Color Groups, Stains and the Staining Mechanism

The chemical mechanism by which biological stains impart color to specific cellular components and tissues is poorly understood in many instances, although it has been the subject of numerous publications and books. The student whose interest or curiosity lies in this area is directed to the references given in Appendix V.

Students frequently hear or read that certain dyes are either basic or acidic, and that certain structures are basophilic or acidophilic. A detailed account of these and other terms can be found in *H. J. Conn's Biological Stains,* by R. D. Lillie, cited in the references. A very brief explanation seems appropriate here, and a discussion of both a synthetic and a natural dye follow.

Known atomic groupings in molecules related to color are called *chromophores.* These atomic groupings include the azo group (N═N), the azin group $\left(\text{N—N}\right)$, and the indamine group (N═), and are known as the basic chromophores. The nitro group ($NO_2$) and the quinoid benzene ring with its C═C groups comprise the important acidic chromophores. Other chromophores are not usually of biological interest. All of the so-called coal tar or synthetic dyes are derivatives of benzene, an important organic compound capable of combining in an infinite number of ways with radicals and elements to form complex compounds. Benzene compounds to which chromophores are combined are known as *chromogens.* Chromogens, although colored, are not dyes until they possess other end groups which permit them to form a chemical union with tissue acidic or basic end groups. Synthetic dyes are prepared so that the essential part of the dye is either acid (anionic) or basic (cationic) in its chemical behavior. Dye solutions are prepared from dye salts which, when placed in water, yield by dissociation either hydroxyl ($OH^-$) ions and act as cations (basic dyes) or hydrogen ($H^+$) ions and act as anions (acidic dyes). A cationic or basic dye is a salt (usually chloride) of a chromogen base and will stain the nucleic acids of the nucleus and cytoplasm, whereas an anionic or acid dye is a salt (usually sodium) of a chromogen acid and will stain the cytoplasm of cells (except cytoplasmic ribonucleoprotein) and certain other tissues. A basic dye has an affinity for nuclei, which are then termed basophilic structures and an acid dye has an affinity for non-nucleic acid-containing cytoplasm and other tissues, which are then termed acidophilic structures.

Eosin Y is an anionic or acid (synthetic) dye in spite of the fact that a solution of the sodium salt of eosin is basic in reaction. It is important to recognize that eosin is an acid or anionic dye because the significant part or chromogen of the dye which forms the union with cellular or tissue cationic or basic end

410

groups is anionic or acidic. When eosin is employed as a tissue stain the acidophilic structures are sometimes referred to as eosinophilic.

Hematoxylin is a natural dye extracted from the logwood tree *Hematoxylin campechium,* found in Central and South America. The extract from the heartwood is not a dye until it undergoes oxidation into hematein, which is an acid chromogen. In this form hematein is only a weak dye with little affinity or specificity. Mordanting is essential to the conversion of this dye to a base, which will then combine actively and strongly with acidic nucleic acids. Mordants most commonly used in tissue staining are salts of aluminum, chromium, iron, potassium and tungsten.

Another kind of staining reaction is metachroming, in which a dye, such as toluidine blue, will react with certain components of cells and tissues and have a different hue from its original blue color. Metachromatic staining is seen in mast cell granules, cartilage and goblet cell mucus, which will appear red-purple when stained with toluidine blue. The nuclei of these cells appear blue, the same color as the original dye solution. The principal reason for metachromatic staining is found in the chemical nature of the components of these cells and tissues which contain a predominance of strongly acidic sulfated protein polysaccharides.

Additional comments about stains and staining reactions are given in the legends of some of the illustrations in this atlas.

# Appendix V: References

## Technique

Davenport, H. A.: *Histological and Histochemical Technics.* 1960, Philadelphia, W. B. Saunders Co.

Drury, R. A. B., and Wallington, E. A.: *Carleton's Histological Technique.* 4th ed., 1967, New York, Oxford University Press.

Emmel, V. M., and Cowdry, E. V.: *Laboratory Technique in Biology and Medicine.* 1964, Baltimore, The Williams & Wilkins Co.

Gatenby, J. B., and Painter, T. S. (Eds.): *Bolles Lee's Microtomists Vade-Mecum,* 10th ed., 1937, New York, McGraw-Hill Book Co.

Glick, D.: *Techniques of Histo- and Cytochemistry.* 1949, New York, Interscience Publishers, Inc.

Humason, G. L.: *Animal Tissue Techniques.* 1962, San Francisco, W. H. Freeman and Co.

Jones, R. M.: *McClung's Handbook of Microscopical Technique.* 3rd ed., 1950, New York, Paul B. Hoeber, Inc., Medical Book Department of Harper and Row Publishers.

Lillie, R. D.: *Histopathologic Technic and Practical Histochemistry,* 3rd ed., 1965, New York, Blakiston Div., McGraw-Hill Book Co.

Luna, L. G. (Ed.): *Manual of Histologic Staining Methods of the Armed Forces Institute of Pathology.* 2nd ed., 1960, New York, Blakiston Div., McGraw-Hill Book Co.

McManus, J. F. A., and Mowry, R. W.: *Staining Methods. Histologic and Histochemical.* 1960, New York, Paul B. Hoeber, Inc., Medical Div., Harper and Row Publishers.

Nassar, T. K., and Shanklin, W. M.: Staining neuroglia with silver diamminohydroxide after sensitizing with sodium sulfite and embedding in paraffin. *Stain Tech.* 26:13–18, 1951.

Nauta, W. J. H., and Ebbesson, S. O. E. (Eds.): *Contemporary Research Methods in Neuroanatomy.* 1970, Berlin, Springer-Verlag.

Pease, D. C.: *Histological Techniques for Electron Microscopy,* 2nd ed., 1964, New York, Academic Press.

Sanderson, A. R., and Stewart, J. S. S.: Nuclear sexing with aceto-orcein. *Brit. Med. J.* ii:1065–1067, 1961.

Windle, W. F. (Ed.): *New Research Techniques of Neuroanatomy.* 1957, Springfield, Charles C Thomas Publishers.

## Histology

Andrew, W.: *Microfabric of Man, A Textbook of Histology.* 1966, Chicago, Year Book Medical Publishers, Inc.

Arey, L. B.: *Human Histology.* 3rd ed., 1968, Philadelphia, W. B. Saunders Co.

Beresford, W. A.: *Lecture Notes of Histology.* 1969, Oxford, Blackwell Scientific Publishers.

Bloom, W., and Fawcett, D. W.: *A Textbook of Histology.* 9th ed., 1968, Philadelphia, W. B. Saunders Co.

Coërs, C., and Woolf, A. L.: *The Innervation of Muscle, A Biopsy Study.* 1959, Oxford, Blackwell Scientific Publication.

Copenhaver, W. M., Bunge, R. P., and Bunge, M. B.: *Bailey's Textbook of Histology.* 16th ed., 1971, Baltimore, The Williams & Wilkins Co.

Cruickshank, B., Dodds, T. C., and Gardner, D. L.: *Human Histology.* 2nd ed., 1968, London, E. & S. Livingstone Ltd.

Elias, H., and Pauly, J. E.: *Human Microanatomy.* 3rd ed., 1966, Philadelphia, F. A. Davis Co.

Fallis, B. D., and Ashworth, R. D.: *Textbook of Human Histology.* 1970, Boston, Little, Brown and Co.

Greep, R. O. (Ed.): *Histology.* 2nd ed., 1966, New York, Blakiston Div., McGraw-Hill Book Co.

Greep, R. O., and Weiss, L. (Eds.): *Histology.* 3rd ed., 1973, New York, Blakiston Div., McGraw-Hill Book Co.

Ham, A. W.: *Histology.* 5th ed., 1965, Philadelphia, J. B. Lippincott Co.

Leeson, C. R., and Leeson, T. S.: *Histology.* 1966, Philadelphia, W. B. Saunders Co.

Zacks, S. I.: *The Motor Endplate.* 1964, Philadelphia, W. B. Saunders Co.

## Neuroanatomy

Boyd, I. A., Eyzaguirre, C., Matthews, P. B. C., and Rushworth, G.: *The Role of the Gamma System in Movement and Posture.* 1964, New York, Assoc. Aid Crippled Children Publication.

Brodal, A.: *Neurological Anatomy.* 2nd ed., 1969, Oxford, Oxford University Press.

Chusid, J. G.: *Correlative Neuroanatomy and Functional Neurology.* 14th ed., 1970, Los Altos, California, Lange Medical Publication.

Crosby, E. C., Humphrey, T., and Lauer, E. W.: *Correlative Anatomy of the Nervous System.* 1962, New York, Macmillan Co.

Elliot, H. C.: *Textbook of Neuroanatomy.* 1963, Philadelphia, J. B. Lippincott Co.

Everett, N. B.: *Functional Neuroanatomy.* 1965, Philadelphia, Lea and Febiger.

Ingram, W. R.: *A Student's Introduction to Neurology.* 1964, Iowa City, University of Iowa Publication.

Truex, R. C., and Carpenter, M. B.: *Human Neuroanatomy.* 6th ed., 1969, Baltimore, The Williams & Wilkins Co.

## Physiology

Davson, H.: *A Textbook of General Physiology.* 3rd ed., 1964, Boston, Little, Brown and Co.

Guyton, A.: *Textbook of Medical Physiology,* 4th ed., 1971, Philadelphia, W. B. Saunders Co.

Mountcastle, V. B. (Ed.): *Medical Physiology.* 12th ed., 1968, Saint Louis, C. V. Mosby Co.

Ruch, T. C., and Patton, H. D. (Eds.): *Physiology and Biophysics.* 19th ed., 1965, Philadelphia, W. B. Saunders Co.

## Miscellaneous

Bradbury, S.: *The Microscope, Past and Present.* 1968, Oxford, Pergamon Press Ltd.

*Dorland's Illustrated Medical Dictionary,* 24th ed., 1965, Philadelphia, W. B. Saunders Co.

Lillie, R. O.: *H. J. Conn's Biological Stains.* 8th ed., 1969, Baltimore, The Williams & Wilkins Co.

Skinner, H. A.: *The Origin of Medical Terms.* 2nd ed., 1961, Baltimore, The Williams & Wilkins Co.

# Index

# INDEX

# INDEX